Prodrugs

DRUGS AND THE PHARMACEUTICAL SCIENCES

A Series of Textbooks and Monographs

edited by

James Swarbrick
School of Pharmacy
University of North Carolina
Chapel Hill, North Carolina

Prodrugs

Topical and Ocular Drug Delivery

edited by
Kenneth B. Sloan

University of Florida
Gainesville, Florida

Marcel Dekker, Inc.   New York • Basel • Hong Kong

R M 301, 57

P 76

1992

Library of Congress Cataloging-in-Publication Data

Prodrugs, topical and ocular drug delivery / edited by Kenneth B.
Sloan.
　　p.　cm. -- (Drugs and the pharmaceutical sciences ; v. 53)
Includes bibliographical references and index.
ISBN 0-8247-8629-7　(alk. paper)
　1. Prodrugs.　2. Transdermal medication.　3. Ocular pharmacology.
I. Sloan, Kenneth B.　　II. Title: Topical and ocular drug
delivery.　III. Series.
[DNLM: 1. Administration, Topical.　2. Drug Administration Routes.
3. Prodrugs.　W1 DR893B v. 53 / WB 340 P964]
RM301.57.P76　1992
615'.6--dc20
DNLM/DLC
for Library of Congress　　　　　　　　　　　　　　　　92-4455
　　　　　　　　　　　　　　　　　　　　　　　　　　　　CIP

This book is printed on acid-free paper.

MARCEL DEKKER, INC.
270 Madison Avenue, New York, New York 10016

Current printing (last digit):
10　9　8　7　6　5　4　3　2　1

PRINTED IN THE UNITED STATES OF AMERICA

Preface

Topical application of drugs is an important route of drug administration. Since this route encompasses the application of drugs to all external membranes, any discussion of the topical application of drugs generally includes dermal and ocular applications but not, for example, buccal or rectal applications. Topical application to treat various disease states is older than the concept of a drug itself. It has probably always seemed a natural thing to do to apply something to an external site whereby the effectiveness or ineffectiveness of the application could be easily monitored. However, the use of topical application of drugs has now progressed well beyond the treatment of topical or local disease states only. For example, transdermal delivery of drugs (delivery *through* the dermal membrane) to treat systemic conditions is fast becoming an important partner with dermal delivery (delivery *into* the dermal membrane) to treat a topical or local condition. In fact, most in vitro experiments such as diffusion cell experiments, which are used to evaluate dermal delivery of drugs, actually measure their transdermal delivery. The results of the transdermal delivery experiments are then extrapolated to the conditions where dermal delivery can be evaluated.

Because the physicochemical properties of the drugs themselves are usually not optimal for their delivery into or through topical membranes, the topical administration of drugs is not always effective. There are several approaches that can be taken in dealing with this problem. The first approach is to use a different formulation with which to deliver the drug. In this approach, various penetration enhancers and topical barrier modifiers can be used to enhance permeation into and through a topical membrane. The second approach is to make a new drug analog or homolog of the original drug. In this approach, entirely new molecules exhibiting the desired physicochemical properties are used; but changes in the pharmacological profile, as compared to the original drug, may result, and this could demand further expensive biological testing. The third approach is to make a transient derivative—a prodrug of the drug—which imparts to the drug the desired transient change in its physicochemical properties. This last approach has many advantages. First, the changes in the physicochemical properties and the pharmacological profile of the drug are transient, so that once the prodrug has delivered the drug, one is left with a well-characterized and well-understood molecule with which to work. Second, the breadth of the possible transient changes is limited only by the imagination and resourcefulness of those responsible for designing the prodrug.

This book is the result of our attempts to organize the available information on the use of prodrugs to enhance dermal, transdermal, and ocular delivery so that it will be easier for the interested reader to take full advantage of what is known. Chapter 1 provides an overview of the mechanisms of topical (dermal and transdermal) delivery and the physicochemical parameters that control it: partition coefficient, water solubility, molecular weight (volume or size), and polarity. In addition, the authors provide a hypothetical example of how to design a promoiety for a specific type of parent drug. Chapter 2 provides an overview of the prodrug approaches that have actually been used to improve dermal and transdermal delivery from a functional group perspective. This chapter is divided into sections on each common type of functional group—acidic or basic amine, thiol, carboxylic acid, hydroxyl, carbonyl—which are further divided into types of promoieties that have been used in combination with each functional group—e.g., acyloxymethyl, dialkylaminomethyl, acyl, thiazolidine. Chapters 3, 4, and 5 develop mathematically and thermodynamically based approaches to predicting and optimizing topical delivery with prodrugs. In each of these chapters the theoretical basis for the approach is established for a wide variety of parent drugs and then it is extrapolated to the situation for prodrugs. Chapter 6 presents an analysis of how effective the prodrug approach has been at enhancing topical (dermal and transdermal) delivery relative to traditional formulation approaches. This chapter balances the more optimistic conclusions of Chapter 2. Finally, Chapter 7 provides an overview of prodrug approaches to enhancing ocular delivery and it delineates the interactions between the different physiological and biological requirements for ocular delivery and the potential for the use of prodrugs to enhance ocular delivery.

We believe that the full potential for the use of prodrugs for optimizing all kinds of topical and ocular delivery has yet to be realized. Part of the reason that this potential has not been realized is that few consensus positions have been reached by the experts in the use of prodrugs to optimize topical and ocular delivery. This fact, which is emphasized in Chapter 6, is not necessarily a negative observation, but merely a reflection of the fact that the use of prodrugs to optimize topical and ocular delivery is not a mature technology. Thus, our goal for this book is not to present consensus but, instead, to present the different approaches to the use of prodrugs for optimizing topical delivery taken by various experts in the area. It presents this information in a forum where the scientific community and readers interested in the area can readily assess the maturity and appropriateness of the technology and compare the different approaches. However, we hope that this book will stimulate the types of productive discussions that will eventually lead to consensus positions.

Kenneth B. Sloan

Contents

Contributors

Bradley D. Anderson, Ph.D. Professor, Department of Pharmaceutics and Pharmaceutical Chemistry, The University of Utah College of Pharmacy, Salt Lake City, Utah

Hans Bundgaard, Ph.D., D.Sc. Professor, Department of Pharmaceutical Chemistry, The Royal Danish School of Pharmacy, Copenhagen, Denmark

Richard H. Guy, Ph.D. Professor, Departments of Pharmacy and Pharmaceutical Chemistry, School of Pharmacy, University of California, San Francisco, California

Jonathan Hadgraft, D.Sc., FRSC Professor, The Welsh School of Pharmacy, University of Wales, College of Cardiff, Cardiff, Wales

William J. Lambert, Ph.D.* Pharmaceutical Research and Development, The Upjohn Company, Kalamazoo, Michigan

Gerald B. Kasting, Ph.D. Staff Scientist, Hair and Skin Care Technology Division, Miami Valley Laboratories, The Procter & Gamble Company, Cincinnati, Ohio

---

Current affiliation:
*Pfizer Central Research, Groton, Connecticut

Vincent H. L. Lee, Ph.D.   Gavin S. Herbert Professor and Chairman, Department of Pharmaceutical Sciences, John Stauffer Pharmaceutical Sciences Center, University of Southern California, Los Angeles, California

David W. Osborne, Ph.D.*   Pharmaceutical Research and Development, The Upjohn Company, Kalamazoo, Michigan

Russell O. Potts, Ph.D.   Associate Director of Biophysical Research, Cygnus Therapeutic Systems, Redwood City, California

Kenneth B. Sloan, Ph.D.   Associate Professor, Department of Medicinal Chemistry, University of Florida, Gainesville, Florida

Ronald L. Smith, Ph.D.   Staff Scientist, Biopharmaceutics Section, Health Care Technology Division, Miami Valley Laboratories, The Procter & Gamble Company, Cincinnati, Ohio

Current affiliation:
*Group Leader, Skin Care Department, Calgon Vestal Laboratories, St. Louis, Missouri

1

Percutaneous Penetration Enhancement: Physicochemical Considerations and Implications for Prodrug Design

Richard H. Guy
University of California, San Francisco, California

Jonathan Hadgraft
University of Wales, College of Cardiff, Cardiff, Wales

INTRODUCTION

The drug development process selects for molecules having the optimal pharmacological activity in the biological assay of choice. However, this evaluation does not take into account other important facets of drug delivery, such as the compatibility of the drug with the formulation or the compound's inherent permeability across membranes separating the dosage form from the site of action. These additional factors are of particular relevance in transdermal and topical drug delivery, for which vehicle selection and percutaneous absorption must be optimized for effective therapy (Fig. 1) (1).

The successful delivery of a drug from a topical formulation into and/or through the skin requires the following sequential steps (2):

1. Dissolution (if necessary), and then diffusion of drug molecules in the vehicle to the vehicle/skin interface
2. Partitioning of the drug from the vehicle into the stratum corneum (SC) (the skin's outermost and least permeable layer)
3. Diffusion of drug through the SC
4. Partitioning of drug from the lipophilic SC into the underlying (and much more aqueous in nature) viable epidermis
5. Diffusion through the viable epidermis and upper dermis
6. Uptake of drug by the cutaneous microcirculation

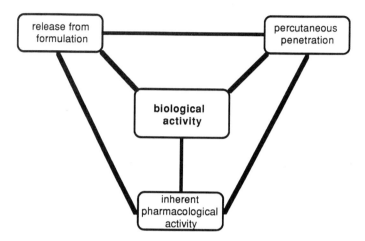

Figure 1 The critical criteria necessary for the biological activity of a topically applied medication. (From Ref. 1.)

It is generally accepted that transport across the SC is the principal rate-limiting step in the percutaneous absorption process (3). Furthermore, the major enzymatic activity in the skin resides in the viable epidermis (4). Therefore, if the target of drug action is the epidermis, the dermis, or the systemic circulation, it follows that a sensible strategy to optimize bioavailability could involve the synthesis of a precursor which would (a) transport efficiently across the SC, and (b) undergo rapid (metabolic) activation in the viable epidermis to the active drug species.

In this chapter, we address the physicochemical factors which are pertinent to the design of topical prodrugs. Our assumption is that the need for a prodrug is established by the fact that the drug itself, while active in the appropriate biological screening assay, is ineffective when administered by the topical route. The objective, therefore, is to propose a menu of considerations which may be taken into account in designing a prodrug of enhanced skin permeability, and formulation compatibility.

MECHANISM OF PERCUTANEOUS ABSORPTION

The most typical reason for the inactivity of a putative topical drug is that it is unable to penetrate the skin at a sufficient rate to maintain an effective concentration at the site of action. Usually, the rate-limiting resistance resides in the SC (3). Hence, if we are to optimize and enhance drug delivery into or through the skin, we must understand (a) the structure and composition of the SC, and (b) the mechanism(s) by which drugs transport across this membrane.

The SC is a thin layer (~10 μm) of terminally differentiated keratinocytes. The cells are flattened and completely filled with keratin. The intercellular spaces contain a complex and unique lipid mixture arranged in multilamellar bilayers. The principal lipid components are ceramides, cholesterol and cholesterol esters, and free fatty acids (5). At physiological temperature, which is below the gel-to-liquid crystalline phase transition temperature, the lipids are highly ordered (6).

The following routes of penetration of drugs across the SC have been suggested (Fig. 2) (3):

1. *Transcellular*: The permeant crosses the SC by the most direct route, and repeatedly partitions between, and diffuses through, the cornified cells and the extracellular lipid bilayers.
2. *Intercellular*: The solute remains in the lipid domains and permeates via a tortuous pathway. Within this lipid domain, the drug has to cross repetitively complete lipid bilayers.
3. *Appendageal*: The penetrant traverses the SC via a "shunt" pathway: e.g., a hair follicle or a sweat gland. Because of the relative density of hair follicles and sweat glands on the human body, the contribution of the former considerably outweighs that of the latter (3).

A number of experimental observations and interpretations have provided considerable circumstantial support for the importance of the intercellular route of penetration. For example, the in situ precipitation of butanol during its passage

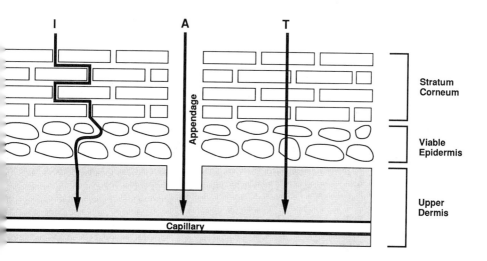

Figure 2 Schematic diagram of the potential routes of drug penetration through the stratum corneum. I = intercellular, T = transcellular, A = appendageal. (From Ref. 12.)

across the SC localized the compound within the intercellular lipid domains (7). Confirmation of this result using other penetrants has been reported (8). The permeability coefficient (K_p) of water across the SC, measured as a function of temperature, is linearly correlated with the infrared spectroscopic assessment of lipid acyl chain disorder (9). Combined with partition coefficient measurements of water specifically into the lipid domain of the SC, it has been further deduced that the pathlength of water transport across the SC is on the order of 100–1000 µm, a value consistent only with an intercellular mechanism of diffusion (10). This deduction is in agreement with an earlier study of nicotinic ester absorption in vivo, which led to a determination of SC diffusion pathlength of about 350 µm, and the conclusion, once again, that these permeants were transporting within the SC lipids (11).

Although the transcellular route appears most favored on geometric grounds (12), there has been no direct evidence presented to provide support for its participation in the SC penetration process. However, the so-called "protein domain" of the SC may represent a region into which topically applied molecules may partition and act as a reservoir (13). Additionally, certain penetration enhancers (e.g., anionic surfactants and alkyl sulfoxides) have been shown to interact with keratin, and induce protein conformational changes (14). The presence of these materials, therefore, could increase the likelihood that permeants access the transcellular route.

The follicular route of permeation is undergoing a renaissance of interest at the present time. While the available surface area for follicular transport is limited on most sites of the body, there have been reports that have implicated the "shunt" pathway as the major contributor to the initial phase of SC permeation (12,15,16). Furthermore, recent experiments using an afollicular animal model have suggested a significant role for the follicular route of transport (17).

In summary, from the available evidence, there is a preponderance of support for the intercellular pathway, and we believe that this represents the major route of transport across the SC. The other possible paths may contribute, but their extent of participation remains ill defined. It follows that the design of prodrugs for topical delivery should be based upon the assumption that the skin involves a lipophilic rate-limiting barrier. At the molecular level, because the lipid domain of the SC consists of multilamellar bilayers, the transporting species must be able to repetitively cross lipid-aqueous phase interfaces. The prodrug must possess an affinity for both lipophilic and hydrophilic environments, therefore.

PHYSICOCHEMICAL PARAMETERS IMPORTANT IN THE CONTROL OF PERCUTANEOUS ABSORPTION

The key parameters which control the penetration kinetics of chemicals across the skin are listed in Table 1. In the design of a new prodrug, these physicochemical factors must be optimized to ensure that the delivery of the active drug species

Table 1 The Key Physicochemical Determinants of the Percutaneous Absorption of Drugs

Oil-water partition coefficient
Lipid solubility and aqueous solubility
Solubility parameter
Molecular size and shape
Polarity and charge

achieves the desired level for therapeutic activity. In the following paragraphs, we outline simple guidelines for obtaining the appropriate values of the parameters in Table 1.

Oil-Water Partition Coefficient

It is generally accepted that the oil-water partitioning characteristics of a chemical are crucial to its ability to penetrate the skin (18). Over 35 years ago, it was stated that molecules with "well-balanced" partitioning behavior were expected to transport across the skin most effectively (19). Given the discussion above dealing with the mechanism of penetration, it is reasonable to anticipate that lipid solubility is an important factor for percutaneous absorption (see below, and Chaps. 2 and 3). However, because the epidermal layers beneath the SC are aqueous in nature, it follows that a penetrant must also exhibit measurable water solubility in order to permeate through to the dermal microcirculation.

There have been a limited number of comprehensive studies in which percutaneous permeability (e.g., K_p) has been related to the corresponding oil-water (e.g., octanol-water, P) partition coefficient (20). These "structure-activity" relationships have shown characteristic patterns. First, they all reveal an essentially linear region, in which, as predicted by Fick's 1st law for a lipophilic membrane, log K_p increases with log P. Second, as log P becomes large, the relationship reaches a limiting value and then, in some cases, declines (21–23). Fig. 3 illustrates this type of behavior for a series of salicylates and other non-steroidal anti-inflammatory drugs (21). In general, when a parabolic relationship has been observed, the maximum permeability measurement is typically attained at a log P value in the range 2.0–2.5.

The limiting value of skin permeability has been explained on the basis of a shift in the rate-determining step from diffusion across the SC to transport through the underlying aqueous tissue, the latter representing a process which would be predicted to be independent of log P (24). Alternatively, the same independence of log K_p on log P can be rationalized by changing the rate-controlling step through the multilamellar bilayers of the SC from diffusion through the hydrocarbon lipid

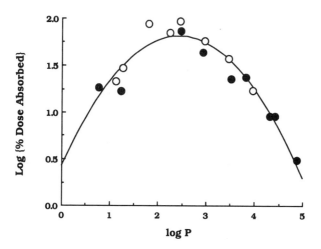

Figure 3 Percutaneous penetration of a series of salicylates (open symbols) and of other nonsteroidal anti-inflammatory drugs (filled symbols), plotted as a function of log P (21).

acyl chains to slow transport at the lipid-aqueous interfaces (25). These explanations, though, cannot explain the diminishing aspect of the parabolic curves seen in the most extensive investigations. The interpretation of these observations requires that one accepts a change in the boundary conditions of the experiment. For very lipophilic compounds, uptake into the SC is rapid and a "reservoir" of chemical throughout this layer is quickly achieved. "Release" of the drug from the lipid phase into the aqueous tissue is impeded, however, because of the high log P and relatively low aqueous solubility of these compounds. The constraints of the system now are that one has a lipophilic reservoir of drug, a lipid-water interface, and an aqueous "sink." Transport across the interface now controls the "efflux" of chemical into the viable epidermis, and this process is inversely dependent upon the lipid-aqueous phase partition coefficient (i.e., as the partition coefficient increases, the interfacial kinetics become progressively slower) (26).

With respect to prodrug design and penetration enhancement, therefore, the target molecule should clearly show affinity for the SC. However, it should also possess sufficient water solubility to ensure that its transport does not become limited by "escape" from the lipophilic regions of the skin. In other words, as far as oil-water partitioning is concerned, it is possible to have too much of a good thing! From a practical standpoint, the engineering of a molecule with suitable partitioning behavior can be achieved through the use of available computer software for log P calculation [e.g., Medchem (27)]. The group contribution approach used by these packages can provide reasonable assessments of the partition coefficient, and can certainly be used to focus the selection of a prodrug structure.

Solubility and Solubility Parameter

Determination of a suitable partition coefficient for a potential prodrug does not guarantee optimum penetration characteristics. The oil-water partition coefficient ($K_{o/w}$) may be defined as follows:

$$K_{o/w} = S_{oil}/S_{water}$$

where S_{oil} and S_{water} are the prodrug's saturation solubilities in oil and water, respectively. Because the partition coefficient is the ratio of solubilities, a $K_{o/w}$ of 2, for example, can also be exhibited by a molecule which is very insoluble in both oil and water. It follows that such a compound will be capable of developing only a very small driving force across the skin, and will penetrate rather slowly. The solubility parameter may give an indication of compounds which are likely to dissolve well in the SC lipids (28). This subject is discussed fully in Chap. 5.

A simple approach to address this issue is to use a standard thermodynamic relationship to relate lipid solubility to melting point. For example, it has been shown, for an unrelated series of chemical structures, that a linear relationship exists between the steady-state flux through excised human epidermis and the reciprocal melting point (Fig. 4) (2,29). It is sensible, therefore, to design prodrugs which have melting points as low as possible.

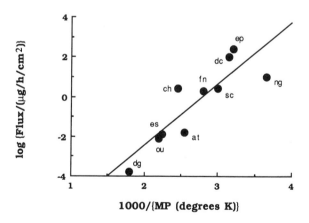

Figure 4 An inverse relationship between drug flux at steady state through excised human skin and penetrant melting point (MP) (2,29). Key: dg = digitoxin, ou = ouabain, es = estradiol, at = atropine, ch = chlorpheniramine, fn = fentanyl, sc = scopolamine, ng = nitroglycerin, dc = diethylcarbamazine, ep = ephedrine.

Molecular Dimensions

There is an ongoing debate concerning the importance of molecular weight (MW), and hence size, on the percutaneous penetration process. The subject is addressed in detail in Chap. 3. At the present time, most of the skin absorption literature relates to the permeation of chemicals whose molecular weights are in the range of 100–400 Da. This fourfold spread in MW is relatively small compared to the very broad (several orders of magnitude) span of oil-water partition coefficients and lipid solubilities exhibited by this same group of compounds. For this reason, in prodrug design (assuming that one is not going to synthesize a molecule larger than, say, 1000 Da), we believe that molecular weight is likely to involve a second-order effect compared to partitioning and solubility.

A further comment about the influence of molecular dimensions on skin permeation is pertinent to previous discussions on the mechanism of percutaneous transport. It has been suggested that a "polar" pathway exists across the SC (24,30). This claim has been justified on the basis of observations that the permeability of polar compounds (log P < –1) is independent of partition coefficient. Typically, data from small and very water-soluble compounds (e.g., glucose, urea, water, methanol) are used to support this thesis (30). Statistically, however, we have shown that the separation of these compounds from those exhibiting the classic linear dependence of permeability upon log P cannot be justified (18). In addition, analysis of a subset of the same data (for the n-alkanols) (24) using the combined lipid solubility/molecular volume approach of Kasting et al. (31) can more than adequately linearize the results (Table 2; Fig. 5).

Table 2 Alkanol Physicochemical Properties and Permeability Coefficients Through Human Skin In Vitro

Alkanol	log P[a]	MV (Å^3)[a]	log $\{K_p(\text{cm/h})\}$[b]
Water	–1.38	10.6	–0.301
Methanol	–0.76	21.7	–0.301
Ethanol	–0.24	31.9	–0.097
Propanol	0.29	42.2	0.146
Butanol	0.82	52.0	0.398
Pentanol	1.35	63.0	0.778
Hexanol	1.88	72.9	1.114
Heptanol	2.41	83.0	1.505
Octanol	2.94	93.0	1.716
Nonanol	3.47	103.0	1.778

[a]From Ref. 27.
[b]From Refs. 24 and 35.

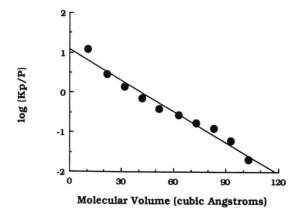

Figure 5 A plot of log {K_p/P} versus molecular volume (MV) for a series of n-alkanols (24). The linearity of the results[log {K_p/P} = (1.09 − 0.026) (MV); r^2 = 0.97] is predicted by the lipid membrane rate-limiting interpretation of Kasting et al. (31).

Molecular weight and volume do not necessarily account for the possible effect of shape on skin transport. Recent work on skin penetration enhancement has shown that the shape of putative promoters can dramatically affect their ability to interact and disorder SC structure (32). Experiments have been conducted in which the penetration-enhancing abilities of the *cis*- and *trans*-isomers of 11-octadecenoic acid were compared. It was found that the *cis*-form (vaccenic acid) was able to enhance significantly the flux of salicylic acid across porcine epidermis, whereas the *trans*-isomer did not. Furthermore, (a) using Fourier transform infrared spectroscopy, it was shown that vaccenic acid increased the overall disorder of the SC lipid domains, and (b) using differential scanning calorimetry, the same *cis*-isomer induced a significant lowering of the intercellular lipid gel-to-liquid crystalline phase transition temperature; the *trans*-isomer had no effect on either of these biophysical measurements. Similar results for oleic acid (*cis*-9-octadecenoic acid) have been reported (33). The conclusion from this work is that the "kinked" structure of the *cis*-unsaturated fatty acids (relative to the essentially "straight" *trans*-isomers) (see Fig. 6) is responsible for their ability to disrupt SC lipid organization and, as a result, to enhance drug flux.

It follows that, as we understand more about the relationships between enhancer structure and function, and with the advent of advanced molecular graphics techniques, it may prove possible to design prodrugs which are capable of enhancing their own penetration across the skin.

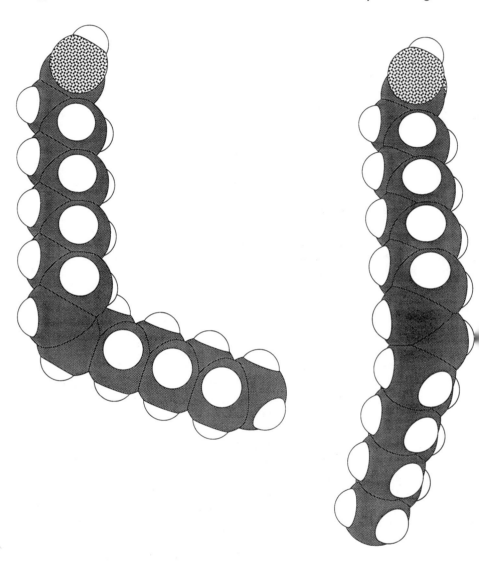

Figure 6   Molecular graphics depictions of the *cis*- and *trans*-isomers of 9-octadecenoic acid.

Polarity and Charge

As stated earlier, polar molecules are poor penetrants through the lipophilic SC. Therefore, prodrug design should minimize the presence of very polar substituents (e.g., hydroxyl and amine groups). The classic work of Scheuplein et al. (35), using corticosteroids of very similar structure but differing in the number of hydroxyl substituents, nicely illustrates this point (Fig. 7). Detailed discussion of the role of functional group contributions in prodrug design is presented in Chaps. 2 and 3.

Given the considerable resistance that the SC presents to the penetration of polar compounds, it is obvious that the skin is extremely impermeable to charged species. Presently, however, there is renewed and intense interest in the use of iontophoresis as a percutaneous penetration enhancement technique (36,37). The possibility exists, therefore, for the development of a strategy of prodrug design that would be based upon the synthesis of a charged precursor of an active drug to be delivered by iontophoresis. One could then take advantage of the anticipated delivery control provided by the iontophoretic procedure to present the prodrug to the activation site in the epidermis or the systemic circulation. At this time, however, no specific examples to illustrate this idea have been reported.

PRODRUG DESIGN TO ENHANCE PERCUTANEOUS PENETRATION

With knowledge of the mechanism of skin permeation and of the major physicochemical factors which influence the kinetics of drug transport, it is possible to identify two approaches that may prove useful in the design of prodrug candidates for topical administration.

1. As indicated above, there are now biophysical techniques available which can be used to deduce the mechanism of penetration enhancer action on the rate-limiting barrier of the SC. Although there have been a number of modes of action of enhancers proposed in the literature (38), few of these are supported by firm experimental data. In most cases, the proposed mechanism has been inferred indirectly; rarely have the data been derived from studies specifically intended to ask mechanistic questions. For example, a typical approach would involve the assessment of an enhancer's effect on the skin penetration of a selection of drugs of different physicochemical properties. If, for instance, the enhancer was found to increase the flux of polar compounds more than that of lipophilic species, then it may be (and, indeed, has been) concluded that the enhancer acts specifically on the polar route through the SC. It may even be speculated that the enhancer action is specific to the protein domains of the barrier (38). Such extrapolations are inappropriate for obvious reasons. First, the experiments have not been designed to probe mechanism. Second, because the skin is such an excellent barrier to polar substances, it is reasonable to expect that the relative enhancement will be greater

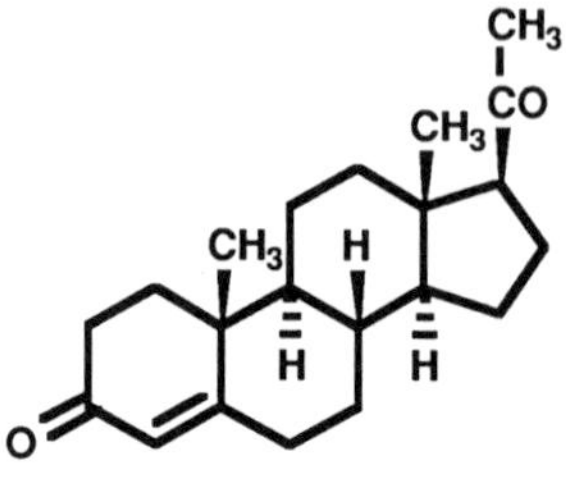

progesterone (1500)

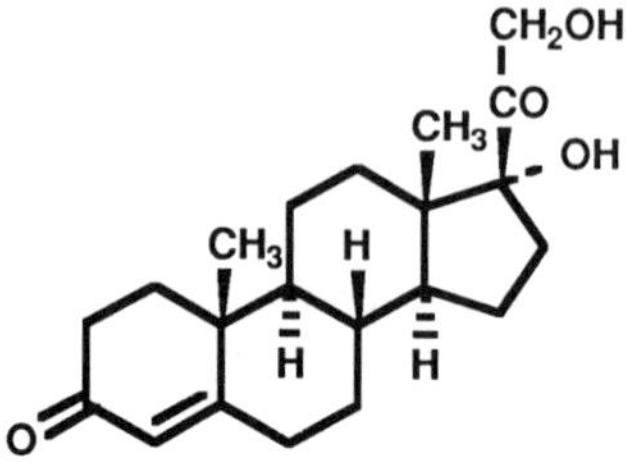

cortexolone (75)

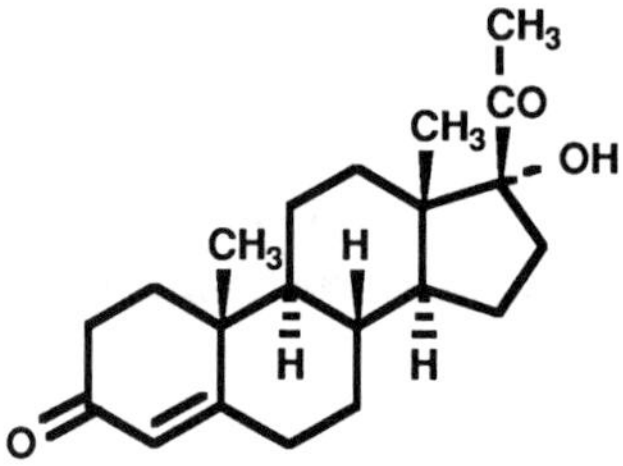

hydroxy-progesterone (600)

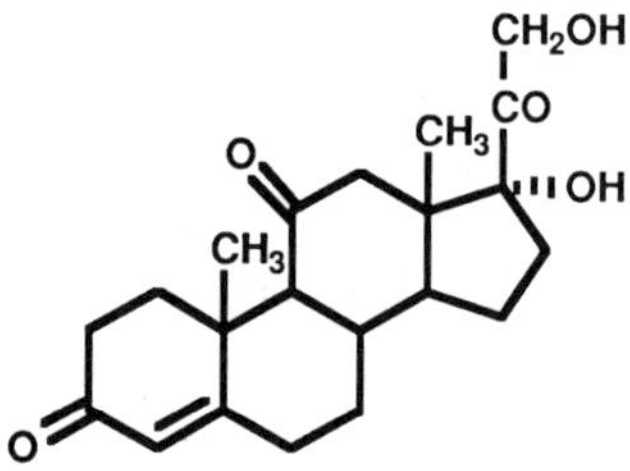

cortisone (10)

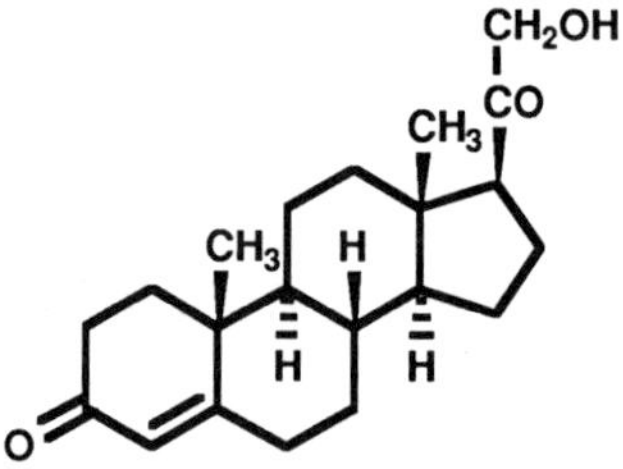

cortexone (450)

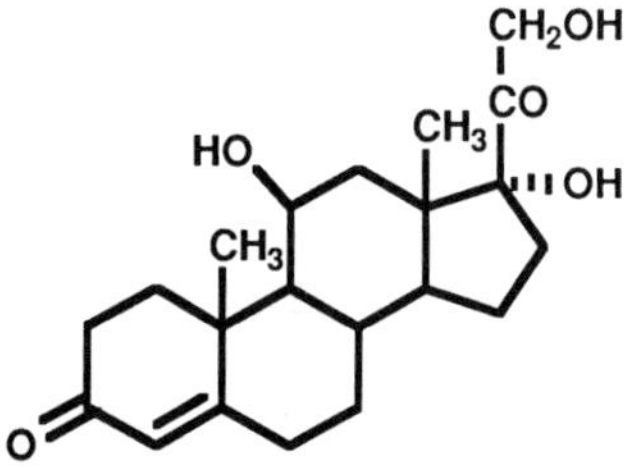

cortisol (3)

Figure 7 The relationship between steroid structure and polarity and percutaneous permeability. The value in parentheses below each analogue is the experimentally determined permeability coefficient ($\times 10^6$ cm/h) across human epidermis in vitro (35).

for less permeable (i.e., polar) compounds, particularly as enhancement (E) is typically defined as the ratio

$$E = \frac{\text{drug flux in the presence of enhancer}}{\text{drug flux in the absence of enhancer}}$$

and one can expect the term in the denominator to be very small (relative to a more lipophilic drug). An example of appropriate mechanistic investigation is the biophysical study of fatty acid penetration enhancers briefly described above (32). In this case, the techniques were intelligently applied and the results were interpreted in a fashion consistent with the membrane biophysics literature. With the information obtained, it is an acceptable hypothesis that the *cis*-unsaturated long-chain fatty acids elicit their action through disruption, in some way, of the SC intercellular lipid domains (32–34). As implied earlier, therefore, one strategy for prodrug design would be to derivatize the active species with a structural feature which possesses inherent enhancing ability (e.g., to synthesize an oleate ester). Naturally, such an approach is not as straightforward as it might seem at first glance. The partitioning and solubility characteristics of the new chemical entity would need to meet appropriate criteria, and the compatibility with, and stability in, the administered formulation or delivery system would have to be acceptable. Nevertheless, this approach could reasonably be characterized as an example of rational (pro)drug design.

2. From the discussion above, we have established that the major physico-chemical influences on percutaneous penetration are the partitioning and solubility characteristics of the penetrant. Therefore, we can envisage that a prodrug synthesized with improved partitioning and solubility features should demonstrate enhanced permeation properties. The question then arises as to how might one design such a prodrug. In recent analyses of the physico-chemical aspects of percutaneous penetration and its enhancement (18,31), it was deduced that (a) the solubility of the permeant in the SC should be maximized in order that the maximum transdermal flux be achieved, and (b) the promotion of lipophilic drug penetration may be most significantly affected by an agent which could facilitate the SC-to-viable epidermis transfer of the penetrant. To exemplify a prodrug design strategy which can address both of these points, we consider a hypothetical molecule which consists of a polar parent drug, such as one containing a carboxylic acid functional group, esterified with propylene glycol. The rationale for this choice, and the expected benefits, are as follows:

1. Esterification of a carboxylic acid functional group with one of the hydroxyls of propylene glycol prevents ionization of the polar functional group at pH values above the pK_a, which might be expected to be about 4.
2. Propylene glycol is a common constituent of topical drug formulations. It is an excellent cosolvent and a useful solubilizing agent for drugs of low water

solubility. It appears to penetrate human skin rapidly, and it has been suggested to be capable of "pulling" the drug along through the SC barrier (14). The proposed prodrug may, therefore, (a) improve the overall solubility properties of the parent drug in both the applied phase and the SC, and (b) increase the diffusive transport of drug species through the SC by, at the least, decreasing the sites of interaction between penetrant and skin. If the remaining -OH on the propylene glycol moiety maintains the polarity of the resulting molecule at too high a level, then a further, simple ester derivatization can be performed.

3. Upon reaching the viable epidermis, we expect rapid hydrolysis of the propylene glycol ester prodrug (by nonspecific esterases, which are present in high concentrations [4]). This should release propylene glycol, which will then be available to enhance the solubilization of the parent drug molecules in the viable tissue.

The likelihood that all of these features can be encompassed in one molecule is probably small, and may not be necessary to achieve the desired enhancement. Furthermore, the arguments may be somewhat different if the strategy is attempted with a lipophilic parent compound. Nevertheless, the approach does illustrate, we believe, a possible solution to a particularly challenging problem.

CONCLUSIONS

The discussion in this chapter has focussed upon the percutaneous penetration component of the triangular relationship related to in vivo drug activity (shown in Fig. 1). The key points involved in the skin transport and enhancement process have been addressed. While it is beyond the scope of this paper to consider the other apices of the "triangle," it should be emphasized that the strategies presented here cannot be conducted without due attention to formulation and pharmacological activity questions. Obviously, if one synthesizes a prodrug, a significant amount of which is not metabolized to the active drug in a timely fashion, then optimization of percutaneous penetration is a waste of time. Equally, it is important that the prodrug has physicochemical properties such that its formulation in practical vehicles is possible. Nevertheless, with our increasing knowledge of the percutaneous penetration process at the molecular level, prodrug design offers interesting research opportunities for the future attention of pharmaceutical scientists in topical drug delivery.

ACKNOWLEDGMENTS

Financial support was provided, in part, by the U.S. National Institutes of Health (HD-23010, HD-27839).

REFERENCES

1. J. Hadgraft, *Nonsteroidal Anti-inflammatory Drugs*, (C. Hensby and N. J. Lowe, eds.), Karger, Basel, 1989, pp. 21–43.
2. R.H. Guy and J. Hadgraft, *Transdermal Drug Delivery: Developmental Issues and Research Initiatives* (J. Hadgraft and R.H. Guy, eds.), Marcel Dekker, New York, 1989, pp. 59–81.
3. B.W. Barry, *Dermatological Formulations: Percutaneous Absorption*, Marcel Dekker, New York, 1983, pp. 95–126.
4. D.A.W. Bucks, *Pharm. Res.*, 1, 148–153 (1984).
5. P.W. Wertz and D.T. Downing, *Transdermal Drug Delivery: Developmental Issues and Research Initiatives* (J. Hadgraft and R.H. Guy, eds.), Marcel Dekker, New York, 1989, pp. 1–22.
6. R.O. Potts, *Transdermal Drug Delivery: Developmental Issues and Research Initiatives* (J. Hadgraft and R.H. Guy, eds.), Marcel Dekker, New York, 1989, pp. 23–57.
7. M.K. Nemanic and P.M. Elias, *J. Histochem. Cytochem.*, 28, 573–578 (1980).
8. H.E. Bodde, M.A.M. Kruithof, J. Brussee, and H.K. Koerten, *Int. J. Pharm.*, 53, 13–24 (1989).
9. R.O. Potts and M.L. Francoeur, *Proc. Natl. Acad. Sci. USA*, 87, 3871–3873 (1990).
10. R.O. Potts and M.L. Francoeur, *J. Invest. Dermatol.*, 96, 495–499 (1991).
11. W.J. Albery and J. Hadgraft, *J. Pharm. Pharmacol.*, 31, 140–147 (1979).
12. R.J. Scheuplein, *J. Invest. Dermatol.*, 45, 334–346 (1967).
13. P.V. Raykar, M. Fung, and B.D. Anderson, *Pharm. Res.*, 5, 140–150 (1988).
14. K.A. Walters, *Transdermal Drug Delivery: Developmental Issues and Research Initiatives* (J. Hadgraft and R.H. Guy, eds.), Marcel Dekker, New York, 1989, pp. 197–246.
15. J.C. Keister and G.B. Kasting, *J. Controlled Release, 4, 111–117 (1986)*.
16. G. Nicolau, R.A. Baughman, A. Tonelli, W. McWilliams, J. Schlitz, and A. Yacobi, *Xenobiotica*, 17, 1113–1120 (1987).
17. H. Schaefer, F. Watts, J. Brod, and B. Illel, *Prediction of Percutaneous Penetration: Methods, Measurements, Modelling* (R.C. Scott, R.H. Guy, and J. Hadgraft, eds.). IBC Technical Services, London, 1990, pp. 163–173.
18. R.H. Guy and J. Hadgraft, *Pharm. Res.*, 5, 753–758 (1988).
19. J.W. Hadgraft and G.F. Somers, *J. Pharm. Pharmacol.*, 8, 625–634 (1956).
20. R.H. Guy and J. Hadgraft, *Percutaneous Absorption*. 2nd Ed. (R.L. Bronaugh and H.I. Maibach, eds.). Marcel Dekker, New York, 1989, pp. 95–109.
21. T. Yano, A. Nakagawa, A., M. Tsuji, and K. Noda, *Life Sci.*, 39, 1043–1050 (1986).
22. T.A. Roy, J.J. Yang, and M.H. Czerwinski, *In Vitro Toxicology: Approaches to Validation* (A.M. Goldberg, ed.). Mary Ann Liebert, New York, 1987, pp. 471–482.
23. R.B. Stoughton, *J. Invest. Dermatol.*, 35, 337–341 (1960).
24. B. Idson and C. R. Behl, *Transdermal Delivery of Drugs*. Vol. 3. (A.F. Kydonieus and B. Berner, eds.). CRC Press, Boca Raton, 1987, pp. 85–151.
25. W.J. Albery and J. Hadgraft, *J. Pharm. Pharmacol.*, 31, 129–139 (1979).
26. J. Hadgraft, *Int. J. Pharm.*, 2, 177–194 (1979).
27. MedChem Release 3.54, DAYLIGHT Chemical Information Systems, Inc., Claremont, California, 1989.

28. K.B. Sloan, *Topical Drug Delivery Formulations* (D.W. Osborne and A.H. Amann, eds.). Marcel Dekker, New York, 1990, pp. 245–270.

29. A.S. Michaels, S.K. Chandrasekaran, and J.E. Shaw, *A.I.Ch.E. J.*, 21, 985–996 (1975).

30. G.L. Flynn, *Percutaneous Absorption*. 2nd Ed. (R.L. Bronaugh and H.I. Maibach, eds.). Marcel Dekker, New York, 1989, pp. 27–51.

31. G.B. Kasting, R.L. Smith, and E.R. Cooper, *Skin Pharmacokinetics* (B. Shroot and H. Schaefer, eds.). Karger, Basel, 1987, pp. 138–153.

32. G.M. Golden, J.E. McKie, and R.O. Potts, *J. Pharm. Sci.*, 76, 25–28 (1986).

33. M.L. Francoeur, G.M. Golden, and R.O. Potts, *Pharm. Res.*, 7, 621–627 (1990).

34. V.H.K. Mak, R.O. Potts, and R.H. Guy, *J. Controlled Release, 12, 67–75 (1990).*

35. R.J. Scheuplein, I.H. Blank, G.J. Brauner, and D.J. MacFarlane, *J. Invest. Dermatol.*, 52, 63–70 (1969).

36. P. Tyle, *Pharm. Res.*, 3, 318–326 (1986).

37. R.R. Burnette, in *Transdermal Drug Delivery: Developmental Issues and Research Initiatives* (J. Hadgraft and R.H. Guy, eds.). Marcel Dekker, New York, 1989, pp. 247–291.

38. B.W. Barry, *J. Controlled Release*, 6, 85–97 (1987).

2

Functional Group Considerations in the Development of Prodrug Approaches to Solving Topical Delivery Problems

Kenneth B. Sloan
University of Florida, Gainesville, Florida

INTRODUCTION

The term *prodrug* was first introduced by Albert in 1951 (1), to describe compounds which undergo biotransformations prior to exhibiting their pharmacological effects. The use of the term has since been expanded to include compounds which undergo chemical as well as biological transformations (2), but the basic concept has remained the same. The prodrug concept encompasses most synthetic organic chemistry–based approaches to changing the physicochemical, and hence the biological properties of a parent drug in a transient manner to overcome some intrinsic problem associated with the therapeutic use of the parent drug. The particular combination of functional groups introduced into the parent drug to give the prodrug comprises the promoiety.

Prodrugs have been developed to overcome bad taste, poor aqueous as well as lipid solubility, inadequate chemical and enzymatic stability, incomplete absorption across a variety of biological membranes, and premature metabolism to inactive species, to name only a few of the problems that have been addressed (3). In many of these cases the problem associated with the bad taste, poor solubility, etc., can be traced to a particular functional group in the parent drug, and the solution to the problem involves transiently covering or masking that functional group with a functional group from the promoiety (4). The combination of the two functional groups results in the formation of a new functional group which usually exhibits quite different physicochemical properties compared to its component functional groups, but which must be capable of reverting to those components in vivo. For this discussion we will call this combination an enabling functional group because it enables the derivative that has been formed to function as a prodrug. For example, the combination of an alcohol functional group in a parent drug with a carboxylic acid (carbonyl) functional group in a promoiety gives an ester functional group (the enabling functional group) which can be readily hydrolyzed to its components in vivo by esterases.

Often overlooked in this analysis is the alkyl or aryl functional group that is attached to the promoiety side of the enabling functional group, and which itself may contain additional functional groups. In many cases, the additional functional group is actually responsible for imparting the desired property to the promoiety, and hence to the prodrug. For example, in the case of hemisuccinate ester prodrugs, the desired enhanced water solubility of the prodrug derives from the free carboxylic acid functional group that is not involved in forming the ester with the parent drug. Thus, the entire promoiety and not just the enabling functional group must be considered in designing a prodrug to exhibit certain targeted physicochemical properties.

Of the many problems addressed with prodrug approaches, incomplete absorption or poor partitioning across a biological membrane presents one of the more challenging problems to overcome. Besides the usual constraints on prodrug design such as the prodrug being stable until the absorption process is complete, a prodrug that has been designed to overcome poor partitioning properties usually has been designed to achieve enhanced aqueous as well as enhanced lipid solubility compared to the parent drug. Often such enhanced biphasic solubility is difficult to accomplish. In addition, many biological membranes are difficult to isolate for in vitro experimentation.

Topical membranes, and especially the skin, are exceptions to the later problem in that they are readily accessible to experimentation. Thus, a systematic delineation of the factors involved in optimizing delivery by prodrugs should be more readily accomplished for topical delivery than for other routes of delivery. In this chapter, the discussion of topical delivery will be limited to include only dermal and transdermal delivery. Chapter 7 will cover ocular delivery which is also considered a form of topical delivery. A discussion of the biology, physiology, etc., of the skin is not presented here either. The interested reader is referred to more general texts for those discussions (5).

Regardless of the ease of access to skin for experimentation and the desirability of developing optimized prodrug approaches to enhancing topical delivery, progress has been relatively slow. It was not until 1985 that a book chapter dedicated to "Prodrugs and skin absorption" appeared (6). Since then one other chapter (7) on the use of "Prodrugs in transdermal delivery" and two reviews on "Prodrugs for dermal delivery" have been published (8,9). Not surprisingly, the number and spectrum of prodrug approaches to enhancing topical delivery has also expanded significantly since 1985.

One of the reasons for the previous lack of systematic investigations of prodrugs for topical delivery may in part be due to the general assumption that a good formulation approach can always be developed to solve topical delivery problems, and that a formulation approach can solve the problem easier, faster, and with fewer problems associated with U.S. Food and Drug Administration (FDA) approval of the formulation approach than of a prodrug approach. The bases for this assumption appear to be (a) that there is no theoretical limit to the improvement in topical delivery that can be obtained using a formulation approach, and (b) that increased improvement in topical delivery with a formulation approach can be achieved without causing irreversible damage to the skin.

In fact, there may be no bases for the assumption. A number of papers have been published which suggest that there is indeed a theoretical limit to the rate of transdermal delivery of polar drugs that can be achieved—at least using simple one component vehicles—without causing irreversible damage to hairless mouse skin (10–13). The analysis of the relationship between flux (J), partition coefficient (K), and permeability coefficient (P) on one hand, and the solubility of the drug in the vehicle (C_v) on the other hand (eq. 1) suggests that there is a parabolic relationship between log K or log P and the polarity of the vehicle. The form of the relationship derives from its basis in regular solution theory (eq. 2). The general result is simply that the more soluble the drug is in the vehicle the lower the permeability coefficient for the transdermal delivery of the drug from that vehicle. Thus, in many instances where an order of magnitude improvement in topical delivery may be necessary to achieve a required therapeutic endpoint, a simple formulation approach may not be adequate and a prodrug or a combination prodrug-formulation approach may be required.

$$J = K \, C_v(D/h)$$

$$P = J/C_v = K(D/h) \tag{1}$$

$$\log K = [(\delta_i{-}\delta_v)^2 - (\delta_i{-}\delta_s)^2] \, V_i/2.3 \, RT \tag{2}$$

The implications of this type of analysis of solute-solvent interactions for predicting and/or optimizing topical delivery will be discussed in Chap. 5 (14). However, for the purpose of these discussions, it should be noted that among the variables in equation 1, this analysis assumes that the diffusion coefficient (D) and the membrane thickness (h) remain constant unless the vehicle changes the properties of the membrane. Thus, $P = K \bullet$ constant. In equation 2, the solubility parameter values for the drug or prodrug (δ_i), vehicle (δ_v), and skin (δ_s), and molar volume of the drug or prodrug (V_i) can be calculated from group contribution methods (15,16), or can be determined experimentally (16,17). Thus, K, and hence P, can be calculated and J can be predicted if C_v is known.

A single solution to the general problem of optimizing prodrug approaches to enhance topical delivery does not exist. An obvious complication is that a promoiety that works for one class of parent drugs may or may not work for a different class containing a different set of functional groups and exhibiting entirely different initial physicochemical properties. In addition, in some situations, absorption through the entire skin to elicit a systemic effect—transdermal delivery—is desired, whereas in other situations absorption only through the stratum corneum and into the epidermis—dermal delivery—is desired. Transdermal delivery would be an undesired side effect in the latter situation. A prodrug approach that optimized transdermal delivery may not necessarily lead to optimization of dermal delivery.

However, a strategy for identifying the best solution to a particular problem of optimizing a prodrug approach to enhance topical delivery does exist. In order to optimize transdermal delivery with a particular type of prodrug that has been synthesized, it is necessary to evaluate results from a minimum of three kinds of experiments. It is necessary to: (a) determine the solubilities of the homologous series of the prodrugs in aqueous and lipoidal solvents, (b) determine the stabilities of the prodrugs to chemical and enzymatic hydrolysis, and (c) determine the rates of delivery of the parent drug by the prodrugs through a membrane in diffusion cell experiments. Trends in results from the latter experiments can then be evaluated to determine which direction changes in the solubilities and stabilities need to take to optimize delivery with that particular type of prodrug. Then other series of prodrugs analogous to the first series can be synthesized, characterized, and their delivery properties evaluated. The cycle can be repeated as necessary to achieve optimization. Alternatively, results from the third experiment may suggest that an entirely different type of prodrug containing different types of functional groups is necessary to give the desired physicochemical properties, and hence the desired rate of transdermal delivery.

On the other hand, in order to optimize dermal delivery, results from an additional, fourth kind of experiment need to be evaluated. In this experiment, rates of delivery into the target epidermal cells are determined from in vivo biological responses. Generally, it has been assumed that increased transdermal delivery correlates with increased dermal delivery. Although there are data to support this assumption for particular cases (18,19), the evidence is certainly not compelling enough to allow one to extrapolate to the general case. Stella and Himmelstein have addressed this issue for the general case (20). If the prodrug regenerates the parent drug slower than its transfer into the target cells, the conversion of the prodrug to the parent drug must be faster than the rate of clearance of the parent drug from the target cell if enhanced delivery into the cell is to be achieved. On the other hand, if the prodrug regenerates the parent drug faster than its transfer into the target cell, high intercellular levels of parent drug build up, and those increased levels must lead to higher intracellular levels of the parent drug—possibly through a passive diffusion process—if enhanced delivery into the cell is to be achieved.

Although data from all four of the above experiments are necessary to confidently optimize dermal delivery by a particular type of prodrug, usually data from only two or three of the different experiments is available for analysis. Often the report of a new type of prodrug describes the synthesis of an homologous series of representatives of the new type, their characterization by partition coefficients, solubilities, stabilities in buffers and biological media, and the ability of one or two members of the series to deliver the parent drug through skin from one vehicle in diffusion cell experiments. Only recently have the effects of different vehicles on topical delivery of a parent drug by a prodrug been described, and only recently have an entire series of homologous prodrugs been characterized in diffusion cell experiments.

In this chapter, we hope to describe results from most of the prodrug approaches that have been used to increase transdermal delivery, and to suggest the implications of those results for the development of other prodrug approaches to enhance dermal and transdermal delivery. Owing to the importance of functional groups in dictating both the problems of the parent drug and the solutions to the problems embodied in the promoiety, the chapter is organized according to functional groups in the parent drugs that are the point of attachment of the promoieties. Each section is then divided into subsections on types of reported prodrug approaches for transiently masking that functional group. This organizational approach will enable the reader to: (a) assess the suitability of using different types of promoieties that have been used for a specific functional group to mask the same functional group in analogous drugs, (b) assess the suitability of using a specific promoiety that has been used for one type of functional group to mask different types of functional groups, and (c) assess the suitability of developing new promoieties from the components of other successful promoieties.

FUNCTIONAL GROUPS

Most prodrugs can be divided into two general types. The first general type is one in which one of the functional groups that gives the promoiety its characteristic physicochemical and biological properties is directly attached to the functional group in the parent drug that is to be transiently masked. The second general type of prodrug is one in which that functional group in the promoiety is separated from the functional group in the parent drug by a methylene group or vinylogous methylene group.

For the first general type of prodrug, the point of attachment of the functional group in the promoiety to the parent drug is through a heteroatom such as nitrogen, oxygen, or sulfur. This heteroatom is a part of the functional group in the parent drug that is to be masked. The combination of the two functional groups is the enabling functional group referred to in the previous section. Thus, the generic formula for this first type of prodrug may be represented simply by 1. In this case, X is the functional group and associated heteroatom from the parent drug, and R is the promoiety which contains the functional group(s) that are responsible for the change in the properties of Drug-XH: the parent drug.

Drug-X-R
1

Table 1 gives examples of the XH functional groups in parent drugs that have been the object of transient modification to enhance the topical delivery of drugs containing those functional groups. Some of the functional groups are simple— either a heteroatom or a carbonyl group. Others are complex—combinations of one or two heteroatoms with a carbonyl group. Table 2 gives representative examples of R that have been used as promoieties for both general types of prodrugs: R contain one or more functional groups. However, not every R can be combined with every Drug-XH. Obviously, R based on the first three examples listed in Table 2 would normally function as promoieties only if attached to a carboxylic acid type Drug-XH functional group, or if a high-energy oxidative metabolic pathway was available to regenerate the parent drug. Table 3 gives a nonexhaustive list of potential Drug-X-R combinations. Cyclic examples are also possible, especially for carbonyl type Drug-XH (entries 18–22), but they are not listed.

For the second general type of prodrug, both the functional group in the promoiety and the functional group in the parent drug are attached to a methylene or a vinylogous methylene group through a heteroatom such as NR', oxygen, or sulfur. Thus, the generic formula for this second type of prodrug may be represented simply by **2**, where X and R have the same definitions as before, but now Z can be NR', oxygen, or sulfur as well. In certain cases, Z may also be sulfinyl or sulfonyl. This ensures that the promoiety is enzymatically or chemically labile due to the chemically labile nature of Drug-X-CH$_2$-ZH after R has been chemically or enzymatically removed (4). This second type of prodrug is a soft alkyl derivative

Table 1 Drug-XH Functional Groups

Structure	Name
1. Drug-NH	Secondary Amine
2. Drug-NH$_2$	Primary Amine
3. Drug-SH	Thiol
4. Drug-OH	Hydroxy
5. Drug-C=O	Carbonyl (aldehyde or ketone)
6. Drug-(C=O)-OH	Carbonylhydroxy (carboxylic acid)
7. Drug-(C=O)-NH$_2$	Carbonylamine (amide)
8. Drug-(C=O)$_2$-NH	Dicarbonylamine (imide)
9. Drug-(O=S=O)-NH$_2$	Sulfonylamine (sulfonamide)

Table 2 R Promoieties

Structure[a]	Name
1. $-CH_2-R'$	Alkyl
2. $-CH=CH-R'$	Alkenyl
3. $-C_6H_4-R'$[b]	Aryl
4. $-(C=O)-R'$	Alkylcarbonyl
5. $-(C=O)-OR'$	Alkoxycarbonyl
6. $-(C=O)-NR'_2$	Dialkylaminocarbonyl
7. $-(C=O)-SR'$	Alkylthiocarbonyl
8. $-S-R'$	Alkylsulfenyl
9. $-(S=O)-R'$	Alkylsulfinyl (sulfoxide)
10. $-(O=S=O)-R'$	Alkylsulfonyl (sulfone)
11. $-(P=O)(O-R')_2$	Dialkylphosphonyl

[a]$R' = (CH_2)_nH$ and $n = 0, 1, 2 \ldots$

[b]$C_6H_4 = $

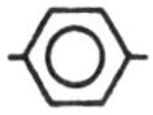

(21). It also increases the types of functional groups that can be introduced into a promoiety for use in combination with any specific functional group in the parent drug to serve as the enabling functional group.

$$\text{Drug-X-CH}_2\text{-Z-R}$$
$$\textbf{2}$$

For example, in Table 3 there are six entries for Drug-X-R combinations where the original functional group in the parent drug is a hydroxy group. In Table 4 is a nonexhaustive list of possible Drug-X-CH$_2$-Z-R combinations, where X is oxygen. The number of possibilities has increased by almost a factor of three because of the flexibility derived from the use of CH$_2$-Z, where Z can be O, NR', or S. Moreover, this analysis does not take into account the possibility of substitution on the methylene group ($-CH_2-$) by alkyl, aryl or electron withdrawing groups such as CCl$_3$, (C=O)R', (C=O)OR', (C=O)NR$_2'$, etc., or the possibility of using a vinylogous methylene group instead of a methylene itself in Drug-X-CH$_2$-Z-R. The last entry in Table 4 describes one example of the latter possibility.

Also, none of the above analyses take into account the possibility of introducing other functional groups into the R' group. An example where a second carboxylic acid group was introduced into R' to impart enhanced water solubility to the promoiety has already been mentioned—a hemisuccinate ester, Drug-O-(C=O)CH$_2$CH$_2$(C=O)OH. Generally, R' has been defined as (CH$_2$)$_n$H, but it could also be defined as (CH$_2$)$_n$–Z(CH$_2$)$_m$H or (CH$_2$)$_n$R. In the former case, if Z = NR'

Table 3 Drug-X]-[R Combinations

Drug-XH	Structure[a]	Compound
1. Drug-NH	Drug-N]-[R'	Alkylamine
2. Drug-NH	Drug-N]-[(C=O)-R'	Alkylcarbonylamino (amide)
3. Drug-NH	Drug-N]-[(C=O)-OR'	Alkoxycarbonylamino (carbamate)
4. Drug-NH	Drug-N]-[(C=O)-NR$_2'$	Dialkylaminocarbonylamino (urea)
5. Drug-NH	Drug-N]-[(C=O)-SR'	Alkylthiocarbonylamino
6. Drug-NH	Drug-N]-[(O=S=O)-R'	Alkylsulfonylamino (sulfonamide)
7. Drug-OH	Drug-O]-[R'	Alkyl ether
8. Drug-OH	Drug-O]-[(C=O)-R'	Alkylcarbonyloxy (ester)
9. Drug-OH	Drug-O]-[(C=O)-OR'	Alkoxycarbonyloxy (carbonate)
10. Drug-OH	Drug-O]-[(C=O)-NR$_2'$	Dialkylaminocarbonyloxy (carbamate)
11. Drug-OH	Drug-O]-[(C=O)-SR'	Alkylthiocarbonyloxy
12. Drug-OH	Drug-O]-[(O=S=O)-R'	Alkylsulfonyloxy
13. Drug-(C=O)OH	Drug-(C=O)-O]-[R'	Alkyloxycarbonyl (ester)
14. Drug-(C=O)OH	Drug-(C=O)-O]-[NR$_2'$	Dialkylaminooxycarbonyl
15. Drug-(C=O)OH	Drug-(C=O)-O]-[(C=O)-R'	Alkylcarbonyloxycarbonyl (anhydride)
16. Drug-(C=O)OH	Drug-(C=O)-O]-[(C=O)-OR'	Alkoxycarbonyloxycarbonyl
17. Drug-(C=O)OH	Drug-(C=O)-O]-[(C=O)-NR$_2'$	Dialkylaminocarbonyloxycarbonyl

18. Drug C=O   Drug-C] $\overset{\diagup OR'}{\diagdown OR'}$ Acetal or ketal

19. Drug C=O   Drug-C] $\overset{\diagup NR_2'}{\diagdown OR'}$

20. Drug C=O   Drug-C] $\overset{\diagup OR'}{\diagdown SR'}$ Hemithioacetal or hemithioketal

21. Drug C=O   Drug-C] $\overset{\diagup NR_2'}{\diagdown SR'}$

22. Drug C=O   Drug-C] $\overset{\diagup SR'}{\diagdown SR'}$ Thioacetal or thioketal

---

[a]R' = (CH$_2$)$_n$H and n = 0, 1, 2 . . .

Table 4   Drug-X]-CH$_2$-Z-[R Combinations

Structures[a]

1. Drug-O-]-CH$_2$-O-[R'
2. Drug-O-]-CH$_2$-NR'-[R'
3. Drug-O-]-CH$_2$-S-[R'
4. Drug-O-]-CH$_2$-(S=O)-[R'
5. Drug-O-]-CH$_2$-(O=S=O)-[R'

6. Drug-O-]-CH$_2$-O-[(C=O)-R'
7. Drug-O-]-CH$_2$-NR'-[(C=O)-R'
8. Drug-O-]-CH$_2$-S-[(C=O)-R'

9. Drug-O-]-CH$_2$-O-[(C=O)-OR'
10. Drug-O-]-CH$_2$-NR'-[(C=O)-OR'
11. Drug-O-]-CH$_2$-S-[(C=O)-OR'

12. Drug-O-]-CH$_2$-O-[(C=O)-NR$_2'$
13. Drug-O-]-CH$_2$-NR'-[(C=O)-NR$_2'$
14. Drug-O-]-CH$_2$-S-[(C=O)-NR$_2'$

15. Drug-O-]-CH$_2$-C$_6$H$_4$-O-[(C=O)-R'[b]

[a]R' = (CH$_2$)$_n$H and n = 0, 1, 2, . . .

[b]C$_6$H$_4$ =

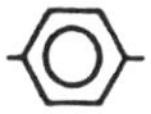

and R' = alkyl, then the effect would be to greatly enhance the water-solubilizing potential of the promoiety.

  The idea in this section has been to illustrate the immense number of combinations that exist for putting together functional groups from the promoiety and the parent drug to form a prodrug. Some of the combinations given as examples may be very difficult to synthesize, some may be too stable or too unstable to be given much consideration for further evaluation, and finally other examples may not impart the desired physicochemical properties to the prodrug. However, we have only begun to scratch the surface of what may be possible. In the next section, we will see what levels of performance are possible from the combinations that have been evaluated.

DRUG-NH

In this section, only a few examples of prodrug approaches to enhancing the delivery of a parent drug containing basic-NH groups will be discussed. Most of the examples will be of drugs containing acidic-NH groups. A basic-NH functional group usually imparts good lipid as well as good water solubility to any molecule to which it is attached. This kind of biphasic solubility characteristic results in molecules that cross biological membranes fairly well without the need of further chemical modification. In fact, there are examples of molecules that contain a basic amine group which purportedly function as penetration enhancers (22–24), and we will see examples later where the incorporation of a promoiety containing a basic amine group into a drug molecule (N-Mannich bases) has improved the transdermal delivery of that drug (25–27).

On the other hand, drugs containing acidic-NH functional groups usually exhibit high melting points and poor solubility characteristics, especially in lipoidal solvents but also in water as well because of their tendency to form intermolecular hydrogen bonds. Among the typical functional groups that can be classed as acidic-NH groups are imides, sulfonamides, amides, carbamates, ureas, etc., although the acidic pK_as of the latter three are quite high—in the region of 15–17. Also included as drugs that contain acidic-NH groups are the various heterocyclic type drugs. In the case of heterocycles, there are frequently no readily identifiable carbonyl functional groups adjacent to or conjugated with the NH groups that are responsible for the acidic nature of the heterocycle, but they behave as acidic groups nonetheless.

α-(Acyloxy)alkyl Derivatives of Acidic-NH Groups: Drug-N-CHR'-O(C=O)-R'

One of the more carefully investigated prodrug approaches to enhancing the topical delivery of drugs containing acidic-NH groups is the use of α-(acyloxy)alkyl derivatives to change the physicochemical properties of the parent drug. These derivatives are formally alkyl derivatives so that their attachment to a heteroatom—in this case nitrogen—does not radically change the electron density on the heteroatom the way attachment of an acyl group would. α-(Acyloxy)alkyl derivatives belong to the second general type of prodrug mentioned above: Drug-X-CH$_2$-Z-R. In this case, X contains a nitrogen atom, Z is oxygen, and R contains a carbonyl functional group which together with Z forms an ester-enabling group—3. So in many ways α-(acyloxy)alkyl derivatives are very similar to the more traditional and familiar O-acyl type of prodrugs in that the enabling functional group is an ester group in both cases, and its esterase-mediated or chemical cleavage is responsible for regeneration of the parent drug. However, in the case of α-(acyloxy)alkyl derivatives, an intermediate, 4, is formed first, which then must spontaneously disassociate into the parent drug and a molecule of an aldehyde, or on rare occasions a ketone (4). This latter reaction is usually very fast for fairly acidic molecules or where the methylene group is substituted, but it can be so slow for a typical amide, for instance, that 4 can undergo oxidation to a formyl derivative before dissociation takes place (28).

DRUG-N-CH$_2$O(C=O)R' $\xrightarrow{\text{ESTERASE}}$ DRUG-N-CH$_2$OH

3   **4**

DRUG-NH + CH$_2$=O   Scheme 1

Theophylline

The α-(acyloxy)alkyl derivatives of theophylline have a historical significance in any discussion of prodrug approaches to enhancing topical delivery. The first examples of α-(acyloxy)alkyl derivatives described as prodrugs were of nitrofurantoin in 1964 (29) and of benzylpenicillin in 1965 (30), but it was not until the 1977 publication of the patent on α-(acyloxy)alkyl derivatives of theophylline that their use to enhance topical delivery was first mentioned (31). The complete description of the theophylline derivatives was finally published in 1982 (18), and was notable for several reasons. First, not only were the results from diffusion cell experiments with several members of a well-characterized homologous series of prodrugs reported, but their effect on inhibiting epidermal deoxyribonucleic acid (DNA) synthesis was reported as well. Second, trends in relationships between the solubilities of the prodrugs in lipoidal solvents and in water, and their ability to deliver the parent drug through skin were observed which have provided a starting point from which subsequent conclusions about optimization of other approaches to enhancing topical delivery with prodrugs have been drawn.

Theophylline exhibits solubility properties that are typical of many heterocycles—it is not very soluble in lipoidal vehicles. Thus, it has been suggested that theophylline does not permeate the lipoidal domains of the skin very well. Interest in increasing the lipid solubility, and hence its topical delivery, derives from its ability to modulate cyclic adenosine monophosphate (cAMP) levels which can affect psoriasis (32).

The acyloxymethyl derivatives of theophylline that were described in 1982 are shown in Table 5. This still represents one of the more diversified groups of this type of prodrug derivatives reported in one publication. Besides the homologous series of simple R' = alkyl acyloxymethyl derivatives, there are two examples of substituted R' where the substituent [R' = CH$_2$N(CH$_3$)$_2$ and R' = CH$_2$CH$_2$(C=O)N(C$_2$H$_5$)$_2$] was designed to impart increased water solubility to the prodrug. There is also an example of an α-(alkoxycarbonyloxy)alkyl prodrug, **16**, which was designed to exhibit entirely different stability and solubility properties compared to the α-(alkylcarbonyloxy)alkyl examples because of the substitution of a carbonate functional group for an ester functional group. Finally, there is an example of a hydroxymethyl prodrug, **7**, which is chemically (4) as opposed to enzymatically labile. This is the only description of the use of a hydroxymethyl derivative as a prodrug to enhance transdermal delivery.

Table 5   Selected Physicochemical Properties of Acyloxymethyl Derivatives of Theophylline

Compound, R =	MP°C	C_v^a		K^b
		H$_2$O	heptane	
5, H, Theophylline	270-274	8.3	—^{c}	—
6, CH$_3$, Caffeine	238	21.8	—	—
7, CH$_2$OH	260-262(d)	—	0.008	—
8, CH$_2$O(C=O)CH$_3$	163-166	3.74	0.03	0.14
9, CH$_2$O(C=O)C$_2$H$_5$	142-144	—	—	—
10, CH$_2$O(C=O)C$_3$H$_7$	102-105	3.89	0.65	0.16
11, CH$_2$O(C=O)C$_5$H$_{11}$	79-82	0.71	2.26	2.4
12, CH$_2$O(C=O)C$_7$H$_{15}$	65-68	0.12	0.52	16.7
13, CH$_2$O(C=O)C(CH$_3$)$_3$	108-109.5	2.01	1.55	0.9
14, CH$_2$O(C=O)CH$_2$N(CH$_3$)$_2$	112-113	>1000	<0.02	—
15, CH$_2$O(C=O)CH$_2$CH$_2$(C=O)N(C$_2$H$_5$)$_2$	100-103	26.3	0.17	0.04
16, CH$_2$O(C=O)OC$_2$H$_5$	126-127	3.87	0.18	0.034

^{a}Solubility in mg/ml at 23 ± 1°C.
^{b}Partition coefficient between water and heptane determined at 23 ± 1°C.
^{c}Could not be determined.
Source: Data from Ref. 18.

In Table 5, the effect of increasing the alkyl chain length of the acyl portion of the simple R′ = alkyl derivatives (**8–13**) can be readily seen. As expected, all of the acyloxymethyl derivatives exhibit lower melting points and lower water solubilities than theophylline. The acetyloxymethyl, **8**, and the butyryloxymethyl, **10**, derivatives exhibit the highest water solubilities in the series, but then the water solubility falls off rapidly for the higher members of the series. However, those solubilities are considerably lower than those exhibited by the derivatives containing basic amine (**14**) or tertiary amide (**15**) functional groups, or the solubility expected for the hydroxymethyl derivative, **7**, based on analogy to other hydroxymethyl derivatives (33,34). Also as expected, the lipid solubilities of the derivatives are all significantly higher than that of theophylline. However, the lipid solubilities seem to peak for the hexanoyloxymethyl derivative, **11**, in heptane and fall off with the octanoyloxymethyl derivative, **12**, even though the melting point of the octanoyloxymethyl derivative continues the trend to lower melting points with longer acyl chains.

In view of the observed lipid and water solubilities of the prodrugs, the results from the diffusion cell experiments in Table 6 were unexpected at that time. Both of the acyloxymethyl derivatives that were evaluated in diffusion cell experiments were more effective at delivering theophylline from an isopropyl myristate (IPM) vehicle than theophylline itself. The particular derivatives (**10** and **13**) that were selected for evaluation were selected because they were two of the more lipid-soluble derivatives which retained significant water solubility compared to theophylline. So the performance of **10** and **13** was not unexpected. What was unexpected was that the hyroxymethyl derivative, **7**, was the best prodrug evaluated for enhancing transdermal delivery. The hydroxymethyl derivative, although much more soluble in IPM than theophylline, was still much less soluble than either **10** or **13**. On the other hand, **7** should be much more soluble in water than theophylline, and hence than any of the simple R′ = alkyl acyloxymethyl derivatives. Comparisons of **7** with **10** or **13** should not be overanalyzed because they represent totally different types of prodrugs, but the comparison does suggest a similar trend in the comparison of **10** with **13**. In that comparison, the more water-soluble derivative **10** is marginally better at enhancing the transdermal delivery of theophylline. Thus, the unexpected result was that water solubility as well as enhanced lipid solubility is an important factor to consider in any attempt to optimize a particular prodrug approach to enhancing topical delivery. In the case of the acyloxymethyl derivatives of theophylline, potentially the best derivatives, **8** and **9**, were not even evaluated.

Although **10** and **13** were effective at enhancing the transdermal delivery of theophylline, the more important question from a therapeutic point of view was whether the prodrugs delivered more theophylline to the target epidermal cells. The results from the inhibition of epidermal DNA synthesis (35) by selected

Table 6 Transdermal Delivery of Theophylline by Hydroxymethyl and Acyloxymethyl Derivatives

Compound	C_v[a]	J[b]	log P[c]
5	0.04	0.017 (0.0001)	–0.37
7	0.63	0.11 (0.030)	–0.75
10	5.40	0.073 (0.00064)	–1.87
13	4.04	0.059 (0.00092)	–1.84

[a]Solubility of compounds in equivalent mg of theophylline/ml of isopropyl myristate (IPM) at 23 ± 1°C.
[b]Flux in mg/cm^2/h (± SD) from an IPM suspension through hairless mouse skin with a receptor phase temperature of 32°C.
[c]Permeability coefficient in cm/h determined from J/C_v.
Source: Data from Ref. 18.

acyloxymethyl derivatives of theophylline suggest that there is a correlation between enhanced delivery of theophylline through skin and its ability to inhibit DNA synthesis in the skin (Table 7). Prodrug 10 delivers more theophylline through the skin from IPM than 13, and 10 is more effective at inhibiting epidermal DNA synthesis than 13 when applied in the same vehicle. Furthermore, the result was the same regardless of whether IPM or propylene glycol (PG) was used.

5-Fluorouracil

5-Fluorouracil (5-FU) is another typical polar heterocycle which exhibits a high melting point and poor lipid solubility. Whereas a clinical usefulness for topically delivered theophylline has not been identified, the clinical usefulness for topical 5-FU preparations is well established (36). 5-FU is useful in treating actinic keratoses and basal cell carcinomas, but an improved topical delivery of 5-FU would be valuable for treating actinic keratoses on less permeable areas such as the arm (37). The first type of prodrug of 5-FU that was evaluated for its potential to enhance the topical delivery of 5-FU is the acyloxymethyl type.

In Table 8 are listed the various 1-mono, 3-mono, and 1,3-bis derivatives that have been synthesized (38,39). Ozaki et al. also synthesized some examples of α-(acyloxy)alkyl derivatives of 5-FU where the methylene group is substituted

Table 7 Inhibition of Epidermal DNA Synthesis in Mice by Acyloxymethyl Derivatives of Theophylline

Treatment[a]	% Concentration	CPM[b]/10 mg DNA	% Inhibition
Nonirradiated		270 ± 93	
IPM control		647 ± 95	
15/IPM	10	653 ± 262	0
13/IPM	10	462 ± 365	49
10/IPM	10	311 ± 155	89
Nonirradiated		230 ± 44	
PG control		623 ± 66	
15/PG	10	569 ± 90	14
13/PG	10	414 ± 77	53
10/PG	10	254 ± 88	94
10/PG	1	641 ± 86	0
FA/PG[c]	1	210 ± 79	105
FA/PG[c]	0.1	389 ± 81	60

[a]Mice irradiated at 254 nm for 5 min at 40 cm, treated with drug/vehicle five times/48h, injected with [3H] thymidine after 53h, sacrificed after 56h.
[b]Counts per minute.
[c]Fluocinolone acetonide in PG.
Source: Data from Ref. 18.

Table 8 Acyloxymethyl Derivatives of 5-FU

$$\begin{array}{c} O \\ R-N \overset{\displaystyle\frown}{} F \\ O \overset{\displaystyle\diagdown}{} N \\ \underset{R'}{|} \end{array}$$

Compound	MP°C[a]	pK$_a$
16, R = R' = H	280-284	8.0, 13.0
17, R = H, R' = CH$_2$O(C=O)CH$_3$	127-128 (122-123)[b]	7.3[b]
18, R = H, R' = CH$_2$O(C=O)C$_2$H$_5$	105-106 (100-102)[b]	7.3[b]
19, R = H, R' = CH$_2$O(C=O)C$_3$H$_7$	96-98 (92-93)[b]	7.3[b]
20, R = H, R' = CH$_2$O(C=O)C$_4$H$_9$	91-92	
21, R = H, R' = CH$_2$O(C=O)C$_5$H$_{11}$	95-96	
22, R = H, R' = CH$_2$O(C=O)C$_6$H$_{13}$	109-110	
23, R = H, R' = CH$_2$O(C=O)C$_7$H$_{15}$	112-113	
24, R = H, R' = CH$_2$O(C=O)C$_8$H$_{17}$	111-112	
25, R = H, R' = CH$_2$O(C=O)C$_9$H$_{19}$	115-116	
26, R = H, R' = CH$_2$O(C=O)C$_{10}$H$_{21}$	93	
27, R = H, R' = CH$_2$O(C=O)C(CH$_3$)$_3$	(158-160)[b]	7.3[b]
28, R = R' = CH$_2$O(C=O)CH$_3$	110-111 (105-106)[b]	
29, R = R' = CH$_2$O(C=O)C$_2$H$_5$	69-70	
30, R = R' = CH$_2$O(C=O)C$_4$H$_9$	Oil	
31, R = R' = CH$_2$O(C=O)C$_5$H$_{11}$	42-44	
32, R = R' = CH$_2$O(C=O)C$_7$H$_{15}$	57-58	
33, R = R' = CH$_2$O(C=O)C(CH$_3$)$_3$	113-114 (102-104)[b]	
34, R = CH$_2$O(C=O)CH$_3$, R' = H	(158-159)[b]	8.0[b]
35, R = CH$_2$O(C=O)C(CH$_3$)$_3$, R' = H	135-137	

[a]From Ref. 38.
[b]From Ref. 39.

with an alkyl or aryl group (38). They are not listed in Table 8. Their physicochemical properties were similar to the acyloxymethyl derivatives and were not further evaluated. Two fairly extensive series of acyloxymethyl derivatives are listed—the 1-mono and the 1,3-bis derivatives. In each case the melting points follow the same trend. The melting point for the first member of each series is fairly high, subsequent members of the series exhibit decreasing melting points until the butyryloxymethyl member is reached, and then the melting points start to increase again. This type of trend has been observed for almost all of the other acyloxymethyl series as well. Although not available for this complete series, generally the trend in lipid solubilities is the inverse of the melting point trend with higher melting points corresponding to lower solubilities and vice versa.

Bundgaard and coworkers (39) have thoroughly evaluated the physicochemical properties of a few representatives of each series of acyloxymethyl derivatives of 5-FU (Table 9). The first member(s) of the two mono series exhibit higher water solubilities than 5-FU while also exhibiting greater lipophilicity than 5-FU as shown by their higher partition coefficient values. The acyloxymethyl derivatives are quite stable in pH 7.4 buffer. The shortest alkyl chain member exhibits the shortest half-life and the longer alkyl chain members exhibit longer half-lives. As expected, the order of stability is reversed in plasma with the longer alkyl chain butyryloxymethyl derivative, **19**, exhibiting the shorter half-life and the shortest alkyl chain acetyloxymethyl derivative, **17**, the longer half-life. The more sterically hindered pivaloyloxymethyl derivative, **27**, is the most stable under either condition. Again, these types of trends are seen with almost all of the other acyloxymethyl series of prodrugs as well.

The results from the diffusion cell experiments are given in Table 10 (40). Only two derivatives were evaluated. The solubilities of the derivatives in PG were not determined so it is not clear that the derivatives were evaluated at the same thermodynamic activity. The butyryloxymethyl derivative, **19**, delivers only 5-FU, whereas the pivaloyloxymethyl derivative, **27**, delivers 5-FU and intact prodrug. Prodrug **19** is almost 2.4 times more effective than 5-FU at delivering 5-FU through human skin, whereas **27** is only about half as effective. Prodrug **27**

Table 9 Selected Physicochemical Properties of Acyloxymethyl Derivatives of 5-FU

Compound	log K^a	C_v^b	Half-lives (h)^c buffer	Half-lives (h)^c 80% plasma
16	−0.83	11.1		
17	−0.67	43.1	70	14.0
18	−0.11	33.6	90^d	9.6
19	0.47	9.6	140^d	2.3
27	0.90	2.3	700^d	40
28	−0.37	4.3	20	0.29
33	2.54	0.045	60^d	1.1
34	−0.42	20.0	—	3.0

^{a}Octanol–pH 4 acetate buffer partition coefficient at 22°C.
^{b}Solubility in mg/ml in pH 4 acetate buffer at 22°C.
^{c}Half-lives determined at 37° in 0.05 M phosphate buffer at pH 7.4. Plasma was human plasma.
^{d}Estimated from data obtained at pH > 8.
Source: From Ref. 39.

Table 10 Transdermal Delivery of 5-FU by Acyloxymethyl Derivatives

Compound	$C_v{}^a$	J^b	Half-lives^c (h)
16, R = R' = H	16.5	0.00072^b	
19, R = H, R' = CH$_2$O(C=O)C$_3$H$_7$	—	0.00172^b	32
27, R = H, R' = CH$_2$O(C=O)C(CH$_3$)$_3$	—	0.00043^b	210
		0.00077^d	

^{a}Solubility in mg/ml of propylene glycol at 23 ± 1°C from Ref. 12.
^{b}Flux in mg of 5-FU/cm^2/h through human abdominal skin at 37°C from a 12% propylene glycol in ethanol solution after the ethanol had evaporated.
^{c}Half-lives (h) in pH 7.4 phosphate buffer exposed to dermis side of human skin for 90 h in diffusion cell.
^{d}Total of 5-FU and intact prodrug in terms of equivalent mg of 5-FU/cm^2/h.
Source: From Ref. 40.

is about as effective as 5-FU if total 5-FU delivered through the skin is taken into account. These results are consistent with **27** being more stable to hydrolysis than **19** (see Tables 9 and 10), so it was more likely to permeate intact. On the other hand, the relative effectiveness of the two derivatives at delivering total 5-FU through skin is consistent with the trend observed for acyloxymethyl derivatives of theophylline. The more water-soluble member of a series of more lipid-soluble derivatives is the more effective derivative at enhancing transdermal delivery. Thus, the trend that is observed for the acyloxymethyl derivatives of theophylline is also observed for the acyloxymethyl derivatives of 5-FU, regardless of the fact that different vehicles (IPM [18] and PG [40]) are used in the two studies.

If the apparent trends observed for theophylline and 5-FU acyloxymethyl derivatives are correct, then there are several other acyloxymethyl derivatives of 5-FU that also should be evaluated for their ability to deliver 5-FU through skin. On the bases of the observed water solubilities and partition coefficients reported in Table 9, the 1-acetyloxymethyl, **17**, and 1-propionyloxymethyl, **18**, derivatives as well as the 3-acetyloxymethyl, **34**, derivative should be evaluated in diffusion cell experiments. All three are much more water soluble than 5-FU or the two derivatives that were evaluated (Table 10), yet they are also more lipid soluble than 5-FU.

Bundgaard and coworkers have also reported the synthesis and characterization of a few 1- and 3-mono, and 1,3-bisalkoxycarbonyloxymethyl derivatives as well (41). Their solubilities and stabilities are listed in Table 11. Although only a limited number of examples were characterized, there are several observations that can be made that may have implications for their use to enhance topical delivery. First, if we assume that the 3-ethoxycarbonyloxymethyl derivative, **39**, is roughly equivalent to the 1-butyryloxymethyl derivative, **19**, then the fact that

Sloan

Table 11 Selected Physicochemical Properties of Alkoxycarbonyloxymethyl
Derivatives of 5-FU

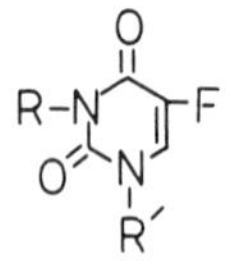

				Half-lives (min)^c	
Compound	MP°C	log K^a	C$_v^b$	buffer	80% plasma
16, R = R' = H	280–284	–0.83	11.1	—	—
36, R = H, R' = CH$_2$O(C=O)OC$_6$H$_5$	145–147	—	—	2.0	2.6
37, R = H, R' = CH$_2$O(C=O)OC$_2$H$_5$	Oil	–0.04	—	120	120
38, R = CH$_2$O(C=O)OC$_6$H$_5$, R' = H	154–157	1.11	1.0	980	10
39, R = CH$_2$O(C=O)OC$_2$H$_5$, R' = H	137–140	0.15	8.0	21000	120
40, R = R' = CH$_2$O(C=O)OC$_6$H$_5$	68–72	—	—	—	—
41, R = R' = CH$_2$O(C=O)OC$_2$H$_5$	Oil	—	—	—	—

^{a}Octanol–pH 4 acetate buffer partition coefficient at 22°C.
^{b}Solubility in mg/ml in pH 4 acetate buffer at 22°C.
^{c}Half-lives determined at 37°C in 0.05 M phosphate buffer at pH 7.4. Plasma was human plasma.
Source: From Ref. 41.

39 is almost as water soluble as **19** suggests that **39** should be as effective
as **19** at delivering 5-FU through skin. Second, the 3-ethoxycarbonyloxymethyl
derivative, **39**, is apparently less lipophilic (more polar) than **19** based on their
respective partition coefficient values, whereas the corresponding 1-ethoxy-
carbonyloxymethyl derivative, **37**, is apparently even more polar than **39** based on
its even lower partition coefficient value. However, on that same basis both **37** and
39 are more lipophilic than 5-FU. Thus, **37** may be even more effective than **39**
at delivering 5-FU through skin, since it may be the more water soluble of the
two. Third, the rates of hydrolysis of the alkoxycarbonyloxymethyl (carbonate)
esters in plasma (see Table 11) are comparable to the rates of hydrolysis of the
simple esters listed in Table 9, so they should function as prodrugs under normal
conditions.

6-Mercaptopurine

6-Mercaptopurine (6-MP) is perhaps one of the more interesting and challenging
polar heterocycles for which acyloxymethyl derivatives have been synthesized.
6-MP is challenging from a synthetic point of view because there are so many

possible sites and combinations of sites available for modification. It is theoretically possible to monoalkylate the 1-, 3-, 7-, and 9-nitrogen as well as the sulfur in the 6-position. Then there are also eight possible dialkyl derivatives of 6-MP: S^6,1-, S^6,3-, S^6,7-, S^6,9-, 1,7-, 1,9-, 3,7-, and 3,9-. Only a few examples of these 13 possible acyloxymethyl derivatives have actually been synthesized and characterized (42–44), and even fewer yet can be synthesized efficiently in usable quantities. 6-MP is interesting from a therapeutic point of view because the possibility exists for greater improvement in the topical performance of 6-MP than for either theophylline or 5-FU. Theophylline and 5-FU exhibit some topical activity before their transient modification, 6-MP does not (45).

There are numerous examples of acyloxymethyl derivatives of the acidic-NH groups in 6-MP, but almost all of them are in combination with acyloxymethyl derivatives of the thiol group in the 6-position (43). Those will be discussed later. The only examples of monoacyloxymethyl derivatives of an acidic-NH group in 6-MP are the 9-acyloxymethyl derivatives (44). Only two members of that series (the acetyloxymethyl and pivaloyloxymethyl) were synthesized and characterized. Both members exhibit much higher melting points than the corresponding S^6-acyloxymethyl derivative. The 9-pivaloyloxymethyl derivative is almost 70 times less soluble in IPM and delivers about 40 times less 6-MP through hairless mouse skin from an IPM suspension than the corresponding S^6-pivaloyloxymethyl derivative. In fact, the 9-pivaloyloxymethyl derivative delivers only a third as much 6-MP through hairless mouse skin as 6-MP itself does. Based on the poor performance of the one 9-acyloxymethyl derivative that was evaluated, the authors concluded that it was more important to mask the thionamide functional group rather than the imidazole functional group in order to improve the topical delivery of 6-MP.

Arabinofuranosyladenine (Ara-A)

For this discussion, purine and pyrimidine bases as well as their corresponding nucleosides which contains exocyclic amine groups have been classed as drugs containing acidic-NH or acidic-NH_2 groups. Thus cytosine-, adenine-, or guanine-based drugs fall into this class. The exocyclic amine functional groups [R(C=N)-NH_2] of these molecules exhibit properties similar to that of amides in that they exhibit basic pK_as of -3 to -1 for R(C=N)-$NH_3^{\oplus} \rightleftharpoons$ R(C=N)-NH_2 + H^+ (46). More important to this discussion, they also reversibly form hydroxymethyl adducts with their exocyclic amine groups (46). It has already been shown that hydroxymethyl adducts themselves may enhance the topical delivery of a polar heterocyclic drug (18) (see above), but so far that possibility has not been explored for this class of drugs. One reason for this is the unstable nature of the adducts.

One way to stabilize the hydroxymethyl adducts is to acylate the hydroxy group. Acylation prevents ionization of the hydroxy group and the subsequent spontaneous disassociation of the oxyanion to the amide anion and the aldehyde (4). The rate of the disassociation depends on the acidity of the amide: The more acidic the amide, the faster the rate of disassociation. Not only does acylation of the hydroxy group stabilize the hydroxymethyl adduct, but the resulting acyloxymethyl derivative should exhibit increased lipophilicity and hydrophilicity if an appropriate acyl group is introduced. Thus, the potential for the use of this approach is fairly promising, especially since there are so few other approaches available to transiently modify these exocyclic amine groups.

So far only one example of the use of acyloxymethyl-type prodrugs of the exocyclic amine group in cytosine-, adenine-, or guanine-based drugs to enhance the topical delivery of the parent drug has been reported (46). Alexander has described the synthesis of O-acyl derivatives of a hydroxymethoxymethyl (instead of the expected hydroxymethyl) adduct with 2',3',5'-triacetylara-A (47). The reason that Alexander obtained the hydroxymethoxymethyl adduct in his reaction between aqueous formaldehyde and ara-A may be that he did not depolymerize his formaldehyde before using it as McGhee and von Hippel had (47). Regardless of the value of n in such intermediate adducts [Drug-N-CH_2-O-(CH_2-O)$_n$H], the mechanism of the decomposition of the acyloxymethyl type prodrugs would remain the same—hydrolysis of the ester group in the prodrug to regenerate the adduct which would spontaneously disassociate on ionization of the adduct as shown below (4). Although the prodrugs have been patented to enhance skin permeability, the products of the acylation were only characterized as oils or hygroscopic foams (no solubility data) and no data showing relative rates of transdermal delivery have been published.

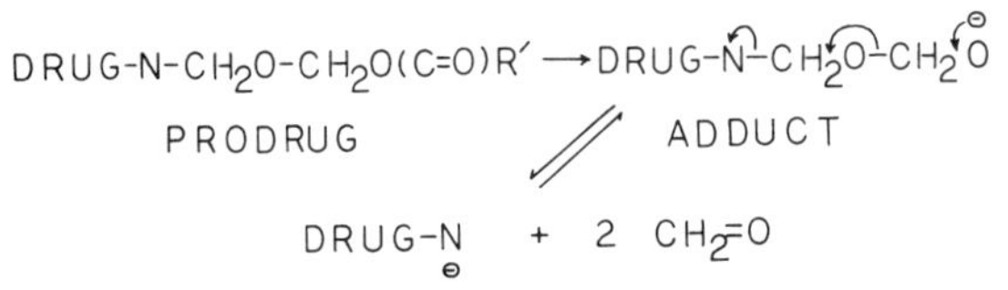

$$DRUG-N-CH_2O-CH_2O(C=O)R' \longrightarrow DRUG-\overset{\frown}{N}-CH_2\overset{\frown}{O}-CH_2\overset{\ominus}{O}$$

PRODRUG   ⫽   ADDUCT   Scheme 2

$$DRUG-\underset{\ominus}{N} \quad + \quad 2 \quad CH_2{=}O$$

α-(Acyloxy)alkyl Derivatives of Basic Drug-NH Groups: Drug-N-CHR'-O(C=O)-R'

The situation for the α-(acyloxy)alkyl derivatives of basic Drug-NH groups is somewhat similar to that for the purines and pyrimidines in the last section in that only one example has been synthesized and characterized for the express purpose of enhancing topical delivery, and so far no results from its use for that purpose have been published. As discussed earlier, molecules containing basic amine groups seem to permeate skin better than molecules containing many other functional groups. However, the effect of making an acyloxymethyl derivative of a basic amine would be to decrease its basicity similar to the effect of the benzamidomethyl group on the amine portion of an N-Mannich base (4). In some cases, a decrease of 2 to 3 pK_a units of the amine portion of the N-Mannich base is observed. The effect of the decrease in basicity of the prodrug compared to the parent drug would tend to present greater amounts of the more permeable free base form of the molecule at the vehicle-membrane interface and lesser amounts of the polar protonated form of the molecule. This tendency, along with enhanced lipophilicity imparted by the promoiety, should result in enhanced permeation.

However, the stability of α-(acyloxy)alkyl derivatives of basic amines is problematic; they may be too labile. Generally, it has been found that α-(acyloxy)alkyl derivatives of less basic amines, such as aziridine (48) and imidazole (49), are more stable than those of the more basic amines such as piperidine, pyrrolidine, and simple alkyl-substituted amines. Although very little study of the hydrolysis of α-(acyloxy)alkyl derivatives of basic amines has been done, by analogy to the N-Mannich bases (4), it may be assumed that the stability of the derivatives is inversely proportional to the ability of the unshared pair of electrons on the amine to stabilize the incipient positive charge developing on the methylene group (carbocation) as the carboxylate group leaves during solvolysis.

$$\text{Drug-N==CHR}' \overset{\oplus}{} \cdots \cdots \overset{\ominus}{} O(C{=}O)R'$$

There are three potential ways to overcome the stability problem of α-(acyloxy)alkylamines. First is to incorporate the carboxylate group and the proaldehyde group into the same molecule so that the proximity effect holds the two groups together. Thus, the reaction of 3-hydroxy-1(3H)-isobenzofuranone, **42**, with any basic secondary amine gives the corresponding 3-dialkylamino derivative, **43**, which is the cyclic analogue of an α-(acyloxy)alkylamine (50,51). Second is to substitute a vinylogous methylene group between the carboxylate group and the amine group. The carbocation stabilizing effect of the unshared pair of electrons on the basic amine is not as strong when it has to be transmitted through two double bonds. This type derivative has been easily synthesized by the O-acylation of 4-dialkylaminomethylphenols or by the alkylation of secondary amines with 4-acyloxybenzyl halides (52). Third is to substitute a carbonate or a carbamate type functional group, which are poorer leaving groups, for the carboxylate functional group. The only example of this approach is one that combines a carbonate functional group with the substitution of a vinylogous methylene group to give N-(2-oxo-1,3-dioxol-4-yl)methylamine derivatives, **44**, which can hydrolyze as shown below (53).

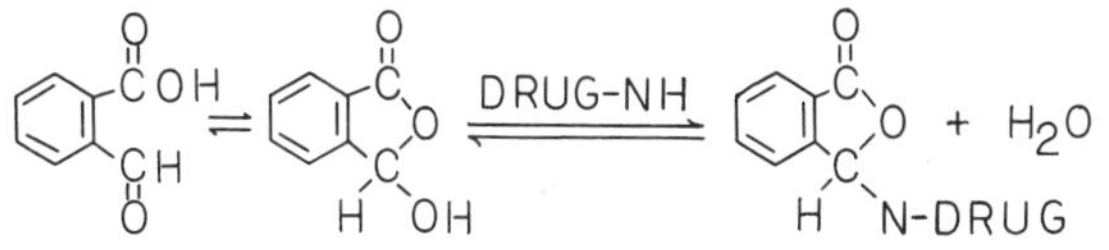

42   **43**

Scheme 3

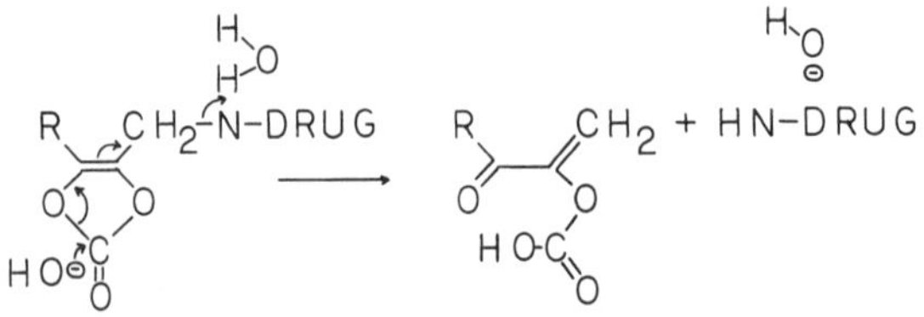

Scheme 4

44

The one example of an α-(acyloxy)alkyl type derivative of a basic amine that has been synthesized for the purpose of evaluating its ability to enhance topical delivery is the benzoyloxymethyl derivative of the 1a-N-position of mitomycin C (48). The nitrogen in the 1a position of mitomycin C is part of an aziridine group which usually exhibits a pK_a of about 1.5. Thus, the stability of the acyloxymethyl prodrug derives from the relative inability of the aziridine nitrogen to stabilize an incipient carbocation in the transition state for its hydrolysis. Although the benzoyloxymethyl derivative exhibited lipophilicity and partition coefficient values that were comparable to the acyl derivatives that were evaluated, it was not evaluated in diffusion cell experiments. This was probably because the derivative could only be obtained in 3% yield. The major product from the reaction of mitomycin C with benzoyloxymethyl chloride was the N-benzoyl derivative rather than the N-benzoyloxymethyl derivative. This result is typical of these reactions between acyloxymethyl halides and amines (49).

α-(Dialkylamino)alkyl Derivatives of Acidic Drug-NH Groups: Drug-N-CHR'-NR$_2'$

α-(Dialkylamino)alkyl, or N-Mannich base, type derivatives of molecules containing acidic drug-NH groups have been known for quite some time. More recently these N-Mannich base derivatives have been shown to be useful (4) for promoting the water solubility of amides, imides, and carbon acids, and their dissolution in water. On the other hand, since the α-(dialkylamino)alkyl group also masks a polar imide or partially masks a polar amide group, the N-Mannich base that results exhibits enhanced lipid solubility compared to the parent compound as well. The fact that N-Mannich bases exhibit enhanced biphasic solubility characteristics makes them ideal candidates to evaluate for use in enhancing topical delivery.

The physicochemical properties of these N-Mannich base derivatives depend on the type of R' substituents on the -NR$_2'$ and -CHR'- groups. All of the derivatives are at least partially ionized at physiological pH because of the incorporation of the basic tertiary amine group (-NR$_2'$) into the promoiety. However, the pK_a of the tertiary amine derivative is 2–3 pK_a units lower than that of the corresponding secondary amine (54). For example, morpholine, which exhibits a pK_a of 8.33, when incorporated into a benzamide N-Mannich base as -NR$_2'$ exhibits a pK_a of

5.6. This means that potentially much more of the morpholinyl group will exist in the free base form at physiological pH, and the prodrug will be much more likely to partition across the vehicle-membrane interface than the N-Mannich base prodrug derived from a more basic amine. In addition to the effect of the substituents on pK_a, the chain length of the R' group also affects the lipophilicity of the prodrug, although, as will be shown later, it is not a continuous function of increasing chain length.

The mechanism for the hydrolysis of the N-Mannich base prodrugs apparently involves their rate-limiting unimolecular cleavage to give the amide or imide anion and a stabilized carbocation as shown below, **45**, for hydrolysis under basic conditions (54–56). An alternative mechanism involving the formation of the corresponding hydroxymethyl derivative as an intermediate does not operate, since the hydroxymethyl derivative hydrolyzes to give the parent amide or imide slower than does the N-Mannich base (54). A comparison of the rates of hydrolysis of N-Mannich bases of various amides and imides shows that the rates depend on the pK_a of the amide or imide under basic conditions: The lower the pK_a of the amide or imide, the more stable the negative charge on the amide or imide nitrogen and the faster the rate of hydrolysis (54). This direct correlation supports the suggested mechanism.

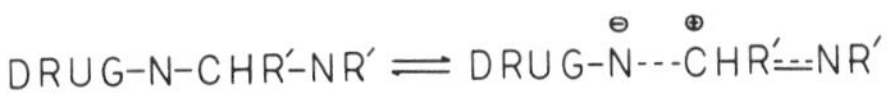

$$\text{DRUG-N-CHR'-NR'} \; \rightleftharpoons \; \text{DRUG-N}^{\ominus} \text{---} \overset{\oplus}{\text{C}}\text{HR'}\text{---}\text{NR'}$$

45

Scheme 5

The substituents on $-NR_2'$ and $-CHR'-$ also affect the rates of hydrolyses of the N-Mannich base prodrugs. A comparison of the rates of hydrolysis of N-Mannich bases derived from the same amide but from different amines shows that the rates depend on the pK_a of the amine, which in turn depends on R': The lower the pK_a of the $-NR_2'$ part of the N-Mannich base, the less stable the positive charge on the carbocation ($\oplus$ CHR-NR_2') and the slower the rate of hydrolysis under basic conditions (54). This direct correlation emphasizes the importance of the availability of the unshared pair of electrons on the amine to stabilize the incipient positive charge on $-CHR'-$ which is generated during the cleavage of the bond between the amide or imide nitrogen and the carbon in $-CHR'-$. On the other hand, under acidic conditions N-Mannich base derivatives derived from amines exhibiting lower pK_a values tended to hydrolyze faster than under basic conditions, whereas those derived from amines exhibiting higher pK_a values tended to hydrolyze slower than under basic conditions. This result suggests the possibility that **46** may be an intermediate in the hydrolysis of the N-Mannich bases under acidic conditions (56), and that transfer of a proton from the protonated amine to the amide carbonyl is less difficult for less basic amines. However, there was no correlation between pK_a values of the amine portion of N-Mannich bases and rates of their hydrolyses under acidic conditions.

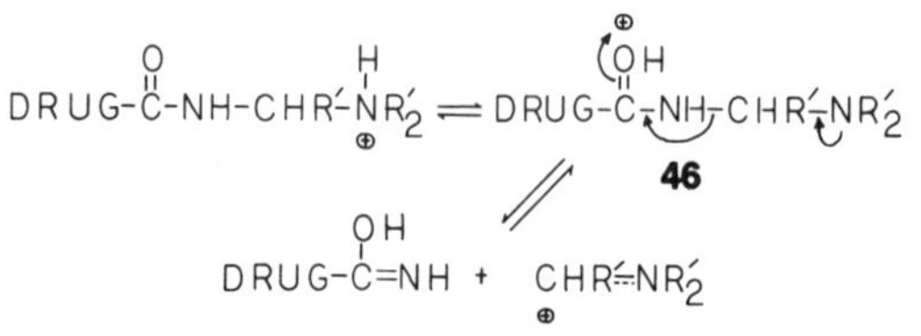

$$\underset{\oplus}{\text{DRUG-}\overset{O}{\overset{\|}{C}}\text{-NH-CHR}'\text{-NR}'_2} \rightleftharpoons \text{DRUG-}\overset{\overset{\oplus}{(\text{OH}}}{\underset{\smile}{C}}\text{-NH-CHR}'\text{-NR}'_2$$

46

$$\underset{\oplus}{\text{DRUG-}\overset{OH}{\overset{|}{C}}\text{=NH} \; + \; \text{CHR}'\text{=NR}'_2}$$

Scheme 6

The incorporation of a substituent into the methylene group (-CHR'-,R' = H) generally has the effect of increasing the rate of hydrolysis of the N-Mannich base. This result is observed regardless of whether R' is an electron-withdrawing or an electron-donating group. In the former case, the substituent might be expected to destabilize the incipient positive charge at the methylene carbon, and hence stabilize the N-Mannich base. Since that result is not observed (52), the effect of -CHR'- in Drug-N-CHR'-NR$'_2$ most likely arises from the tendency of the methylene group to seek relief from steric compression by changing from tetrahedral in the intact prodrug to trigonal hybridization in the carbocation.

All of the N-Mannich bases hydrolyze quite rapidly in water and in most protic solvents. Bundgaard and coworkers have developed equations that predict the rates of hydrolyses of N-Mannich bases derived from particular amines and from amides and imides exhibiting quite different pK$_a$s (54). For instance, the half-life of hydrolysis of the piperidine N-Mannich base of an amide with a pK$_a$ of 15 should be 63 min, whereas that of an imide with a pK$_a$ of 12 should be 0.2 s. In spite of their inherent aqueous instability, N-Mannich bases are usually formed in, and isolated from, aqueous solutions, and are often reported to have been recrystallized from alcohols. The formation of the N-Mannich base is frequently driven to completion by its precipitation from the reaction mixture, in effect limiting its contact with the water which is formed as a byproduct of the reaction.

Although on first inspection the use of N-Mannich bases to enhance topical delivery may seem limited by their stability and by the R' substituents that have been used in -CHR'- and -NR$'_2$, the possibilities are actually quite large. The stabilities of the N-Mannich bases can be increased by using amines exhibiting lower pK$_a$s. Besides the cyclic amines—morpholine, piperazine, and substituted imidazoles, derivatives of acyclic secondary amines such as di(hydroxyethyl)amine and sarcosine amide provide an as yet untapped source of low pK$_a$ secondary amines that can be used to form more stable N-Mannich bases. The stability of the N-Mannich bases during their topical applications can be increased by using aprotic formulations containing vehicles such as IPM, dimethylformamide (DMF), triacylglycerides, etc., in which they are stable. Thus, the fact that N-Mannich bases must be formulated in an aprotic vehicle makes them uniquely suitable for use in enhancing topical delivery, since such vehicles can actually be used in real formulations for topical delivery but not for other routes of administration. Finally, although only a limited number of aldehydes can be used to form stable, isolable, and characterizable hydroxymethyl derivatives, a far greater number of aldehydes can be combined with secondary amines to form stable N-Mannich bases. Thus, there is considerable flexibility in the choice of R' in -CHR'- for N-Mannich bases which is not readily available even for α-(acyloxy)alkyl derivatives, especially if the goal is to introduce a basic tertiary amine into the promoiety. For instance, the synthesis of the generic N-Mannich base (Drug-N-CHR'-NR$_2$) is much simpler than the synthesis of the corresponding generic α-(acyloxy)alkyl derivative (Drug-N-CHR'-O(C=O) (CH$_2$)$_n$NR$_2'$). For example, see the synthesis of the latter type prodrug of allopurinol (57).

Theophylline

The use of N-Mannich bases of theophylline and 5-FU to enhance their trans-dermal or dermal delivery was first reported in 1984 (25). That study only evaluated one example of an N-Mannich base for each parent drug in diffusion cell experiments. No correlations between solubilities and rates of topical delivery can be deduced, but it is apparent that the approach has merit, since the pyrroli-dinylmethyl derivative, **54**, of theophylline is 6.9 times better than theophylline at delivering theophylline from IPM through hairless mouse skin, whereas 1,3-bis(4'-morpholinylmethyl)-5-FU, **56**, is 5.5 times better than 5-FU. Although neither series was optimized, both N-Mannich bases, (**54** and **56**) are more effective than the best acyloxymethyl derivatives evaluated for their respective parent drugs (see above).

A more complete evaluation of N-Mannich base derivatives of theophylline and 5-FU was eventually published in 1988 (58). The melting points, solubilities, and abilities of the N-Mannich bases of theophylline to deliver theophylline through hairless mouse skin are given in Table 12. The correlation between the melting points and IPM solubilities in the homologous series of dialkylamine-derived N-Mannich bases and in those derived from cyclic amines is expected: The lower the melting points, the higher the lipid solubilities. No attempt was made to determine their water solubilities, although aqueous solubilities have been reported for some N-Mannich bases under acidic conditions (59). Water solubilities obtained at low pH where the N-Mannich base is completely protonated (and in some cases relatively more stable, see above) may exaggerate their water solubilities at pH 7.4 compared to the parent drug. However, it is generally assumed that these N-Mannich bases should exhibit enhanced water solubilities compared to the acidic parent Drug-NH.

Among the homologous series of prodrugs, the diethylaminomethyl, **48**, and dipropylaminomethyl, **49**, derivatives are marginally better than the other deriva-tives at delivering theophylline through skin: about 9 times better than theo-phylline itself. Although all of the derivatives are more soluble in IPM than theophylline (100–1000 times), neither **48** nor **49** is the most lipid-soluble deriva-tive in the homologous series that was evaluated. On the other hand, among the derivatives derived from the cyclic amines, the more lipid-soluble derivatives are indeed the more efficient ones at delivering theophylline. However, the cyclic

Table 12 Physicochemical Properties of Theophylline N-Mannich Bases and Their Rates of Transdermal Delivery of Theophylline

Compound	MP°C	$C_v{}^a$	J^b	P^c
5, R = H	270–274	0.062	0.041 (0.0037)	0.66
47, R = CH$_2$-N(CH$_3$)$_2$	121–123	8.71	0.21 (0.010)	0.024
48, R = CH$_2$-N(C$_2$H$_5$)$_2$	122–124	21.76	0.37 (0.11)	0.017
49, R = CH$_2$-N(C$_3$H$_7$)$_2$	72–73	77.59	0.36 (0.019)	0.0046
50, R = CH$_2$-N(C$_4$H$_9$)$_2$	62–64	86.13	0.30 (0.021)	0.0035
51, R = CH$_2$-N(CH$_2$)$_5$	115–116	11.42	0.16 (0.014)	0.014
52, R = CH$_2$-N(CH$_2$CH$_2$)$_2$O	175–178	1.05	0.11 (0.020)	0.10
53, R = CH$_2$-N(CH$_2$CH$_2$)$_2$NCH$_3$	131–133	2.84	0.090 (0.0082)	0.032
54, R = CH$_2$-N(CH$_2$)$_4$	114–115	8.47	0.23 (0.014)	0.027

^{a}Solubility of compounds in equivalent mg of theophylline/ml of IPM at 23 ± 1°C.
^{b}Flux in mg/cm^2/h (± SD) from an IPM suspension through hairless mouse skin with a receptor phase temperature of 32°C.
^{c}Permeability coefficient in cm/h determined from J/C$_v$.
Source: From Ref. 58.

series is composed of such disparate members that the significance of that result is not clear. The pyrrolidinylmethyl and piperidinylmethyl derivatives (**54** and **51**) are more lipid soluble and are the more efficient members, whereas the morpholinylmethyl and piperazinylmethyl derivatives (**52** and **53**), which contain an extra heteroatom in the ring, are the less lipid soluble and less efficient members of the series. The effect of the extra heteroatom in **52** and **53** is possibly confounding.

In both series, when solubility is factored out by comparing the permeability coefficients (P) for the delivery of theophylline by the N-Mannich bases, a consistent trend is observed. The highest value for P is observed for the derivative that is least soluble in the vehicle and the lowest P is observed for the derivative that is most soluble in the vehicle. Assuming that permeability coefficient is directly proportional to partition coefficient (K) (see eq. 1 above), the observed trend suggests that the ability of the prodrugs to partition into the skin is inversely proportional to the solubility of the prodrug in the vehicle. This result is reasonable if one considers that the rational activity coefficient is inversely proportional to the mole fraction solubility. Hence, the more soluble the prodrug is in a particular vehicle, the lower its escaping tendency.

5-Fluorouracil

The melting points, solubilities, and abilities of the N-Mannich bases of 5-FU to deliver 5-FU through hairless mouse skin are given in Table 13 (58). The number of compounds that were isolated, characterized, and evaluated in this series is quite small. It was actually possible to synthesize other members of the cyclic amine series and some members of the acyclic series, but in each case those members would not crystallize and could not be purified. Regardless, the correlations between decreased melting point and increased lipid solubilities are evident for this series of N-Mannich bases as well. However, because of the wide variations in the properties of the amines from which the N-Mannich bases were derived, it is not surprising that there are no correlations between solubilities and fluxes or permeability coefficients.

Among all the heterocycles for which prodrugs have been evaluated, 5-FU is the only one for which commercial formulations are available. In Table 14, the abilities of the commercial formulations (comprising mainly PG) to deliver 5-FU through hairless mouse skin are compared with the abilities of either 5-FU or **56** to deliver 5-FU from IPM (60). The results are interesting in that the prodrug is much more efficient than any of the commercial formulations at delivering 5-FU, and that among the commercial solution formulations the 2% solution is the most efficient. Since the solubility of 5-FU in PG is about 1.6%, the better performance by the 2% formulation compared to the 1% formulation is expected, since the 1% solution is not close to being at saturation where the maximum in thermodynamic activity of 5-FU in the solution would be expected. Similarly, the 5% solution would be expected to be less efficient from a thermodynamic

Table 13   Physicochemical Properties of 5-FU N-Mannich Bases and Their Rates of Transdermal Delivery of 5-FU

$$R-N \underset{O \diagdown N}{\overset{O}{\bigcirc}} F$$
$$\underset{R'}{|}$$

Compound	MP°C	C_v[a]	J[b]
16, R = R' = H	280–284	0.0051	0.022 (0.0088)
55, R = R' = CH_2N(CH_2)_5	96–98	6.98	0.076 (0.0030)
56, R = R' = CH_2N(CH_2CH_2)_2O	136–139	2.53	0.11 (0.013)
57, R = R' = CH_2N(CH_2CH_2)_2NCH_3	117–120	4.27	0.013 (0.010)

[a]Solubility of compounds in equivalent mg of 5-FU/ml of IPM at 23 ± 1°C.
[b]Flux in mg/cm^2/h (± SD) from an IPM suspension through hairless mouse skin with a receptor phase temperature of 32°C.
Source: From Ref. 58.

Table 14 Transdermal Delivery of 5-FU Through Hairless Mouse and Human Skin by Vehicles and a Prodrug of 5-FU

Formulation	Source of skin	J^a	h^b	P^c
Fluoroplex, 1% Solution	Mouse	0.0082 (0.0031)	4.7	0.00082
Fluoroplex, 1% Solution	Human	0.00042 (0.00001)	6.8	0.000042
Efudex, 2% Solution	Mouse	0.017 (0.0046)	3.7	0.00084
Efudex, 2% Solution	Human	0.0022 (0.0025)	7.6	0.00011
Efudex, 5% Solution	Mouse	0.0072 (0.0042)	4.0	0.00016
Efudex, 5% Solution	Human	0.00071 (0.00018)	13.6	0.000016
5-FU/IPM, 4% Suspension	Mouse^d	0.022 (0.0088)	15.1	4.3^e
5-FU/IPM, 4% Suspension	Human	0.0011 (0.00052)	13.6	0.22^e
56/IPM, 10% Suspension	Mouse^d	0.11 (0.013)	0.7	0.043^f
56/IPM, 10% Suspension	Human	0.0166 (0.0032)	9.9	0.0067^f

^{a}Flux in mg/cm^2/h ($\pm$ SD) with a receptor phase temperature of 32°C.
^{b}Lag-time in hours.
^{c}Permeability coefficient in cm/h determined from J/C_v.
^{d}From Ref. 58.
^{e}Solubility of 5-FU in IPM is 0.0051 mg/ml.
^{f}Solubility of 56 in IPM is equivalent to 2.53 mg of 5-FU/ml.
Source: From Ref. 60.

point of view because of the excess solubilizing capacity of such a solution comprising mainly PG.

A comparison between human and hairless mouse skin is also presented in Table 14. Although human skin is consistently about 10 times less permeable to all the 5-FU/vehicle combinations and the lag time for development of steady-state flux is always greater using human skin, the prodrug is again by far the most effective approach to delivering 5-FU through skin. The same authors also evaluated apparent damage to the human skin by measuring the fluxes from the application of a standard drug/vehicle after the initial application of 5-FU/vehicles. According to that criterion, the application of 56 in IPM caused no more damage to the human skin samples than the commercial formulations comprising mainly PG.

As was pointed out earlier, diffusion cell experiments are useful predictors of transdermal delivery as long as interspecies differences and the unnatural hydration state of skin in the diffusion cells are taken into account. However, for topical delivery of 5-FU the target organ is the epidermis—dermal delivery. It has been assumed that increased transdermal delivery correlates with increased dermal delivery, but verification of increased dermal delivery must ultimately be accomplished by measuring some in vivo change in the target organ. In the case of 5-FU and other antiproliferative agents, decreased epidermal DNA synthesis correlates with increased epidermal cellular delivery. In Table 15 are the results from the topical application of 5-FU in three commercial formulations, and in IPM, and the topical application of **56** in IPM to hairless mice (19). These results, along with those in Table 14, show that increased transdermal delivery (see Table 14) causes increased inhibition of epidermal DNA synthesis (see Table 15). Consequently, there must have been an increase not only in dermal delivery but, more important, also into the epidermal cells.

6-Mercaptopurine

The N-Mannich base derivatives of 6-MP that have been synthesized are listed in Table 16 (27). The N-Mannich bases derived from the lower pK_a amines such as morpholine and 4-methylpiperazine were not evaluated because pure derivatives could not be isolated. The melting points and solubilities of the homologous acyclic series given in Table 16 fit the previously observed correlation: Lower melting points result in higher IPM solubilities. However, in this case, **60** exhibits the lowest melting point but only the second highest solubility. A larger series

Table 15 Inhibition of Epidermal DNA Synthesis by 5-FU in Vehicles and by a Prodrug of 5-FU

Treatment	CPM/Disc		% Inhibition
	Upper dorsal (local effect)	lower dorsal (systemic effect)	
Control	1310 ± 552	1316 ± 219	
IPM/Control	4133 ± 1121	1656 ± 384	−250[a]
5-FU/IPM	2124 ± 669	1280 ± 307	37[b]
56/IPM	561 ± 168	1317 ± 203	83[b]
PG Control	1687 ± 489	1552 ± 181	
Fluoroplex, 1% Solution	1219 ± 161	1380 ± 359	12[c]
Efudex, 2% Solution	990 ± 263	1228 ± 214	19[c]
Efudex, 5% Solution	932 ± 252	1249 ± 339	25[c]

[a]An increase in epidermal DNA synthesis caused by IPM, calculated from (upper dorsal cpm/lower dorsal cpm) × 100.
[b]Calculated from [(lower dorsal cpm × 2.5)–upper dorsal cpm]/(lower dorsal cpm × 2.5) × 100.
[c]Calculated from [(lower dorsal cpm–upper dorsal cpm)/(lower dorsal cpm)] × 100.
Source: From Ref. 19.

Table 16 Physicochemical Properties of 6-MP N-Mannich Bases and Their Rates of Transdermal Delivery of 6-MP

Compound	MP°C	$C_v{}^a$	J^b	P^c
58, R = H	314	0.0030	0.00066 (0.00004)	0.22
59, R = CH$_2$N(CH$_3$)$_2$	231	0.0058	0.023 (0.007)	3.97
60, R = CH$_2$N(C$_2$H$_5$)$_2$	178	0.042	0.120 (0.030)	2.86
61, R = CH$_2$N(C$_3$H$_7$)$_2$	184	0.077	0.0059 (0.00020)	0.077
62, R = CH$_2$N(C$_4$H$_9$)$_2$	193	0.018	0.0034 (0.0016)	0.19
63, R = CH$_2$N(CH$_2$)$_5$	220	0.0050	0.0021 (0.0008)	0.42
64, R = CH$_2$N(CH$_2$)$_4$	195	0.0024	0.0041 (0.0008)	1.71
58, R = H		14.5^d	0.0038 (0.0007)^e	0.00026
59, R = CH$_2$N(CH$_3$)$_2$		9.1^d	0.011 (0.0010)^e	0.0012
61, R = CH$_2$N(C$_3$H$_7$)$_2$		27.4^d	0.010 (0.00090)^e	0.00036

^{a}Solubility of compounds in equivalent mg of 6-MP/ml of IPM at 23 ± 1°C.
^{b}Flux in mg/cm^2/h (± SD) from an IPM suspension through hairless mouse skin with a receptor phase temperature of 32°C.
^{c}Permeability coefficient in cm/h determined from J/C$_v$.
^{d}Solubility of compounds in equivalent mg of 6-MP/ml of DMF at 23 ± 1°C.
^{e}Flux in mg/cm^2/h (± SD) from a DMF suspension through hairless mouse skin with a receptor phase temperature of 32°C.
Source: From Ref. 27.

probably needs to be examined. As expected, **59** and **61** are 2000 and 300 times, respectively, more soluble in DMF than they are in IPM and the lower melting derivative **61** is the more soluble derivative. For the prodrugs derived from the two cyclic amines, the higher melting compound exhibits the higher lipid solubility.

The fluxes and permeability coefficients of the homologous series **59–62** generally fit the correlation between solubilities of the derivatives and their abilities to deliver the parent drug from a lipoidal vehicle through skin: The higher the solubility, the lower the flux. Again, **60** is an exception in that it exhibits the second highest solubility and gives the highest rate of delivery of 6-MP. On the other hand, the least soluble derivative **59** gives the second highest flux, and the most soluble derivative **61** gives the second lowest flux. Although the worst N-Mannich base prodrug of 6-MP is only about 4 times more effective than 6-MP itself, the best prodrug, **60**, is about 180 times more effective than 6-MP and about 3 times more effective than any other prodrug approach (using a single promoiety) to increasing the transdermal delivery of 6-MP. This emphasizes the usefulness of incorporating a tertiary amine functional group into a promoiety designed to enhance topical delivery. It also suggests that prodrugs designed to rapidly revert to the parent drug by chemical rather than enzymatic processes may have an advantage in topical delivery.

Later, prodrugs derived from the combination of the N-Mannich base approach and the acyloxymethyl prodrug approach will be discussed. This combination approach is more effective than the N-Mannich base approach alone.

The effect of using a vehicle in which the prodrug is much more soluble can be seen from the experiments in which DMF was used as the vehicle. Even though the prodrugs and 6-MP are much more soluble in DMF than IPM, the results are mixed as far as the performance of the prodrugs are concerned. Only the delivery of 6-MP itself from DMF shows any marked improvement over its delivery from IPM and then it is only a sixfold increase. Thus, it is apparent that using a vehicle in which the prodrug is more soluble can actually lead to a decrease in the effectiveness of its transdermal delivery of the parent drug.

In addition to the potentially detrimental effect on transdermal delivery of using a vehicle in which the prodrug is more soluble, there is the effect on delivery into the skin to be considered. Because all three of the more efficient N-Mannich base prodrugs (**59–61**) underwent decomposition in IPM toward the end of the diffusion cell experiments, the skin accumulation of 6-MP data for those members of this series of prodrugs tend to give lower values than expected based on the corresponding rates of transdermal delivery of 6-MP. Thus, the skin accumulation data for the entire series has not been presented. However, the accumulation of 6-MP in the skin from the application of **59** in DMF is almost half of what it is from the application of **59** in IPM (0.121 vs 0.219 mg, respectively), or from **61** in DMF compared to **61** in IPM (0.074 vs 0.133 mg, respectively) even though **61** was almost twice as effective in delivering 6-MP through the skin from DMF. On the other hand, accumulation of 6-MP in the skin from the application of 6-MP in DMF was about twice that from its application in IPM (0.031 vs 0.018 mg). Thus, using a vehicle in which the prodrug is more soluble may result in decreased dermal delivery as well as decreased transdermal delivery. Finally, although the correlation between transdermal delivery and skin accumulation is not good, all of the prodrugs used cause more 6-MP to accumulate in the skin when applied in IPM than 6-MP in IPM, and **59** is the most efficient—12 times as much 6-MP.

5-Fluorocytosine and 5-Iododeoxycytidine

5-Fluorocytosine (5-FC) (26) and Iododeoxycytidine (5-IDC) (61) are the final two examples of heterocyclic drugs whose transdermal delivery has been enhanced by the application of their N-Mannich bases in IPM. These drugs fall into the same category as ara-A which has already been discussed previously. They all contain exocyclic amine groups which are essentially nonbasic and behave like amides in many reactions. Since pyrimidines or purines (cytosine, adenine, guanine) and their corresponding nucleosides are known to form adducts with formaldehyde, it was an obvious extension to determine if their bases formed

N-Mannich base derivatives. Although they had not been described prior to 1984, Siver and Sloan reported in 1984 that high yields of N-Mannich bases derived from diverse types of secondary amines could be isolated from the simple reaction of the purine or pyrimidine with formaldehyde and a secondary amine in a nonprotic solvent (62).

Further extension of the reaction to 5-FC resulted in the synthesis, characterization, and evaluation in diffusion cell experiments of a limited number of 5-FC N-Mannich base prodrugs (26). A compilation of melting points, solubilities, fluxes, and permeability coefficients for the prodrugs are given in Table 17. There is no correlation between melting points and solubilities of the derivatives, and there are no trends in the relationships between solubilities and either fluxes or permeability coefficients. This result may be simply due to the fact that there really are no data from an homologous series available for evaluation. Regardless of whether there are any trends in the data that might suggest which future derivatives should be made, the results do suggest that this N-Mannich base approach is useful for this type of parent drug, since the dimethylaminomethyl derivative is 9 times more effective than 5-FC itself at delivering 5-FC through hairless mouse skin. This is important, since there are only a limited number of prodrug approaches available for use with the exocyclic amine type of functional group.

Table 17 Physicochemical Properties of 5-Fluorocytosine (5-FC) N-Mannich Bases and Their Rates of Transdermal Delivery of 5-FC

$$\begin{array}{c} \text{NHR} \\ \underset{O}{\overset{N}{\bigcirc}}\!\!\!\!\!\!\!\!\!\!\!\!\overset{N}{\underset{R'}{\bigcirc}}\!\!-F \end{array}$$

Compound	MP°C	$C_v{}^a$	J^b	P^c
65, R = R' = H	295–297	0.0050	0.005 (0.0015)	1.01
66, R = R' = CH₂N(CH₃)₂	136–138	0.12	0.045 (0.0027)	0.37
67, R = R' = CH₂N(C₂H₅)₂	129–131	1.18	—	—
68, R = R' = CH₂N(CH₂)₄	140–142	0.079	—	—
69, R = R' = CH₂N(CH₂)₅	181–183	0.048	0.034 (0.0015)	0.71
70, R = R' = CH₂N(CH₂CH₂)₂O	154–156	0.072	0.015 (0.0010)	0.21
71, R = R' = CH₂N(CH₂CH₂)₂NCH₃	163–165	0.029	0.026 (0.0084)	0.90

[a]Solubility of compounds in equivalent mg of 5-FC/ml of IPM at 23 ± 1°C.
[b]Flux in mg/cm²/h (± SD) from an IPM suspension, through hairless mouse skin with a receptor phase temperature of 32°C.
[c]Permeability coefficient in cm/h determined from J/C$_v$.
Source: From Ref. 26.

The data from the 5-IDC series is even more meager (61). Only two N-Mannich base derivatives of the exocyclic amine group in 5-IDC were synthesized: the morpholinylmethyl and piperidinylmethyl derivatives. Both are much more soluble in IPM than 5-IDC itself, especially since the solubility of 5-IDC in IPM could not be detected by HPLC. In spite of their much more lipidlike nature, the only derivative that was evaluated—the piperidinylmethyl derivative—is only 2.3 times more effective than 5-IDC at delivering 5-IDC through mouse skin. However, its lag time to the point where steady-state delivery is achieved is only about 5 h compared to about 14 h for 5-IDC. Although the N-Mannich base prodrugs of 5-FC are stable in IPM, the piperidinylmethyl prodrug of 5-IDC is not, and the flux of 5-IDC leveled off after about 20 h owing to its decomposition in the donor phase to 5-IDC. However, even this lack of stability should not be a drawback under normal conditions where a topical formulation may be applied two or three times a day.

Acyl Derivatives of Acidic Drug-NH Groups: Drug-N-(C=O)R′

Acyl derivatives of drugs containing acidic-NH groups have only very recently been evaluated for their potential to enhance topical delivery. On one hand, the acyl derivatives of drugs containing an amide functional group (pK_a 12–17) are considered to be too stable, whereas on the other hand, acyl derivatives of drugs containing an imide functional group (pK_a 2–12) are considered to be too unstable to function as prodrugs. However, that analysis is primarily concerned with oral or rectal routes of delivery. In the case of topical delivery, acyl derivatives of imides which ordinarily might be considered too unstable for use as prodrugs can be formulated in aprotic vehicles in which they are stable. Examples of prodrugs which are very unstable in the presence of water or protic solvents but which function as prodrugs in aprotic vehicles such as IPM, DMF, and triacylglycerides have already been given in the discussion of N-Mannich bases. Thus, the greater flexibility available in the choice of formulation vehicles for topical delivery make it possible to use prodrug approaches which are not acceptable for other routes of administration.

In the case of the acyl derivatives of drugs containing high pK_a amide functional groups, there are problems associated with their topical use unless transdermal delivery is the goal. This is especially true for a primary amide which when acylated becomes an imide. Imide-NH groups are much more acidic than amide-NH groups because of the additional electron-withdrawing carbonyl group attached to the nitrogen. The extensive ionization of the imide-NH group that results at physiological pH repulses the approach of hydroxide or other electron-rich nucleophiles which could cause their hydrolysis. Acyl derivatives of secondary amides do not present similar problems because there is no ionizable NH group left. Hence, they are much more amenable to enzymatic or chemical hydrolysis.

The mechanism for hydrolysis of various acyl derivatives of drugs containing low pK_a acidic Drug-NH groups is reported to be specific-base catalyzed and spontaneous (pH independent) or water catalyzed (63–66). Comparing various amides and imides, the rates of hydrolysis should depend on the acidity of the amide or imide: The more acidic the amide or imide, the faster the rate of hydrolysis. Although the above correlation has not been unequivocally established for N-acyl amides or imides, it has been established for the analogous N-acyl derivatives of azoles (67). Comparing the various types of N-acyl promoieties, their rates of hydrolyses should depend on the strength of the N-(C=O) bond and enzymatic specificity. There are five types of N-acyl derivatives that have been previously identified in Table 3 (entries 2–6). They are formed from the combination of R promoieties in Table 2 (entries 4–7 and 10) with the corresponding Drug-XH in Table 1 (entries 7–8). Specific mechanisms for the hydrolysis of each type of N-acyl derivative will be discussed in the appropriate section below.

5-Fluorouracil

The first drug for which N-acyl derivatives have been evaluated for their ability to enhance its topical delivery is 5-FU. 5-FU is a good candidate for improvement by an N-acyl prodrug approach because it is a relatively acidic drug which exhibits pK_as of 8.0 and 13.0 (63). The two acidic Drug-NH functional groups in 5-FU are an imide (3-N) and a secondary amide (1-N), so that even the N-acyl derivative of the amide functional group should be fairly labile. The only aspect of N-acyl derivatives of 5-FU about which some question remains is why the 1-N derivatives are more labile than the 3-N derivatives (65). Usually one expects an N-acyl derivative of an imide to hydrolyze faster than that of an amide because the imide is more acidic: The more acidic the NH group, the more stable the nitrogen anion and the better leaving group the nitrogen anion becomes. The answer may not lie in their respective pK_as. Some authors have reported that the 1-NH ionizes first, while others have reported that the 3-NH predominantly ionizes first (65). In addition, the pK_a of a 1-acyloxymethyl derivative (3-NH ionization) of 5-FU is lower than that of a 3-acyloxymethyl derivative (1-NH ionization) (see Table 8). Thus, there seems to be no simple answer to the question at this point.

Drug-N-(C=O)-NHR'. The first type of N-acyl derivative of 5-FU which has been evaluated for its ability to enhance the topical delivery of 5-FU is the urea type of derivative (Drug-N-(C=O)-NR$'_2$, where one R' = H and the other R' = alkyl). Although one might anticipate that these derivatives would be too stable for use as prodrugs if their hydrolysis occurred by a typical specific base-catalyzed reaction, this particular type of urea derivative undergoes rapid hydrolysis (half-lives of about 10 min; see Table 19) probably because of E1cB-like elimination of the acyl group as an isocyanate (see below) (66). An example, **84**, where both R' are alkyl and the formation of an isocyanate intermediate is not possible, exhibits less than 1% hydrolysis at pH 7.4 and 37°C after 8 h. Under similar conditions, the corresponding amides [R=(C=O)-R'] exhibit half-lives of about 4–6 min (see Tables 23 and 24), and the corresponding carbamates [R=(C=O)–OR'] exhibit half-lives of about 190–550 min (see Table 27). Hydrolyses of both of these latter types of derivatives take place by the expected specific base and spontaneous water-catalyzed mechanisms. So the dialkyl urea derivative fits the expected trend, being the most stable in the series of amide, carbamate, and urea, whereas the alkyl ureas do not, suggesting that a different mechanism is operating.

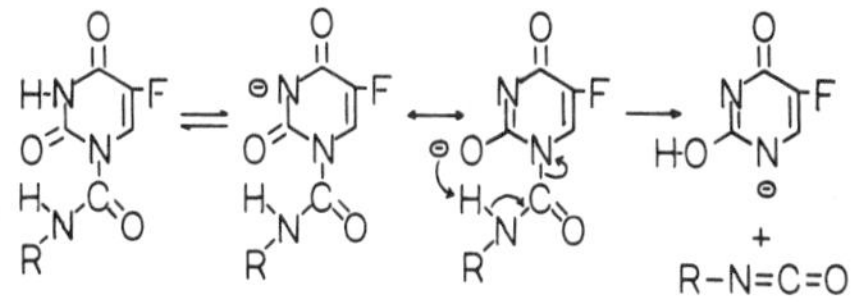

Scheme 7

In Table 18 is a representative list of the various urea-type derivatives of 5-FU that have been synthesized and evaluated for biological activity—mostly for oral administration. One obvious difference between the results obtained by Ozaki's group (68) and by Bundgaard's group (66) is the reported melting points. Both groups recognized the potential for thermal decomposition of one isomer of the derivatives to 5-FU and isocyanate (see **86** below). Although Ozaki verified the decomposition of **72** by differential thermal and gravimetric analysis, the remainder of the reported melting points were apparently obtained using a simple melting point apparatus. On the other hand, all of Bundgaard's melting points were obtained using differential scanning calorimetry. It is interesting that, except for **83**, the melting points reported by Bundgaard are uniformly higher. One possible explanation for the differences in melting points of the derivatives (except for **76**) isolated by the two groups is that different polymorphs have been isolated. Since the amount of hydrogen-bonded isomer **86** compared to non-hydrogen-bonded isomer **85** depends on the solvent (CDCl$_3$ or DMSO-d$_6$ in [^{1}H]nuclear magnetic resonance (NMR) experiments) (68), the use of different crystallization solvents easily could have led to the formation of different crystal forms containing different ratios of **86** to **85**: The greater the amount of hydrogen-bonded isomer **86**, the lower the expected melting point.

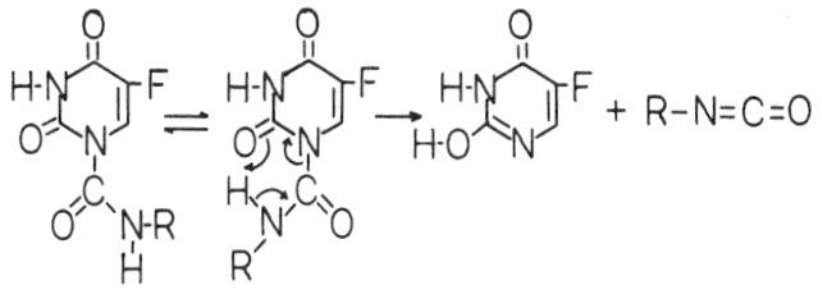

Scheme 8

85   **86**

The water solubilities, partition coefficients, and half-lives of selected members of the urea type of N-acyl prodrug are listed in Table 19 (66). None of the derivatives that were evaluated are more soluble in water than 5-FU itself. There is no correlation between melting points and water solubilities. The first member

Table 18 Alkylaminocarbonyl Derivatives of 5-FU

Compound	MP°C[a]		pK$_a$
16, R = R' = H	280–284		8.0, 13.0
72, R = H, R' = (C=O)-NHCH$_3$	170°	(225–228)[b]	6.7[b]
73, R = H, R' = (C=O)-NHC$_2$H$_5$	165°	(190–196)[b]	6.7[b]
74, R = H, R' = (C=O)-NHC$_3$H$_7$	145		
75, R = H, R' = (C=O)-NHCH(CH$_3$)$_2$	145		
76, R = H, R' = (C=O)-NHC$_4$H$_9$	137	(136)[b]	6.8[b]
77, R = H, R' = (C=O)-NHC(CH$_3$)$_3$	108		
78, R = H, R' = (C=O)-NHC$_5$H$_{11}$	117		
79, R = H, R' = (C=O)-NHC$_6$H$_{13}$	110–111		
80, R = H, R' = (C=O)-NHC$_7$H$_{15}$	103		
81, R = H, R' = (C=O)-NHC$_8$H$_{17}$	98–100		
82, R = H, R' = (C=O)-NHC$_{12}$H$_{25}$	107–108		
83, R = H, R' = (C=O)-NHC$_6$H$_5$	280	(221–224)[b]	
84, R = H, R' = (C=O)-N(CH$_3$)$_2$	194–196	(226–227)[b]	6.7[b]

[a]From Ref. 68.
[b]From Ref. 66.

Table 19 Selected Physicochemical Properties of 1-Alkylaminocarbonyl Derivatives of 5-FU

Compound	log K[a]	C$_v$[b]	Half-lives (min)[c]	
			buffer	80% plasma
16	–0.83	11.1		
72	–0.20	0.62	11.0	20.0
73	0.35	1.5	8.7	22.5
76	1.44	0.82	8.0	53.0
83	—	—	0.07	—
84	–0.37	6.0	—[d]	—

[a]Octanol–pH 4 acetate buffer partition coefficient at 22°C.
[b]Solubility in mg/ml in pH 4 acetate buffer at 22°C.
[c]Half-lives determined at 37°C in 0.05 M phosphate at pH 7.4. Plasma was human plasma.
[d]Less than 1% hydrolyzed after 8 h.
Source: From Ref. 66.

of the series exhibited the highest melting point and is the least soluble. The fact that the most water-soluble derivative is the dimethyl derivative **84** (where both of the hydrogens on nitrogen are replaced by alkyl groups) suggests that the reason the other derivatives (where one of the hydrogens on nitrogen remains) are less water soluble is that there is no net loss of intermolecular hydrogen-bonding NH groups. The prodrugs **72**, **73**, and **76** still have two polar NH groups. However, their melting points are all lower than that of 5-FU; and their partition coefficient values suggest that there is a correlation between melting point and lipid solubility for the series **72**, **73**, and **76**. In addition, the differences in their log K values is as expected based on the π substituent value for a methylene group. According to that criterion, **84** should be more lipophilic than **72** because it contains an extra methyl group, but it is in fact much more polar according to melting point values and log K values. The greater lipophilicity of **72**, **73**, and **76** compared to **84** may be due to the same reason that all the derivatives except **84** undergo facile hydrolysis and thermolysis—the occurrence of intramolecular hydrogen bonding between the urea NH and the 2-C=O in **72**, **73**, and **76** as in **86**.

The half-lives observed for the hydrolysis of the derivatives are short as expected based on an ElcB mechanism of hydrolysis for **72**, **73**, and **76** instead of a specific base-catalyzed mechanism. On the other hand, **84**, which cannot undergo hydrolysis by an ElcB mechanism, is essentially stable at pH 7.4. The half-lives of the series in human plasma are longer than in buffer. This suggests strong protein binding by the derivatives in biological samples.

In Table 20 are listed the melting points, solubilities, and rates of transdermal delivery of 5-FU by the derivatives **76**, **79**, and **81** (69). For these members of the series, the expected correlations between melting points and solubilities are observed. Also, as expected from the previous results obtained for the α-(acyloxy)alkyl derivatives of theophylline (see above) and 5-FU (see above), the least lipid-soluble and most water-soluble member of the series is the most effective at enhancing the transdermal delivery of the parent drug. The results in Table 21 show that not only is **76** the most effective derivative for enhancing the transdermal delivery of 5-FU, it also delivers more 5-FU and intact prodrug into the skin than does 5-FU or the other prodrugs. Thus, there is a correlation between enhanced transdermal and enhanced dermal delivery. This result is not due to increased binding to keratin as can be seen from the last column in Table 21. The most effective prodrug, **76**, binds to keratin least tightly.

The only conclusion that can be reached is that the increased transdermal and dermal delivery attained by the use of **76** is due to a more favorable partition coefficient between skin and vehicle for **76**, and hence a more favorable permeability coefficient (see eq. 1). The more soluble the derivative is in the vehicle (IPM), the lower its partition coefficient into skin unless the vehicle has solubilizing properties similar to skin. But that is hardly ever the case. Alternatively, the lower the solubility of a member of a series of more lipid-soluble derivatives is in water, the lower its biphasic solubility (solubility in aqueous and lipid phases), and

Table 20 Physicochemical Properties of 1-Alkylaminocarbonyl Derivatives and Their Rates of Transdermal Delivery of 5-FU

		$C_v{}^a$			
Compound	MP°C	buffer	IPM	J^b	P^c
16	280–284	11.7	0.0104	0.0043	0.410
76	130–133	0.62	4.95	0.016	0.0032
79	112–113	0.047	5.84	0.014	0.0024
81	92–94	0.0039	6.29	0.0057	0.00091

[a]Solubility in equivalent mg of 5-FU/ml of pH 4 acetate buffer or ml of IPM at 37°C.
[b]Flux in mg/cm^2/h from suspensions in IPM through full thickness shaved abdominal skins from male Wistar albino rats with receptor phase at 32°C.
[c]Permeability coefficients in cm/h calculated from J/C_v.
Source: From Ref. 69.

the less soluble it is in the intercellular spaces in skin through which the prodrug must diffuse. Extension of either explanation to its logical conclusion suggests the methylaminocarbonyl, **72**, ethylaminocarbonyl, **73**, or propylaminocarbonyl, **74**, derivatives may be the more effective members of this type of N-acyl prodrugs for the enhancement of the transdermal delivery of 5-FU and should be investigated. Of these, the ethylaminocarbonyl derivative, **73**, should be the most promising, since it is the most water soluble.

Table 21 Binding of 1-Alkylaminocarbonyl Derivatives of 5-FU to Biological Materials

	Skin accumulation[a]		Binding to keratin[b]	
Compound	5-FU	prodrug	33 mg/ml	83 mg/ml
16	0.091 (0.7)		0	7
76	0.065 (0.5)	0.40 (1.75)	33	50
79	0.033 (0.25)	0.22 (0.85)	66	85
81	0.026 (0.20)	0.26 (0.90)	84	100

[a]Mg of 5-FU or prodrug after 2 h of contact with IPM suspension of prodrug. Value in parenthesis is in micromoles.
[b]Percent of prodrug from 0.1 mM pH 7.4 phosphate buffer solution bound to keratin after contact with keratin suspension. Values are for 33 and 83 mg of keratin/ml of aqueous solution.
Source: From Ref. 69.

Drug-N-(C=O)-R'. Independent of the evaluation of 1-alkylaminocarbonyl derivatives of 5-FU by Sasaki and coworkers (69), this author's group has been evaluating other types of N-acyl derivatives of 5-FU. Based on the correlations between water solubilities of prodrugs and their relative abilities to deliver a parent drug through skin that was observed in previous studies of α-(acyloxy)alkyl derivatives (see above), attention was directed toward types of more lipophilic N-acyl prodrugs which might in addition be more soluble in water than the parent drug. Bundgaard and coworkers (63–65) evaluated the physicochemical properties of a wide variety of types of N-acyl derivatives of 5-FU. Inspection of that data showed that the first members of the 1- and 3-substituted 5-FU series of alkylcarbonyl and alkoxycarbonyl types of N-acyl derivatives were more soluble in water than 5-FU. This suggested that both types of N-acyl derivatives should be evaluated for their ability to deliver 5-FU through skin.

The N-alkylcarbonyl derivatives were examined first. In Table 22 is a partial list of the various 1- and 3-mono, and 1,3-bisalkylcarbonyl derivatives of 5-FU that have been synthesized and characterized by the various research groups (63,70,71). Although many arylcarbonyl derivatives have also been synthesized and characterized (71), the focus of this discussion is on the alkylcarbonyl derivatives because they are more labile (compare **94** with **91–93** in Table 23) and more water soluble than the arylcarbonyl derivatives—the latter because fewer carbons can be introduced with the initial members of the series of alkylcarbonyl derivatives (also see below). Structure assignments have been made based on literature precedents. However, there are inconsistencies in the [1H]NMR and pK$_a$ data that may require reassessment of the structures at a later date (70).

At this point, only partial information is available for all three series, and diffusion cell data are only available for a limited number of the 1-mono and 1,3-bisalkylcarbonyl series. There is no consistent trend in the melting points of the members of each series versus their alkyl chain length for this type of N-acyl derivative. In the two mono series, the butyryl derivative exhibits the highest melting point, whereas in the 1,3-bisalkylcarbonyl series, the melting point goes down consistently as the alkyl chain length increases. No pK$_a$ data are available for the 1-alkylcarbonyl series because of their rapid hydrolysis.

In Table 23 are listed some physicochemical properties of selected 1- and 3-alkylcarbonyl derivatives determined by Bundgaard (63). The 3-derivatives are much more stable than the 1-acetyl derivative, **87**, and the 1,3-bisalkylcarbonyl derivatives. The half-life values for the 1,3-series are not listed in Table 23, but they are even less stable than **87** with half-lives of 2.7 min being exhibited by **95**, **97**, and **98** (63). In each case, the half-life for the hydrolysis of the derivative in the 1,3-series was for hydrolysis to the corresponding 3-alkylcarbonyl derivative. Because of their poor stability in water (and protic solvents as well), the water solubilities of **87** and the 1,3-series were not determined by the same methods used to determine the solubilities of the 3-series. Their partition coefficients

Table 22 Alkylcarbonyl Derivatives of 5-FU

$$\begin{array}{c} O \\ \parallel \\ R-N \diagup \diagdown F \\ \mid \quad \mid \\ O \diagup \diagdown N \diagup \\ \mid \\ R' \end{array}$$

Compound	MP°C	$pK_a{}^c$
16, R = R' = H	280–284	8.0, 13.0
87, R = H, R' = (C=O)-CH₃	126–127[a]	—
88, R = H, R' = (C=O)-C₂H₅	127–128[a]	—
89, R = H, R' = (C=O)-C₃H₇	142–143[a]	—
90, R = H, R' = (C=O)-C₄H₉	117–118[a]	—
91, R = (C=O)-CH₃, R' = H	114–117[b]	7.1
92, R = (C=O)-C₂H₅, R' = H	99–102[b]	7.2
93, R = (C=O)-C₃H₇, R' = H	132–134[c]	7.2
94, R = (C=O)-C₆H₅, R' = H	170–172[b]	6.9
95, R = R' = (C=O)-CH₃	109–110[a]	—
96, R = R' = (C=O)-C₂H₅	97–99[a]	—
97, R = R' = (C=O)-C₃H₇	47.5–48.5[c]	—
98, R = R' = (C=O)-C₆H₅	169–171[b]	—

[a]From Ref. 70.
[b]From Ref. 71.
[c]From Ref. 63.

Table 23 Physicochemical Properties of Selected Alkylcarbonyl Derivatives of 5-FU

Compound	log K[a]	$C_v{}^b$	Half-lives (min)[c]	
			buffer	80% plasma
16	–0.83	11.1		
87	—	—	6.9	—
91	–0.34	42.8	43	4.6
92	0.19	35.3	50	20
93	0.67	—	58	28
94	0.80	1.3	2900	110

[a]Octanol-pH 4 acetate buffer partition coefficient determined at 22°C.
[b]Solubility in mg/ml in pH 4 acetate buffer at 22°C.
[c]Half-lives determined at 37°C in 0.05 M phosphate buffer at pH 7.4. Plasma was human plasma.
Source: From Ref. 63.

between 1-octanol and water were not determined either. Even though the stability of the 3-series is greater than that of the 1- or 1,3-series, their half-lives are still less than 1 h, so their solubilities in water and their partition coefficients had to be determined quickly. Both the 3-acetyl, **91**, and 3-propionyl, **92**, derivatives, are much more soluble in water than 5-FU and are considerably more lipid soluble as well based on their measured partition coefficients. There are no water solubility data given for the 3-butyryl derivative, **93**, but based on the consistent differences in log K values between successive members of the 3-series, the 3-butyryl derivative appears to behave analogously to the other members of the series in spite of the fact that its melting point is considerably higher than that of the 3-propionyl derivative. Thus, based on the information available in Table 23, members of the 3-alkylcarbonyl series appear to be excellent candidates with which to enhance the transdermal delivery of 5-FU. At this point their evaluation awaits further effort.

Instead, the 1- and 1,3-series of alkylcarbonyl derivative were evaluated first. The synthesis of the 3-alkylcarbonyl derivatives requires the initial synthesis of the 1,3-bisalkylcarbonyl derivatives, and their subsequent hydrolysis to give the desired prodrugs. So quantities of the 1,3-series became available first. On the other hand, the 1-series could be synthesized directly from 5-FU, so it was much easier to synthesize than the 3-series. Although both the 1- and 1,3-series have been described as being too unstable for use as prodrugs, they are more stable in water than the N-Mannich bases that were discussed in previous sections. The N-Mannich bases were stable when applied topically in aprotic vehicles, so it was anticipated that the 1- and 1,3-series would be sufficiently stable to be applied topically in aprotic vehicles as well. Finally, although water solubilities and partition coefficient values for the 1-alkylcarbonyl derivatives were not available at the time the decision was made to evaluate them, it was anticipated that their physicochemical properties would be very similar to those of the 3-alkylcarbonyl derivatives, and this would make them good candidates to evaluate as prodrugs to enhance topical delivery. This turned out to be the case.

In Table 24 are listed the solubilities, partition coefficients, and half-lives of the first members of the 1- and 1,3-series (70). All of the prodrugs are much more soluble in IPM, and exhibit much higher IPM:pH 4 acetate buffer partition coefficients than 5-FU. Apparent water solubilities for members of both series were determined from their partition coefficient values and their saturated solubilities in IPM. Using this approach to estimate the water solubilities of easily hydrolyzed derivatives, the 1-acetyl derivative, **87**, is the only derivative of either series that exhibits greater water solubility than 5-FU. Even then, its solubility is only about half that of the 3-acetyl and 3-propionyl derivatives. However, the water solubilities determined by the partition coefficient method may under-estimate the true water solubilities (see below).

The rates of delivery of 5-FU by the 1- and 1,3-series are given in Table 25 (70). The 1-acetyl derivative, **87**, which is by far the most water-soluble deriva-tive, is also by far the most effective member of the series at delivering 5-FU

Table 24 Physicochemical Properties of 1- and 1,3-Bisalkylcarbonyl Derivatives of 5-FU

| Compound | $C_v{}^a$ | | log K^b | Half-lives (min)^c |
	IPM	buffer		
16	0.0064	12.5	–3.29	
87	3.80 (2.87)	20.6 (15.6)	–0.73	4.4
88	6.77 (4.73)	8.9 (6.2)	–0.12	3.0
89	3.48 (2.26)	1.31 (0.85)	0.43	4.0
90	8.39 (5.10)	0.74 (0.45)	1.05	3.7
95	5.60 (3.40)	1.91 (1.16)	0.47	—
96	17.4 (9.35)	0.80 (0.43)	1.34	—

^{a}Solubility at 23 ± 1°C in mg/ml of IPM or pH 4 acetate buffer (equivalent mg of 5-FU/ml). Solubility in buffer determined from partitioning between a saturated IPM solution and a pH 4 acetate buffer, then extrapolating from the K value and the solubility in IPM to a value for the saturated solubility in buffer.
^{b}Partition coefficient between IPM and pH 4 acetate buffer at 23 ± 1°C.
^{c}Half-lives for hydrolysis to 5-FU at 32°C in pH 7.1 phosphate buffer.
Source: From Ref. 70.

Table 25 Rates of Transdermal Delivery of 5-FU by 1- and 1,3-Bisalkylcarbonyl Derivatives of 5-FU and Their Effect on Skin Integrity

Compound	J^a	log P^b	Skin^c accumulation	J^d
16	0.0311 (0.0114)	0.69	0.48	0.215 (0.042)
87	1.213 (0.038)	–0.37	8.85	0.296 (0.008)
88	0.560 (0.015)	–0.93	8.96	0.219 (0.030)
89	0.168 (0.025)	–1.13	1.07	0.185 (0.004)
90	0.133 (0.017)	–1.58	2.08	0.144 (0.005)
95	0.291 (0.063)	–1.07	1.24	0.282 (0.019)
96	0.090 (0.0079)	–2.02	0.51	0.288 (0.047)

^{a}Flux in mg/cm^2/h (± SD) from an IPM suspension through hairless mouse skin with receptor phase at 32°C.
^{b}Permeability coefficient in cm/h calculated from J/C_v equivalent mg of 5-FU/ml.
^{c}Amount of 5-FU in mg leached from hairless mouse skin in the 24 h subsequent to application of 5-FU or prodrug in IPM for 48 h.
^{d}Flux in mg/cm^2/h (± SD) for theophylline/PG after application of 5-FU or prodrug/IPM.
Source: From Ref. 70.

through hairless mouse skin. However, it should also be added that the 1-propionyl, **88**, 1-butyryl, **89**, the 1-valeryl, **90**, and the 1,3-diacetyl, **95** derivatives were all more effective than the previously reported best prodrug of 5-FU at delivering 5-FU through hairless mouse skin: the N-Mannich base **56** in Table 13.

It is apparent that it is not necessary to mask both polar N-H groups in 5-FU to obtain high levels of transdermal delivery. The 1-derivatives are more soluble in water, less soluble in lipids, and much more effective at delivering 5-FU than the 1,3-derivatives. The advantage gained by masking both polar groups is offset by the loss of water solubility engendered by the addition of a second lipophilic promoiety.

There is also a significant increase in accumulation of 5-FU in the skin caused by the topical application of both series of alkylcarbonyl prodrugs compared to the application of 5-FU itself in the same vehicle. Generally, the prodrugs that delivered more 5-FU through the skin are also more effective at causing accumulation of 5-FU in the skin. The most effective prodrug at enhancing transdermal delivery is almost 20 times more effective at causing 5-FU to accumulate in the skin than 5-FU. Finally, it should be pointed out that the prodrugs caused no more damage to the skin than did 5-FU itself in IPM.

Drug-N-(C=O)-OR'. A selection of the various 1- and 3-mono and 1,3-bisalkoxycarbonyl derivatives of 5-FU that have been synthesized is given in Table 26 (64,65,70,72). In the 1-alkoxycarbonyl series there is a good correlation between decreased melting point and increased alkyl chain length until after the hexyl derivative, **103**, when the melting point goes back up again. As already pointed out for the acyloxymethyl prodrugs of 5-FU in Table 8, the pK_as of the 1-derivatives (3-N ionization) are lower than that of the 3-derivatives (1-N ionization).

In Table 27 are listed the physicochemical properties of the 1- and 3-alkoxycarbonyl series of derivatives determined by Bundgaard and coworkers (64,65,72). They observed that only the 1-methoxy- and 3-ethoxycarbonyl derivatives were more soluble in water than 5-FU, and that the 3-derivative was more soluble than the 1-derivative. This is consistent with the trends observed for the alkylcarbonyl derivatives. However, the 3-derivatives are essentially stable to buffer or plasma esterase (64), so they are useless as prodrugs for enhancing dermal delivery. The 1-alkoxycarbonyl derivatives are about an order of magnitude more stable in buffer than the 1-alkylcarbonyl derivatives, but their hydrolyses by plasma esterases is so fast that they can still function as prodrugs for dermal delivery.

In Table 28 are listed some additional physicochemical properties of the 1-alkoxycarbonyl series of derivatives that were evaluated in diffusion cell experiments (70). The order of their solubilities in IPM is expected, but the order of their water solubilities is not. The water solubilities listed were obtained from partitioning experiments, but when the solubilities were determined by the same

Table 26   Alkoxycarbonyl Derivatives of 5-FU

Compound	MP°C	pK$_a$
16, R = R′ = H	280–284	8.0, 13.0
99, R = H, R′ = (C=O)-OCH$_3$	159–160[a]	6.8[a]
100, R = H, R′ = (C=O)-OC$_2$H$_5$	126–128[a]	6.9[a]
101, R = H, R′ = (C=O)-OC$_3$H$_7$	124–126[b]	—
102, R = H, R′ = (C=O)-OC$_4$H$_9$	97–98[b]	6.8[a]
103, R = H, R′ = (C=O)-OC$_6$H$_{13}$	68–69[c]	6.8[c]
104, R = H, R′ = (C=O)-OC$_8$H$_{17}$	97–98[b]	—
105, R = H, R′ = (C=O)-OCH$_2$C$_6$H$_5$	188–190[a]	6.8[c]
106, R = H, R′ = (C=O)-OC$_6$H$_5$	203–204[a]	6.8[c]
107, R = (C=O)-OC$_2$H$_5$, R′ = H	126–128[d]	8.6[d]
108, R = (C=O)-OCH$_2$C$_6$H$_5$, R′ = H	157–158[d]	8.5[d]
109, R = (C=O)-OC$_6$H$_5$, R′ = H	169–170[d]	6.6[d]
110, R = R′ = (C=O)-OCH$_2$C$_6$H$_5$	129–130[d]	—
111, R = R′ = (C-O)-OC$_6$H$_5$	148–149[d]	—

[a]From Ref. 65.
[b]From Ref. 70.
[c]From Ref. 72.
[d]From Ref. 64.

general method as used by Bundgaard and coworkers (65), the solubilities reported by them for **99** and **102** but not **100** were reproduced. Under those conditions **100** exhibits a water solubility of about 52 mg/ml. There does not seem to be a simple explanation for the discrepancy in the reported water solubility. However, the second member of the 1-alkylaminocarbonyl series was also the most water-soluble member of that series.

The previously observed correlation between the relative water solubilities of the members of a series of prodrugs and their abilities to deliver the parent drug through skin seen for the 1-alkylaminocarbonyl and 1-alkylcarbonyl derivatives is seen for the 1-alkoxycarbonyl series as well. In the 1-alkoxycarbonyl series, the most water-soluble derivative is the second member in the series not the first member, but it is by far the most effective member of the series at delivering total 5-FU through hairless mouse skin. In contrast to the 1-alkylcarbonyl type of

Table 27 Physicochemical Properties of Selected Alkoxycarbonyl Derivatives of 5-FU

Compound	log K^a	$C_v{}^b$	Half-lives (min)^c buffer	80% plasma
16	−0.83	11.1		
99	−0.68^d	23.3^d	190^d	—
100	−0.17^d	6.9^d	550^d	2.1^d
102	0.89^d	5.9^d	550^d	3.1^d
103	2.04^e	1.5^e	550^e	2^e
105	1.18^d	0.08^e	150^d	0.8^d
106	0.64^d	0.9^d	18^d	<0.5^d
107	0.11^f	72^f	—^{g}	—^{g}
108	1.42^f	—	—^{g}	—^{g}
109	1.73^f	0.15^f	80h^f	390^f

^{a}Octanol-pH 4 acetate buffer partition coefficient determined at 22°C.
^{b}Solubility in mg/ml in pH 4 acetate buffer at 22°C.
^{c}Half-lives determined at 37°C in 0.05 M phosphate buffer at pH 7.4. Plasma was human plasma.
^{d}From Ref. 65.
^{e}From Ref. 72.
^{f}From Ref. 64.
^{g}No apparent hydrolysis after 4–5 h.

prodrug which delivered only 5-FU, the 1-alkoxycarbonyl series delivers not only 5-FU, but also considerable amounts of intact prodrug as well. The ratio of 5-FU to intact prodrug varies with the particular member of the series. This result is probably the consequence not only of the greater stability of the 1-alkoxycarbonyl series, but also of the fact that so much derivative is being delivered into the skin that the enzyme system is not capable of keeping up: The greater the success of the prodrug, the greater the potential for the latter condition obtaining.

As already seen for the 1-alkylaminocarbonyl and the 1-alkylcarbonyl-5-FU derivatives, the more efficient the 1-alkoxycarbonyl-5-FU derivatives are at delivering 5-FU through the skin, the more efficient they are at causing 5-FU to accumulate in the skin. However, the 1-alkoxycarbonyl derivatives are not nearly as effective as the 1-alkylcarbonyl derivatives. This result may be due to two factors. First, the 1-alkoxycarbonyl derivatives are much more stable than the 1-alkylcarbonyl derivatives. Second, the 1-alkoxycarbonyl derivatives exhibit greater biphasic solubility than 5-FU, which is comparable to that of the 1-alkylcarbonyl derivatives: Compare **100** with **87**. Thus, the 1-alkoxycarbonyl derivatives possess solubility properties that enable them to easily partition into and

Table 28　Physicochemical Properties of 1-Alkoxycarbonyl Derivatives of 5-FU and Their Abilities to Deliver 5-FU Through Hairless Mouse Skin

Compound	$C_v{}^a$ IPM	$C_v{}^a$ buffer	$\log K^b$	J^c	Skin^d accumulation
16	0.0051	12.5	−3.29	0.0311 (0.0114)	0.48
99	0.40 (0.28)	16.0 (11.1)	−1.60	0.34 (0.074)	1.08
100	2.64 (1.70)	35.2 (22.7)	−1.12	0.77 (0.163)	2.38
101	3.28 (1.97)	9.2 (5.54)	−0.44	0.29 (0.029)	0.65
102	7.77 (4.39)	5.4 (3.03)	0.16	0.28 (0.011)	0.54

[a]Solubility at 23 ± 1°C in mg of 5-FU or prodrug/ml of IPM or ml of pH 4 acetate buffer (equivalent mg of 5-FU/ml). Solubility in buffer determined from partitioning between a saturated IPM solution and a pH 4 acetate buffer, then extrapolating from the K value and the solubility in IPM to a value for the saturated solubility in buffer.
[b]Partition coefficient between IPM and pH 4 acetate buffer determined at 23 ± 1°C.
[c]Flux in mg of 5-FU/cm^2/h (± SD) from an IPM suspension through hairless mouse skin with receptor phase at 32°C.
[d]Amount of 5-FU in mg leached from hairless mouse skin in the 24 h subsequent to application of 5-FU or prodrug in IPM for 48 h.
Source: From Ref. 70.

diffuse through biological membranes, but they are so stable that the prodrug is not completely hydrolyzed to the parent drug before it completes the diffusion process.

Theophylline

Although there are no topical formulations of theophylline that are commercially available, there is continuing interest in the topical delivery of theophylline. α-(Acyloxy)alkyl and N-Mannich base derivatives of theophylline provided some of the first examples of the usefulness of those approaches to enhancing the topical delivery of polar heterocycles. Although there are no reports of the use of N-acyl derivatives of theophylline for enhancement of its topical delivery, there are a few reports of the use of its N-acyl derivatives for other purposes. In this section, some pertinent data from those reports on N-acyl derivatives is presented which suggests their possible use for topical delivery.

Drug-N-(C=O)-R' and drug-N-(C=O)-OR'.　7-Alkylcarbonyl derivatives of theophylline were synthesized primarily for use as sustained-release forms of theophylline in which release was dissolution rate controlled (74,76). The 7,7'-succinyldisucceinylditheophylline derivative (not shown in Table 29) was eventually identified as the best candidate for that purpose from among the derivatives that were synthesized. Its high melting point and poor solubility in virtually all

Table 29   7-Alkylcarbonyl Derivatives of Theophylline

Compound	MP°C	Half-life
5, R=H		
112, R=(C=O)-CH$_3$[a]	156–157	40 sec[d]
113, R=(C=O)-C$_2$H$_5$[a]	129–130	
114, R=(C=O)-C$_3$H$_7$[a]	88–90	
115, R=(C=O)-C$_7$H$_{15}$[b]	62–63	
116, R=(C=O)-C$_9$H$_{19}$[b]	71–72	
117, R=(C=O)-C$_{15}$H$_{31}$[b]	92–93	
118, R=(C=O)-CH$_2$CH$_2$(C=O)OC$_2$H$_5$[b]	107–109	
119, R=(C=O)-OC$_2$H$_5$[c]	135–140	

[a]From Ref. 73.
[b]From Ref. 74.
[c]From Ref. 75.
[d]From Ref. 76.

solvents makes it a poor candidate for use as a topical delivery form. However, based on the results with 5-FU, a number of those other derivatives that were synthesized may be more useful. In Table 29 is a list of some of those 7-alkylcarbonyl derivatives and of others selected from the literature (73–75). Because of their very rapid hydrolysis, as evidenced by the half-life of **112** in water (40 s), no water-solubility data are available. However, the water solubility of the more stable 7-alkoxycarbonyl derivative **119** is reported to be one part in 35 parts of cold water (75). All of the derivatives listed should be more lipid-soluble than theophylline based on the previously established relationship between melting point and lipid solubility. Similarly, based on previous results, the first one or two members of the series should be the more effective members at enhancing topical delivery and may in fact be more effective than other types of prodrugs of theophylline if the experience with 5-FU is any indication.

Acyl Derivatives of Basic Drug-NH Groups: Drug-N-(C=O)-R'

Generally, acyl derivatives of basic amines are not particularly good prodrugs of the parent amines. Compared to acyl derivatives of amides, and especially imides where the negative charge can be stabilized by the adjacent carbonyl groups so that the amide or imide anion becomes a good leaving group, acyl derivatives of basic amines are usually very stable because the corresponding anions derived from the basic amines are not stable. There are exceptions to this analysis. N-Acyl derivatives of imidazole, which exhibits a basic pK_a of about 7.05, are very labile to chemical hydrolysis (67). Nonsubstituted aziridine exhibits a pK_a of about 8.01, so it was of interest to determine if N-acyl derivatives of aziridine could, like N-acyl derivatives of imidazole, function as prodrugs. Recently, Sezaki and coworkers (48,77) characterized several series of different types of prodrugs of an alkylating anticancer drug—mitomycin C—which contains an aziridine ring as one of its reactive centers. Among the types of prodrugs evaluated were several types of acyl derivatives of the aziridine ring in mitomycin C (48,77).

Mitomycin C

Mitomycin C is a very polar heterocyclic drug which like many other anticancer agents has potential use for the treatment of topical cancers or psoriasis (78). It is somewhat soluble in water but it is not very soluble in lipids. Derivatives exhibiting enhanced lipid solubilities were targeted for evaluation not only for their potential to enhance topical delivery, but also for incorporation into liposomes and emulsions.

Drug-N-(C=O)-R′ drug-N-(C=O)-OR′. In Table 30 are listed the various types of prodrugs of mitomycin C synthesized and characterized by Sezaki and coworkers (48,78). All of these derivatives except the N-arylcarbonyl derivative, **123**, are more soluble in lipids than mitomycin C. It is not clear why **123** is so much less soluble in lipids and water than mitomycin C or, for that matter, than its N-alkylcarbonyl analogue—the benzylcarbonyl derivative, **124**. None of the derivatives are more soluble in water than mitomycin C. The one acyloxymethyl derivative, **122**, is very unstable in aqueous solutions, reverting to mitomycin C with a half-life of about 3.5 min at pH 7 (77). This lack of stability was considered sufficient cause not to evaluate it any further. However, based on the previous examples of the successful application of chemically labile prodrugs in aprotic solvents to enhance topical delivery, it may have deserved more attention. The series of alkoxycarbonyl derivatives **126–128** were synthesized after the benzyloxycarbonyl derivative, **125**, was found to revert to mitomycin C in 2% rat plasma with a half-life of about 3 min (77). There is no correlation between melting point and lipid solubility or water solubility for **125–128**. Of these N-alkoxycarbonyl derivatives, the previously observed trends would suggest that **125** and **127** should be the more efficient prodrugs in the series for enhancing topical delivery because they are quite lipophilic but retain more water solubility than the other two members of the series.

The results from the diffusion cell experiments are given in Table 31 (78). First, the prediction based on the past correlations between water solubilities and transdermal delivery is verified. Of the derivatives that function as prodrugs, **125** and **127** are by far the more effective delivery forms. The best

Table 30 N-Alkyl and N-Acyl Derivatives of Mitomycin C

Compound	MP°C	$C_v{}^a$	
		water	IPM
120, R=H	>270	2.73	0.019
121, R=CH$_2$C$_6$H$_5$	119–121	1.49	5.67
122, R=CH$_2$O(C=O)-C$_6$H$_5$	112–116[b]	—	—
123, R=(C=O)-C$_6$H$_5$	>270	0.01	0.009
124, R=(C=O)-CH$_2$C$_6$H$_5$	154–156	2.24	0.41
125, R=(C=O)-OCH$_2$C$_6$H$_5$	102–104	0.52	3.28
126, R=(C=O)-OC$_3$H$_7$	203–207	0.33	0.11
127, R=(C=O)-OC$_5$H$_{11}$	89–93	0.59	8.22
128, R=(C=O)-OC$_9$H$_{19}$	139–141	0.00025	12.62

[a]Solubility in mM for water at 25°C and for IPM at 37°C.
[b]From Ref. 48.
Source: From Ref. 78.

derivative for increasing total transdermal delivery is the N-benzyl derivative, **121**, but it did not function as a prodrug. Second, partition coefficient seems to be a rather poor predictor of the ability of a prodrug to enhance topical delivery. Prodrug **123** exhibits about the same log K value as **125**, yet **125** is 300 times more effective at delivering mitomycin C. The difference between **123** and **125** lies in the absolute solubilities exhibited by the two compounds. Prodrug **123** is much less soluble in lipids and in water than is mitomycin C. On the other hand, **125** is more soluble in lipids than mitomycin C yet retains significant water solubility as well. The fact that the two compounds exhibit about the same partition coefficient is meaningless. Absolute solubilities are the important criteria. Third, for these types of prodrugs, lipid solubility may be more important than water solubility when comparing different types of acyl prodrugs. Prodrug **125** (an alkoxycarbonyl type) is almost 8 times more effective than **124** (an alkylcarbonyl type), and **125** is 8 times more soluble in lipids but about 15 times less soluble in water. Thus, the use of N-acyl derivatives of a low pK$_a$ basic amine as prodrugs has some utility in enhancing the topical delivery of the parent drug.

Table 31 Rates of Permeation of Mitomycin C Prodrugs and Their Abilities to
Deliver Mitomycin C Through Rat Skin

Compound	Concentration[a]	log K^b	J^c as parent	as prodrug
120	10	−0.39	9.0 (0.63)	—
121	10	1.59	—	58.6 (18.2)
123	2	1.89	0.01 (0.01)	0.12 (0.03)
124	2	1.54	3.2 (0.57)	2.0 (0.49)
125	6	2.05	37.6 (10.0)	—
126	2	1.51	2.1 (1.2)	0.19 (0.09)
127	10	2.45	30.7 (1.9)	0.10 (0.05)
128	2	3.57	0.19 $(0.11)^d$	—

[a]Initial donor phase concentration in mM of compound suspended in IPM.
[b]Partition coefficient between water and 1-octanol at 25°C.
[c]Flux in nmol/h (± SD) for diffusion cell experiments run at 37°C.
[d]Solution.
Source: From Ref. 78.

β-*Blockers*

β-Blockers typically exhibit pK_a values expected of basic amines—between 9 and
10. Because of the strongly basic nature of the amine groups and the induced local
alkalinity that can result, direct application of β-blockers topically either for
transdermal or ocular delivery can cause severe irritation. Acylation of the basic
amine group would render it nonionizable at physiological pH, and hence much
more compatible with topical membranes. In addition, it was anticipated that
acylation would improve the lipid solubility, and hence the partition coefficients
of the prodrugs. The major drawback with this approach is reversibility of the
derivative. Alexander and coworkers (79,80) have overcome this drawback by
designing N-alkoxycarbonyl derivatives which incorporate an easily hydrolyzed
enabling functional group (an ester group) into the alkoxy portion of the prodrug
to give **129**. Hydrolysis of the ester functional group releases an N-hydroxy-
methoxycarbonyl intermediate, **130**, which spontaneously hydrolyses to give a
carbamic acid, **131**, and formaldehyde. The carbamic acid subsequently loses
carbon dioxide as the final step in a cascade of reactions to regenerate the parent
amine. This type of derivative has been described as a triple prodrug because of
the number of discrete steps in the cascade (8).

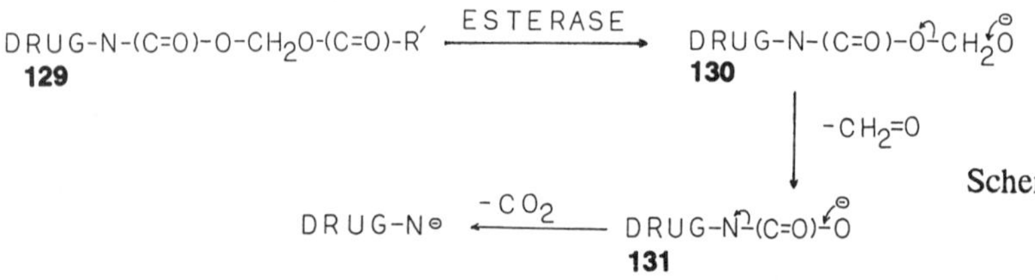

Scheme 9

Drug-N-(C=O)-OR'. In Table 32 is a list of the β-blockers that were investigated by Alexander and coworkers (79) along with the corresponding rates at which they are delivered through fuzzy rat skin from neat films deposited by evaporation of the ethanol solutions of the β-blockers and their respective prodrugs. Theoretically, the thermodynamic activities of all the compounds that were evaluated should have been the same by this method, and there should have been very little solvent effect on the rates of delivery that were observed. All of the prodrugs that were evaluated reverted completely to their parent amines during diffusion through the membranes, since no detectable prodrug was observed in the receptor phases.

Of interest from the standpoint of designing new prodrug approaches and optimizing currently used approaches is the dichotomy of the results obtained for the prodrugs of the various β-blockers. β-Blockers have been previously arbitrarily divided into very lipophilic, lipophilic, and hydrophilic β-blockers based on their partition coefficients (81). Atenolol and pindolol are considered to be hydrophilic, whereas timolol is considered to be lipophilic and propranolol is considered to be very lipophilic. Thus, the rates of transdermal delivery of the hydrophilic β-blockers, atenolol and pindolol, are increased significantly by their application in the forms of their more lipophilic prodrugs, **132** and **133**, whereas the rates of transdermal delivery of the more lipophilic β-blockers, propranolol and timolol, are decreased significantly by their application in the form of their

Table 32 Rates of Delivery of β-Blockers Through Fuzzy Rat Skins
Drug-NR-(C=O)-OCHR'-O(C=O)CH₃

| Compound | J^a | Half-lives (min)^b | | R | R' |
		buffer	plasma		
Atenolol	0.36				
132	2.04	—	—	$CH(CH_3)_2$	CH_3
Pindolol	0.15				
133	2.27	—	—	$CH(CH_3)_2$	CH_3
Propranolol	11.1				
134	3.12	2670	3	$CH(CH_3)_2$	CH_3
Timolol	199				
135	5.3	1410	3	$C(CH_3)_3$	H

^{a}Flux in nmol/cm²/h.
^{b}Half-lives in pH 7.4 phosphate buffer at 37°C. Plasma was rat plasma.
Source: From Ref. 79.

more lipophilic prodrugs, 134 and 135. This suggests that the incorporation of additional lipophilicity into atenolol and pindolol imparted the more balanced lipid and water solubilities that are necessary to improve their partitioning into the skin, and hence their diffusion through the skin. On the other hand, incorporation of more lipophilicity into the already relatively lipophilic propranolol and timolol molecules actually decreased their ability to partition into and diffuse through the skin. Thus, enhanced biphasic solubility should be the target for attempts to enhance or optimize transdermal delivery and not merely enhanced lipid solubility.

Although the suggested trend for the lipophilic prodrug of β-blockers fits the same general trends observed for prodrugs of polar heterocycles, no partition coefficients are reported for this series, so it is not sure how lipophilic the prodrugs are. However, the prodrugs are reported to be oils or glasses, so they should indeed be more soluble in lipids than their parent drugs.

DRUG-SH

In the previous section, prodrugs of a number of different parent drugs were discussed. There are a large number of drug molecules which contain either a basic or an acidic Drug-NH group and which are also candidates for topical administration. The same cannot be said of drug molecules containing an SH group. In this section on Drug-SH functional groups there is really only one drug that is a candidate for topical administration; i.e., 6-mercaptopurine or 6-MP. Examples of α-(acyloxy)alkyl derivatives and N-Mannich base derivatives of 6-MP where an acidic Drug-NH group was masked have already been discussed previously. In this section, α-(acyloxy)alkyl and α-(acylamino)alkyl derivatives of the Drug-SH functional group alone and in combination with derivatives of the acidic Drug-NH functional groups in 6-MP will be discussed. The latter are the only examples of the use of the combination prodrug approach to enhance topical delivery, but the approach may be quite useful when applied to other drugs. In addition, the discussion of the effect of vehicles on prodrug enhancement of transdermal delivery will be expanded upon from the results already discussed previously.

α-(Acyloxy)alkyl Derivatives of Drug-SH Groups: Drug-S-CHR′-O-(C=O)-R′

α-(Acyloxy)alkyl derivatives are different from acyl derivatives of parent drugs in that the enabling functional group is not directly attached to the functional group in the parent drug that is to be masked. Thus, their stability is not substantially affected by the heteroatom in the parent drug to which they are attached. Instead, their stability is primarily affected by the sensitivity of the ester enabling functional to chemical and enzymatic hydrolysis and only secondarily to the chemical stability of the intermediate α-hydroxyalkyl derivative of Drug-XH that results after the ester group is cleaved. That analysis assumes the hydrolysis of the α-(hydroxy)alkyl intermediate does not become the rate-limiting step in the regeneration of the parent drug. In the case of α-(acyloxy)alkyl derivatives of Drug-SH groups, little is known about the stability of that intermediate, Drug-S-CHR'-OH. Attempts to synthesize the intermediate for study by allowing 6-MP to react with aqueous formaldehyde yields a complex mixture of products comprised mainly of 7-hydroxymethyl and S^6, 3-bishydroxymethyl-6-MP (82). However, if one assumes that the hydrolysis of a formaldehyde adduct with a thionamide functional group depends on the same mechanism for hydrolysis that defines the relative stabilities of formaldehyde adducts with the usual amides or imides, then the half-life of the intermediate should be less than 0.2 sec (4). Thus, α-(acyloxy)alkyl derivatives of 6-MP should function as prodrugs of 6-MP.

6-Mercaptopurine

Drug-S-CHR'-O(C=O)-R'. A representative number of S^6-acyloxymethyl derivatives have been synthesized, characterized and evaluated in diffusion cell experiments (83). Since the first few members of any homologous series representing a particular prodrug approach have been observed to be the more efficient members of the series at enhancing topical delivery, the authors have found that n=1–7 or 8 in R' =$(CH_2)_nH$ is usually sufficient to define most series. The melting points of the derivatives and their solubilities in water are given in Table 33. The water solubilities decrease with increasing chain length, whereas the melting points plateau at 144–154°C for the butyryloxymethyl, **138**, through the octanoyloxymethyl, **141**, derivatives (n=3–7). The lipid solubilities plateau as well for the same derivatives as shown in Table 34 by the fairly constant solubilities in IPM. On the other hand, the solubilities of the derivatives in PG increase gradually up to the valeryloxymethyl derivative, **139**, and then fall off gradually.

The rates of delivery of 6-MP by the S^6-acyloxymethyl-6-MP series from suspensions in either IPM or PG are given in Table 34. Since Bundgaard has shown that the stability of the acyloxymethyl derivatives to esterases is sensitive to the drug portion of the prodrug (84), the stabilities of the acetyloxymethyl, **136**, and butyryloxymethyl, **138**, derivatives in buffer and in buffer which had been in contact with the dermis of hairless mice in diffusion cells were compared. The acetyloxymethyl derivative is half as stable (half-life = 114 h) in buffer but 6 times more stable (half-life = 12 h) in buffer which had been in contact with hairless mouse dermis. Thus, the prodrugs are sufficiently stable that if they were diffusing through the skins intact they could have been detected in the receptor phase. In all the diffusion cell experiments, only 6-MP was observed in the receptor phase; no intact S^6-acyloxymethyl-6-MP was detected.

There are three notable extensions of previously observed trends that are apparent in the results of Tables 33 and 34. First, regardless of the vehicle in which the prodrug is applied, the highest rates of delivery of 6-MP are observed for the

Table 33 Physicochemical Properties of S^6-Acyloxymethyl Derivatives of 6-MP

Compound	MP°C	$C_v{}^a$
58, R = H (6-MP)	314	0.17
136, R = CH$_2$O-(C=O)-CH$_3$	192.5–194.5	1.61 (1.09)
137, R = CH$_2$O-(C=O)-C$_2$H$_5$	163–165	0.96 (0.62)
138, R = CH$_2$O-(C=O)-C$_3$H$_7$	152–154	0.51 (0.31)
139, R = CH$_2$O-(C=O)-C$_4$H$_9$	146.5–148.5	0.21 (0.12)
140, R = CH$_2$O-(C=O)-C$_5$H$_{11}$	149.5–151	0.067 (0.036)
141, R = CH$_2$O-(C=O)-C$_7$H$_{15}$	144–148	0.0075 (0.0037)
142, R = CH$_2$O-(C=O)-C(CH$_3$)$_3$	195–196	—

[a]Solubility in mg/ml of water (equivalent mg of 6-MP/ml) at 23 ± 1°C.
Source: From Ref. 83.

Table 34 Rates of Delivery of 6-MP by S^6-Acyloxymethyl Derivatives of 6-MP Through Hairless Mouse Skin

	IPM		Skin[c]	PG	
Compound	$C_v{}^a$	J^b	accumulation	$C_v{}^a$	J^b
58	0.0034	0.60 (0.30)	0.018	6.2	0.093 (0.0060)
136	0.24 (0.16)	30.8 (8.8)	0.150	20.9 (14.2)	0.55 (0.22)
137	0.55 (0.35)	32.5 (14.8)	0.155	29.8 (19.0)	0.54 (0.073)
138	0.83 (0.50)	39.8 (19.7)	0.356	37.6 (22.7)	0.96 (0.17)
139	1.12 (0.64)	33.5 (15.7)	0.333	38.7 (22.1)	0.95 (0.13)
140	1.04 (0.56)	8.3 (3.9)	0.113	20.7 (11.2)	0.48 (0.065)
141	1.28 (0.63)	2.0 (1.1)	0.057	16.7 (8.24)	0.29 (0.024)
142	1.40 (0.80)	9.4 (1.4)	0.119	—	—

[a]Solubility in mg/ml of IPM or PG (equivalent mg of 6-MP/ml) at 23 ± 1°C.
[b]Flux in mg/cm^2/h × 10^3 (± SD) from suspensions in IPM or PG with a receptor phase at 32°C.
[c]Amount of 6-MP in mg leached from hairless mouse skin in the 24 h subsequent to application of 6-MP or prodrug in IPM for 48 h. From unpublished work of R. P. Waranis.
Source: From Ref. 83.

prodrugs that are the more water-soluble derivatives. In this series, the first three members of the series are more soluble in water than 6-MP and the fourth member—the valeryloxymethyl derivative, **139**—is close. The trend is particularly obvious for the delivery of 6-MP from IPM where there is a precipitous fall off in the rate of delivery after the valeryloxymethyl derivative.

Second, increased solubility of the prodrug in the vehicle does not lead to increased transdermal delivery of the parent drug. This trend is especially obvious in the comparison between the rates of delivery of 6-MP from IPM compared to the rates of delivery from PG. The rates are 10–50 times greater from IPM even though the prodrugs are 12–90 times more soluble in PG. Part of this difference in rates of delivery may be due to the greater damaging effect of IPM on hairless mouse skin compared to PG. However, the same sort of trend can be seen in rates of delivery of 6-MP from the same vehicle, IPM. Of the derivatives that are more soluble in IPM (the valeryloxymethyl, **139**, through octanoyloxymethyl derivative, **141**), only the valeryloxymethyl is capable of delivering 6-MP at the same rates as the less lipid-soluble derivatives, and it is the most water soluble of the more lipid-soluble derivatives. Thus, the most important property of a prodrug from which to predict its relative ability to enhance transdermal delivery is its water solubility.

Third, the relative ability of the prodrugs to deliver 6-MP through the skin correlates with the relative accumulation of 6-MP in the skin. Prodrug **138**, which delivers the most 6-MP through the skin, causes the highest accumulation 6-MP in the skin, whereas **141**, which delivers the least amount of 6-MP through the skin, also causes the lowest accumulation of 6-MP in the skin. Similar results were obtained for the accumulation of 6-MP after the topical application of the S^6-acyloxymethyl-6-MP prodrugs in PG (results not given), except that the values are over an order of magnitude lower in keeping with the much lower rates of transdermal delivery of 6-MP obtained using PG as the vehicle.

Combination of Drug-S-CHR′-O(C=O)-R′ with Drug-N-CHR′-O (C=O)-R′. Two series of combinations of S^6-acyloxymethyl with N-acyloxymethyl derivatives were obtained from the reaction of acyloxymethyl chlorides with 6-MP (85). The primary product is the S^6,9-bisacyloxymethyl-6-MP series, whereas the secondary product, and the one usually isolated in lower yield, is the S^6,3-bisacyloxymethyl-6-MP series. From Table 35 it is obvious that the S^6,3-bisacyloxymethyl series is the higher melting and less lipid-soluble series. No water solubilities were determined for the S^6,3-series. In the S^6,9-bisacyloxymethyl series the peak solubility in IPM is observed for the lowest melting member of the series—the bisvaleryloxymethyl derivative, **146**—then decreases as the chain length increases. The water solubilities in the series fall off as the chain length increases, and only the first two members of the series actually exhibit greater water solubility than 6-MP.

Table 35 Physicochemical Properties of S^6, 3- and S^6, 9-Bisacyloxymethyl Derivatives of 6-MP

$$S^6,3- \qquad S^6,9-$$

| Compound | MP°C | $C_v{}^a$ | |
		IPM	H_2O
S^6, 9-			
143, R=R′=CH₂O-(C=O)-CH₃	120.5–122.5	1.56	0.85
144, R=R′=CH₂O-(C=O)-C₂H₅	76–77	10.9	0.54
145, R=R′=CH₂O-(C=O)-C₃H₇	68.5–69.5	32.0	0.069
146, R=R′=CH₂O-(C=O)-C₄H₉	56.5–57.5	66.3	0.018
147, R=R′=CH₂O-(C=O)-C₅H₁₁	70.5–72	20.3	—
148, R=R′=CH₂O-(C=O)-C₇H₁₅	78–79	7.93	—
149, R=R′=CH₂O-(C=O)-C(CH₃)₃	89–91	78.4	—
S^6, 3			
150, R=R′=CH₂O-(C=O)-CH₃	200–204	0.014	—
151, R=R′=CH₂O-(C=O)-C₅H₁₁	167–169	0.16	—
152, R=R′=CH₂O-(C=O)-C₇H₁₅	161–163	0.14	—
153, R=R′=CH₂O-(C=O)-C(CH₃)₃	193.5–195	0.31	—

[a]Solubility in mg/ml determined at 23 ± 1°C.
Source: From Ref. 85.

   In Table 36 are given the rates of delivery of 6-MP by S^6,9-bisacyloxymethyl-6-MP derivatives from a wide variety of vehicles. Only one of the S^6,3-bisacyloxymethyl-6-MP derivatives was evaluated in a diffusion cell experiment (S^6,3-bispivaloyloxymethyl-6-MP, **153**), and it performed much worse than the corresponding S^6,9-derivative, **149** (21), so none of the other S^6,3-derivatives were further evaluated. Among the S^6,9-bisacyloxymethyl prodrugs, the performances of the bisacetyloxymethyl, **143**, and the bispropionyloxymethyl, **144**, derivatives consistently stand out. Regardless of the solubilizing capacity of the vehicle, they are the most effective prodrugs at delivering 6-MP through hairless mouse skin. In the case of vehicles that exhibit solubility parameter values less than 15 (cal/cm³)$^{1/2}$, **143** and **144** are not the most soluble derivatives in those nonpolar vehicles. While for vehicles that exhibit solubility parameter values greater than 15 (cal/cm³)$^{1/2}$, **143** and **144** are the most soluble derivatives in those

Table 36 Rates of Delivery of 6-MP by S^6,9-Bisacyloxymethyl Derivatives of 6-MP Through Hairless Mouse Skin

Compound/vehicle $(\delta_v)^a$	$C_v{}^b$	J^c	J^d	Skin^e accumulation
6-MP/OA (7.6)	0.0030	0.043 (0.021)	—	—
143/OA (7.6)	1.08	5.92 (2.42)	1.66	0.058
144/OA (7.6)	11.3	8.33 (1.52)	1.17	0.069
146/OA (7.6)	69.6	3.35 (0.29)	—^{f}	0.069
6-MP/IPM (8.5)	0.0034	0.60 (0.30)	—	0.018
143/IPM (8.5)	0.80	34.5 (2.8)	4.24	0.431
144/IPM (8.5)	5.11	35.2 (9.9)	0.57	0.352
145/IPM (8.5)	13.8	21.5 (5.4)	—^{f}	0.287
146/IPM (8.5)	26.5	15.5 (7.4)	—^{f}	0.207
147/IPM (8.5)	7.56	1.75 (0.44)	—	—
148/IPM (8.5)	2.60	0.19 (0.014)	—	—
149/IPM (8.5)	31.4	5.48 (0.55)	—^{f}	0.184
6-MP/OCT (10.3)	0.23	18.6 (1.6)	—	0.103
143/OCT (10.3)	1.11	75.4 (2.7)	22.3	—
144/OCT (10.3)	5.57	85.3	2.0	—
145/OCT (10.3)	11.5	25.7	—^{f}	—
6-MP/DEET(10)	4.4	3.2 (0.24)	—	0.057
143/DEET(10)	30.7	10.5 (1.6)	—	—
6-MP/MEG (12.1)	10.0	0.75 (0.10)	—	0.020
143/MEG (12.1)	36.8	2.42 (0.33)	0.41	—
6-MP/PG (14.8)	6.2	0.093 (0.0060)	—	0.004
143/PG (14.8)	2.79	0.58 (0.04)	0.39	0.019
144/PG (14.8)	8.63	1.95 (0.28)	—^{f}	0.025
145/PG (14.8)	9.54	1.60 (0.050)	—	0.020
146/PG (14.8)	8.32	0.77 (0.060)	—^{f}	0.010
147/PG (14.8)	1.71	0.18 (0.045)	—	0.009
6-MP/FOR (17.9)	9.1	1.50 (0.10)	—	0.031
143/FOR (17.9)	15.8	2.59 (0.27)	—	0.038
144/FOR (17.9)	22.3	7.06 (1.13)	—	—
146/FOR (17.9)	6.2	2.00 (0.30)	—	0.023
6-MP/H_2O (23)	0.17	0.36 (0.21)	—	0.005
143/H_2O (23)	0.44	1.58 (0.88)	0.14	0.024
144/H_2O (23)	0.25	1.97 (0.16)	—^{f}	0.019
145/H_2O (23)	0.030	0.81 (0.081)	—	0.008
146/H_2O (23)	0.0071	0.50 (0.12)	—^{f}	0.009

Abbreviations: OA = oleic acid; IPM = isopropyl myristate; OCT = 1-octanol; DEET = diethyltoluamide; MEG = 2-methoxyethanol; PG = propylene glycol; FOR = formamide.
^{a}The δ_v are solubility parameters given in $(cal/cm^3)^{1/2}$.
^{b}The solubilities are given in equivalent mg of 6-MP/ml.
^{c}Flux in mg/cm^2/h $\times$ 10^3 ($\pm$ SD) with a receptor phase at 32°C.
^{d}Flux in mg of S^6,9-bisacyloxymethyl-6-MP/cm^2/h $\times$ 10^3.
^{e}Amount of 6-MP in mg leached from hairless mouse skin in 24 h subsequent to application of 6-MP or prodrug in vehicle for 48 h. From unpublished work of R. P. Waranis.
^{f}Intact prodrug or intermediate hydrolysis products not detected in receptor phase during experiment.
Source: From Ref. 85.

73

polar vehicles. The dominant factor dictating the relative abilities of the members of this series of more lipophilic prodrugs to increase the transdermal delivery of its parent drug is their water solubilities, not their relative solubilities in the vehicles used.

Although intact S^6-acyloxymethyl-6-MP prodrugs were not observed in the receptor phases of the diffusion cell experiments in which they were evaluated (see previous section), in the case of the S^6,9-bisacyloxymethyl-6-MP prodrugs, intact prodrugs were observed in the receptor phases of the diffusion cell experiments, but only when bisacetyloxymethyl, **143**, or bispropionyloxymethyl, **144**, derivatives were applied. Intact bisbutyryloxymethyl, **145**, bisvaleryloxymethyl, **146**, or bispivaloyloxymethyl, **149**, derivatives were never detected in receptor phases. The stabilities of the S^6,9-bisacetyloxymethyl, S^6,9-bispropionyl-oxymethyl, and S^6,9-bisbutyryloxymethyl derivatives were determined in buffer and in buffer which had been in contact with the dermis of hairless mice in diffusion cells (85). The S^6,9-bisacetyloxymethyl derivative is half as stable in buffer (half-life = 4.25 h) but 10 times more stable in buffer which had been in contact with hairless mouse dermis (half-life = 5.6 h) than the S^6,9-bisbutyryl-oxymethyl derivative. The S^6,9-bispropionyloxymethyl derivative is in between. Also, the half-lives are for disappearance of the bis derivatives. Both mono derivatives can be detected by HPLC during the hydrolysis studies, but only intact prodrug and 6-MP can be detected in the receptor phases during diffusion cell experiments. Thus, although both the S^6-series and the S^6,9-series are fairly stable chemically and enzymatically, they are almost completely converted to 6-MP during their diffusion through the skin which attests to the durability of the enzymes in these in vitro systems.

There are three general comments about the results from the use of the S^6,9-bisacyloxymethyl derivatives to enhance the transdermal delivery of 6-MP. First, it seems that it is not important to mask both polar functional groups in a polar heterocycle to obtain significant enhancement of its transdermal delivery. This conclusion was also reached in the comparison of the 1-alkylcarbonyl with the 1,3-bisalkylcarbonyl-5-FU derivatives in a previous section. However, in this case it is clearly more important to mask one polar functional group (the thionamide functional group) than it is to mask the other (the 9-NH functional group) as discussed previously. This can be concluded from the fact that the rates of delivery of 6-MP by S^6,9-bisacyloxymethyl derivatives are no greater than the rates of delivery obtained by the S^6-acyloxymethyl derivatives. Part of the reason for this result is the disproportionately greater lipophilicity imparted by incorporating two acyloxymethyl groups into the prodrug and the concomitant decrease in the prodrug's water solubility.

Second, in all the available comparisons between the rates of delivery by 6-MP from a particular vehicle and the rates of delivery of 6-MP by a S^6,9-bisacyloxymethyl-6-MP prodrug from the same vehicle, the best prodrugs not only deliver more 6-MP through the skin, but also deliver more 6-MP into the skin. Similar to what was observed for the S^6-acyloxymethyl-6-MP derivatives, the greatest increase in amount of 6-MP accumulated in the skin is obtained when IPM is used as the vehicle.

Third, it may have been anticipated that the conversion of a polar heterocyclic drug to a much more lipophilic prodrug would mean that the optimum vehicle for delivering the drug would change, but that does not seem to be the case. Although the rates of delivery of 6-MP from lipoidal vehicles such as oleic acid and IPM have increased dramatically with the rather dramatic increase in solubility of the prodrugs in those vehicles, IPM, in which 6-MP is almost insoluble, is one of the better vehicles with which to deliver 6-MP in the first place. On the other hand, it is obvious that the improvement in the rate of delivery of 6-MP by the prodrugs from the more polar vehicles is not nearly as dramatic as that from the more lipoidal vehicles.

Combination of Drug-S-CHR'-O(C=O)-R' with Drug-N-CHR'-NR$_2'$. Potentially, the combination of a promoiety such as the α-(acyloxy)alkyl type (which is chemically stable but which adds significant lipophilicity when incorporated into a prodrug) with a promoiety such as the N-Mannich base type (which is chemically unstable but which adds significant hydrophilicity) could be an ideal combination. It seems clear that incorporating increased biphasic solubility into the prodrug is the key to optimizing the transdermal delivery of the parent drug. Thus, an approach using two different types of promoieties in a single prodrug, one type that imparts increased lipophilicity and the other type that imparts increased hydrophilicity, could offer a significant advantage over an approach which uses only one type of promoiety. In addition, it is apparent from the discussion in previous sections that little improvement in the performances of the α-(acyloxy)alkyl and N-Mannich base–type prodrug approaches to improving the transdermal delivery of 6-MP should be anticipated.

A series of N-Mannich base derivatives of two S^6-acyloxymethyl-6-MP derivatives were synthesized and evaluated (86,87). The two S^6-acyloxymethyl-6-MP derivatives chosen represented the available extremes in the lipid solubilities of the S^6-acyloxymethyl series: the S^6-pivaloyloxymethyl derivative which was the most soluble in IPM and the S^6-acetyloxymethyl derivative which was the least soluble. The N-Mannich base derivatives of S^6-pivaloyloxymethyl-6-MP, **142**, are all much more soluble in IPM than **142** itself (Table 37), and there is a reasonable correlation between melting point and IPM solubility which includes the homologous acyclic series **154–157** and the cyclic series **158–160** (86). Several members of the acyclic series (**155** and **157**) are actually more soluble in IPM than the most IPM soluble member of the S^6,9-bisacyloxymethyl-6-MP series, S^6,9-bispivaloyloxymethyl-6-MP. However, in spite of their relatively high lipid solubilities, all of the combination derivatives are at least 5 times, and as high as 9 times, more effective than the parent S^6-pivaloyloxymethyl-6-MP derivative at delivering total 6-MP through hairless mouse skin (Table 38). On the other hand,

Table 37 Physicochemical Properties of Dialkylaminomethyl Derivatives of S^6-Pivaloyloxymethyl-6-MP

$$S\,C\,H_2O(C=O)C(C\,H_3)_3$$

Compound	MP°C	$C_{v,j}{}^a$	$C_{v,i}{}^b$
142, R = H	195–196	1.40	0.80
154, R = CH₂N(CH₃)₂	86–88	38.2	17.9
155, R = CH₂N(C₂H₅)₂	70–72	111.3	48.2
156, R = CH₂N(C₃H₇)₂	87–89	56.5	22.7
157, R = CH₂N(C₄H₉)₂	56–60	313.5	117.1
158, R = CH₂N(CH₂CH₂)₂O	134–136	5.6	2.3
159, R = CH₂N(CH₂)₅	91–93	55.2	23.1
160, R = CH₂N(CH₂CH₂)₂N-CH₃	104–106	24.0	9.7

[a]Solubility of derivatives in mg/ml of IPM.
[b]Solubility in equivalent mg of 6-MP/ml of IPM.
Source: From Ref. 86.

Table 38 Rates of Delivery of 6-MP and S^6-Pivaloyloxymethyl-6-MP Through Hairless Mouse Skin by 9-Dialkylaminomethyl-S^6-Pivaloyloxymethyl-6-MP

Compound	$J_i{}^a$	$J_j{}^b$	$J_\Sigma{}^c$	$\log P_\Sigma{}^d$
58	0.6 (0.3)	—	—	—
142	9.4 (1.4)	—	—	—
154	37.0 (0.9)	43.3 (0.3)	80.3	–2.35
155	33.9 (3.2)	18.6 (1.3)	52.5	–2.97
156	24.5 (1.2)	40.0 (1.9)	64.5	–2.55
157	30.3 (3.1)	20.2 (1.2)	50.5	–3.37
158	38.6 (1.8)	16.9 (2.1)	55.5	–1.62
159	33.3 (0.5)	14.6 (3.6)	47.9	–2.68
160	29.0 (7.1)	30.1 (5.2)	59.1	–2.21

[a]Flux of 6-MP in mg/cm²/h × 10³ (± SD) from IPM suspensions of derivatives with a receptor phase of 32°C.
[b]Flux of S^6-pivaloyloxymethyl-6-MP in equivalent mg of 6-MP/cm²/h × 10³ (± SD).
[c]Total flux of 6-MP from $J_i + J_j$.
[d]Total permeability coefficient from $J_\Sigma/C_{v,i}$ in cm/h.
Source: From Ref. 86.

among the acyclic series of derivatives, the member that is the least soluble in IPM (dimethylaminomethyl, **154**) delivers the most 6-MP, and the next to the least soluble member (dipropylaminomethyl, **156**) the next highest amount. Similarly, the morpholinylmethyl derivative, which is by far the least soluble in IPM of the members in the cyclic series, delivers as much total 6-MP as either of the more soluble members. Again, increased IPM solubility—increased solubility in the vehicle—is not the important criterion in determining the best performance.

The trends observed for the N-Mannich base series of derivatives of S^6-acetyloxymethyl-6-MP, **136**, are similar to that observed for essentially the same series of derivatives of S^6-pivaloyloxymethyl-6-MP (87). All of the derivatives are much more soluble in IPM than **136** or even S^6,9-bisacetyloxymethyl-6-MP, **143**, which also has both polar functional groups masked (Table 39). The correlation between decreased melting point and increased lipid solubility is much weaker for the S^6-acetyloxymethyl series than for the S^6-pivaloyloxymethyl series. Similarly, the trend of the least soluble member of a series being the most effective member at enhancing transdermal deliveries is also much weaker for the S^6-acetyloxymethyl series (Table 40). However, the best performance is by a member of the cyclic amine series which are on average less soluble than the acyclic series by an order of magnitude. So, in general, the previously observed correlations can be

Table 39 Physicochemical Properties of Dialkylaminomethyl Derivatives of S^6-Acetyloxymethyl-6-MP

$$S\,CH_2O(C=O)CH_3$$

Compound	MP°C	$C_{v,j}{}^a$	$C_{v,i}{}^b$
136, R = H	192–194	0.24	0.16
161, R = CH$_2$N(C$_2$H$_5$)$_2$	71–72	48.5	23.9
162, R = CH$_2$N(C$_3$H$_7$)$_2$	80.5–81	49.6	22.4
163, R = CH$_2$N(C$_4$H$_9$)$_2$	91–92	30.5	12.7
164, R = CH$_2$N(C$_5$H$_{11}$)$_2$	56.5–57.5	300.0	116.0
165, R = CH$_2$N(CH$_2$CH$_2$)$_2$O	104–106	5.3	2.5
166, R = CH$_2$N(CH$_2$)$_5$	121–122	5.6	2.6
167, R = CH$_2$N(CH$_2$CH$_2$)$_2$N-CH$_3$	134–135	3.0	1.4

[a]Solubility of derivatives in mg/ml of IPM.
[b]Solubility in equivalent mg of 6-MP/ml of IPM.
Source: From Ref. 87.

Table 40   Rates of Delivery of 6-MP and S[6]-Acetyloxymethyl-6-MP Through Hairless Mouse Skin by 9-Dialkylaminomethyl-S[6]-acetyloxymethyl-6-MP

Compound	$J_i{}^a$	$J_j{}^b$	$J_\Sigma{}^c$	Skin[d] accumulation
58	0.6 (0.3)	—	—	0.018
136	30.8 (8.8)	—	—	0.15
161	100 (4.0)	10.5 (2.1)	111	0.87
162	69.0 (13.0)	2.8 (1.2)	72	0.97
163	84.0 (5.9)	6.5 (2.6)	91	0.63
164	55.0 (9.1)	11.3 (3.4)	66	0.64
165	124.0 (31)	23.4 (12.6)	147	0.54
166	25.0 (4.9)	3.1 (0.8)	29	0.27
167	59.0 (6.4)	3.5 (0.6)	63	0.82

[a]Flux of 6-MP in $mg/cm^2/h \times 10^3$ (± SD) from IPM suspensions of derivatives with a receptor phase of 32°C.
[b]Flux of S[6]-acetyloxymethyl-6-MP in equivalent mg of $6\text{-MP}/cm^2/h \times 10^3$ (± SD).
[c]Total flux of 6-MP from $J_i + J_j$.
[d]Amount of 6-MP in mg leached from hairless mouse skin in the 24 h subsequent to application of 6-MP or prodrug in vehicle for 48 h. From unpublished work of K. B. Sloan and H. D. Beall.
Source: From Ref. 87.

extrapolated to combination prodrug approaches to enhancing transdermal delivery which use a combination of acyloxymethyl and N-Mannich base promoieties.

All of the N-Mannich base derivatives of S[6]-acetyloxymethyl-6-MP are much more effective than either 6-MP or S[6]-acetyloxymethyl-6-MP, **136**, at causing 6-MP to accumulate in the skin. In fact, they are also almost twice as effective as the more effective S[6],9-bisacyloxymethyl derivatives (see Table 36) at causing 6-MP to accumulate in the skin. However, as opposed to previous observations, there is no apparent correlation between the ability of the prodrugs to deliver 6-MP through the skin and their ability to deliver 6-MP into the skin.

Combination of Drug-S-CHR'-O(C=O)-R' with N-Ribosyl.   One of the most common types of polar drug molecule is the purine or pyrimidine nucleoside. Many of these molecules exhibit antiproliferative, antiviral, antibacterial, etc., activity, and the capability of using a topical treatment regimen would be advantageous. However, not only do these molecules contain acidic-NH groups, but they also contain multiple hydroxy groups. The combination of these polar groups in one molecule invariably means that they exhibit little activity when applied topically. Traditionally, such nucleoside-type molecules have been simply converted to their corresponding esters in attempts to improve their transdermal delivery, and the polar acidic-NH groups—or in the case of 6-MP, the thionamide functional group—have been ignored. Not unexpectedly, the success of such attempts has been limited.

In the case of 6-MP, an S^6-pivaloyloxymethyl derivative of the 2',3',5'-triacetyl-riboside of 6-MP, **170**, was prepared and its ability to deliver 6-MP through skin was compared with that of 6-MP itself, its riboside, **168**, its 2',3',5'-triacetyl-riboside, **169**,and the corresponding S^6,9-bispivaloyloxymethyl-6-MP, **149** (Table 41) (21). In each case, the predominant species detected in the receptor phase is 6-MP. Approximately 10% of intact **169** and 1% of intact **170** are observed in the receptor phase after their topical application to hairless mouse skin in diffusion cell experiments. No intact **168** or **149** is observed. Not only are the pivaloyloxymethyl promoieties hydrolyzed, but the ribosyl groups are cleaved by nucleoside phosphorylase during the diffusion of the prodrug through the skin.

Based on the above discussions, the poor performances of the riboside, **168**, and the 2',3',5'-triacetylriboside, **169**, of 6-MP are expected. The performance of the S^6-pivaloyloxymethyl-2',3',5'-triacetylribosyl-6-MP, **170**, is consistent with previous results (discussed above) in that **170** and **149** are the only two prodrugs where the thionamide functional group is transiently masked in addition to the 9-NH group, and they are the most effective prodrugs evaluated in the study. The results in Table 41 illustrate the fact that modification of the purine or pyrimidine base portion of a nucleoside in addition to the ribosyl hydroxy groups is essential

Table 41 Transdermal Delivery of 6-MP by Riboside Derivatives of 6-MP

R'S

Compound	MP°C	6-MP in receptor phase[a]
58, R = R₁ = H	>300(d)	0.0026 (0.00049)
168, R = riboside, R₁ = H	221–223	0.0015 (0.0003)
169, R = 2',3',5'-triacetylriboside, R' = H	255–256	0.0022 (0.0011)
170, R = 2',3',5'-triacetylriboside, R' = CH₂-O-(C=O)-C(CH₃)₃	oil	0.033 (0.010)[b]
149, R = R' = CH₂-O-(C=O)-C(CH₃)₃	87–89	0.013 (0.0020)[b]

[a]Cumulative mmole (± SD) of 6-MP in receptor phase 48 h after application of 0.5 ml of 0.01 M suspensions in IPM.
[b]Solutions (0.01M) were applied.
Source: From Ref. 21.

to maximize the transdermal delivery of the purine or pyrimidine. However, it is not clear that using nucleosides to deliver the corresponding purine or pyrimidine is cost effective. Prodrug **170** is only 2.5 times more effective than **149**, but the starting nucleoside (**168** or **169**) is much more expensive than 6-MP which is the starting point in the synthesis of **149**.

α-(Acylamino)alkyl Derivatives of Drug-SH:
Drug-S-CHR'-NR'-(C=O)-R'

In the section on acyl-type derivatives of 5-FU several examples were given of the effect of incorporating amidelike functional groups into promoieties. Some of the results obtained with N-alkylcarbonyl– and N-alkoxycarbonyl–type derivatives (both discussed previously) of 5-FU were quite spectacular, and suggested that the incorporation of an amide functional group into the promoiety be examined for other types of prodrugs. The problem with implementing this course of action is that many drugs do not contain an acidic-NH group that can be transiently acylated. One way to solve the problem is to use a prodrug of the second general type where a methylene group separates the enabling functional group in the promoiety from the functional group in the parent drug that is to be masked. The nitrogen for the amide functional group is introduced as part of the promoiety. The functional group that is to be masked can then contain an oxygen or, in this case, a sulfur atom instead of a nitrogen.

6-Mercaptopurine

Drug-S-CHR'-NR'-(C=O)-OR'. For this type of prodrug an homologous series of prodrugs was synthesized in which all possible combinations of alkyl groups from methyl to butyl on both the nitrogen and the oxygen atoms in the promoiety were obtained (88). However, although all 16 members of the series were synthesized and their physicochemical properties determined, only seven members were actually evaluated in diffusion cell experiments, so only the physicochemical properties of those seven members are given in Tables 42 and 43. Inspection of their IPM solubilities in Table 43 shows that all the prodrugs were at least 5 times more soluble in IPM than 6-MP but does not reveal any correlation with their melting points in Table 42. The only trend in the solubilities (data not given here) is that in every series except the N-butyl series, when the N-alkyl group is kept constant, the O-propyl member is the most soluble in IPM.

The seven members of the series that were evaluated in the diffusion cell experiments were chosen to represent the extremes in the substitution pattern, but with greater weight placed on evaluating members substituted with the shorter alkyl groups both on nitrogen and oxygen. Based on literature precedent, it was anticipated that the later would be the more effective members of the series at enhancing transdermal delivery. Inspection of the results from the diffusion cell experiments in Table 43 shows that the prediction is correct. The

Table 42 Physicochemical Properties of S^6-(N-Alkyl-N-alkoxycarbonyl) aminomethyl-6-MP Prodrugs

$$SCH_2NR(C=O)OR'$$

Compound	MP°C	Half-lives[a]	C_v
58, 6-MP	>300(d)	—	0.22
171, R = CH₃, R' = CH₃	161–164	91	0.23
172, R = CH₃, R' = C₂H₅	150–151	92.7	0.078
173, R = CH₃, R' = C₄H₉	121–122	108	—
174, R = C₂H₅, R' = CH₃	148–149	82	0.011
175, R = C₂H₅, R' = C₂H₅	114–115	82.3	—
176, R = C₄H₉, R' = CH₃	134–135	89	—
177, R = C₄H₉, R' = C₄H₉	87–89	—	—

[a]Half-lives in minutes determined at pH 7.1 at 32°C.
[b]Solubility at 23 ± 1°C in equivalent mg of 6-MP/ml of 10% THF in water.
Source: From Ref. 88.

Table 43 Rates of Delivery of 6-MP by S^6-(N-Alkyl-N-alkoxycarbonyl) aminomethyl-6-MP Prodrugs

Compound	C_v^a	J^b	log P[c]	Skin[d] accumulation
58	0.0034	0.66 (0.40)	−0.73	0.018
171	0.167	3.9 (0.6)	−1.63	0.067
172	0.182	0.58 (0.34)	−2.50	0.016
173	0.167	0.054 (0.014)	−3.49	0.0093
174	0.319	0.058 (0.020)	−3.74	0.0031
175	0.213	0.014 (0.002)	−4.18	0.0030
176	0.730	0.20 (0.07)	−3.56	0.016
177	10.34	0.071 (0.029)	−5.16	0.0058

[a]Solubility at 23 ± 1°C in equivalent mg of 6-MP/ml of IPM.
[b]Flux in mg/cm²/h ± 10³ (± SD) from suspensions of IPM with receptor phase at 32°C.
[c]Permeability coefficients in cm/h calculated from J/C_v.
[d]Amount of 6-MP in mg leached from hairless mouse skin in the 24 h subsequent to application of 6-MP or prodrug in vehicle for 48 h. From unpublished work of K. G. Siver.
Source: From Ref. 88.

N-methyl-O-methyl derivative, **171**, is the only derivative that is more effective than 6-MP at delivering 6-MP through hairless mouse skin. The N-methyl-O-ethyl derivative, **172**, is the next most effective member of the series at delivering 6-MP but it is somewhat less effective than 6-MP itself. Interestingly, only **171** is even as soluble in water as 6-MP, and the next most water-soluble derivative is **172**.

Size or lipid solubility does not seem to be determining factors in predicting the ability of this series of prodrugs to deliver 6-MP. The N-ethyl-O-methyl derivative, **174**, is about the same size as the N-methyl-O-ethyl derivative, **172**. Prodrugs **172** and **174** exhibit almost exactly the same melting point, and **174** is 1.75 times more soluble in IPM than **172**. However, **172** is 7 times more soluble in water than **174**, and it is 10 times more efficient at delivering 6-MP through the skin. Also, a comparison of the physicochemical properties of the members of this series with that of the much more effective S^6-acyloxymethyl-6-MP series shows that the biggest difference is the fact that S^6-acyloxymethyl series are more soluble in water. The first member of the S^6-acyloxymethyl series (the acetyloxymethyl derivative, **136**) exhibits the same solubility in IPM as does the first member of the S^6-(N-alkyl-N-alkyoxycarbonyl)aminomethyl series, **171**. However, **136** is a little over 6 times more soluble in water than **171**, it is almost 8 times more effective at delivering 6-MP through the skin, and it is a little over twice as effective at delivering 6-MP into the skin. Thus, in any comparison of different types of more lipid soluble prodrugs, the type of prodrug which contains a functional group that can impart greater water solubility to the prodrug than the functional groups in the other types will be the more efficient type of prodrug at enhancing transdermal delivery.

For this series of homologues there is a good correlation between the abilities of the members of the series to deliver 6-MP through the skin with their abilities to deliver 6-MP into the skin. In addition, the only prodrug to deliver more 6-MP through the skin is also the only prodrug to deliver more 6-MP into the skin than 6-MP itself.

The hydrolysis of this series of prodrugs of 6-MP is not enzyme mediated. Nevertheless, their rates of chemical hydrolysis are fast enough that no intact prodrug is detected in the receptor phases of the diffusion cell experiments. Thus, although this series is not generally an effective one for enhancing topical delivery, the evaluation of the series shows that these types of derivatives do function as prodrugs of 6-MP.

Drug-S-CHR′-NR′-(C=O)-R′.   Only one other example of an α-(acylamino) alkyl–type derivative of 6-MP has been synthesized and evaluated, and that is S^6-benzamidomethyl-6-MP, **178** (21). This molecule exhibits a much higher melting point (222–223°C) than S^6-acetyloxymethyl-6-MP or S^6-(N-methyl-N-methoxycarbonyl)aminomethyl-6-MP and is much less soluble in IPM and water (0.063 and 0.00045 equivalent mg of 6-MP/ml, respectively) than either of them. In fact, **178** is much less soluble in water than 6-MP itself and not much more soluble in IPM. Thus, it is not surprising that 6-MP delivers over 8 times as much 6-MP through hairless mouse skin as does **178**. The apparent problem is that there is no net decrease in the number of hydrogen-bonding polar groups in **178** compared to 6-MP. The thionamide functional group is merely replaced by a secondary amide functional group.

On the other hand, only 6-MP was detected in the receptor phase of the diffusion cell experiments. Thus, this type of prodrug also functions as a prodrug of 6-MP and the S^6-benzamidomethyl derivative has served as a model for potentially more successful analogues or homologues of this type of derivative where, for example, the NH group in the promoiety is replaced by an N-alkyl group.

DRUG-(C=O)-OH

The majority of the examples of drugs containing carboxylic acid functional groups are found among the nonsteroidal anti-inflammatory (NSAID) and antibiotic types of drugs. Psoriasis, inflammation, ultraviolet-B (UV-B) radiation erythema, atopic eczema, etc., are among the various conditions that have been proposed as being amenable to topical treatment with drugs containing a carboxylic acid functional group. However, carboxylic acids are generally very polar functional groups and tend to be ionized under most of the conditions suitable for their topical application. Also, it has been shown rather conclusively that the ionized form of carboxylic acids tends to diffuse through skin at a much lower rate than the unionized form (89,90). Obviously, one way to overcome the liability of excessive ionization of the parent drug is to transiently replace the ionizable group (H) with an unionizable group (promoiety). Thus, a prodrug approach to enhancing the topical delivery of drugs containing a carboxylic acid functional group is quite attractive.

α-(Acyloxy)alkyl Derivatives of Drug-(C=O)-OH:
Drug-(C=O)-OCHR'-O(C=O)-R'

Simple alkyl esters of drugs containing a carboxylic acid functional group sometimes do not hydrolyze quickly or completely enough to serve as prodrugs because the Drug-carbonyloxyalkyl enabling functional group is not a good substrate for enzymatic hydrolysis (30). One simple solution to this complication is to introduce the carbonyloxyalkyl enabling functional group into the promoiety portion of the prodrug instead of it being part of the drug portion, and design the alkyl group to spontaneously hydrolyze to regenerate Drug-(C=O)-OH after the enabling group is cleaved. α-(Acyloxy)alkyl derivatives of carboxylic acids are one type of prodrug that have resulted from the implementation of this approach. They were first designed and synthesized in 1965 to enhance the oral absorption of penicillins (30). However, there are no reports of their use to treat topical infections. Subsequently, there have been reports on the synthesis of α-(acyloxy)alkyl derivatives of NSAID such as aspirin (91) and indomethacin (92), to name a few representative examples. Although there are no literature reports of the evaluation of α-(acyloxy)alkyl derivatives of these NSAIDs in diffusion cell experiments or of their topical use to treat inflammation, there are numerous patent disclosures claiming such usefulness.

Nalidixic Acid

Nalidixic acid is a relatively high melting solid which is poorly soluble in water and in IPM, but has shown some promise in the topical treatment of psoriasis (93). Bundgaard and coworkers have described the synthesis, characterization, and evaluation in diffusion cell experiments of a number of different types of prodrugs of nalidixic acid designed to enhance its transdermal delivery (Tables 44 and 45) (94). The acyloxymethyl series of prodrugs (182–185) fits the trends observed for the acyloxymethyl derivatives of Drug-SH and Drug-NH functional groups. The first member of the series exhibits the highest melting point, and the melting point for the members of the series decrease as the alkyl chain in the acyl portion of the promoiety increases in length. In the same order, the solubilities of the members decrease in water (0.76 to 0.26) and increase in IPM (0.34 to 2.69 equivalent mg of nalidixic acid/ml of solvent). The first member is the least stable member of the series in buffer but the most stable in plasma. Finally, only nalidixic acid was detected in the receptor phase from the topical application of these prodrugs to

Table 44 Physicochemical Properties of Nalidixic Acid Prodrugs

| Compound | MP°C | Half-lives[a] | |
		buffer	plasma
179, R = H (Nalidixic Acid)	225–231	—	—
180, R = CH₃	154–155	3100	>100[b]
181, R = CH₂(C=O)N(C₂H₅)₂	142–143	3600	>100[b]
182, R = CH₂O(C=O)-CH₃	120–121	87	0.30
183, R = CH₂O(C=O)-C₂H₅	105–106	89	0.15
184, R = CH₂O(C=O)-C₃H₇	104–105	114	0.13
185, R = CH₂O(C=O)-CH(CH₃)₂	105–106	130	0.26

[a]Buffer was sodium carbonate at pH 10–12. Half-lives in h at 37°C extrapolated from pH 10–12 to pH 7.4. Plasma was 80% human plasma.
[b]Less than 5% degradation after 24 h.
Source: From Ref. 94.

Table 45 Rates of Delivery of Nalidixic Acid by Prodrugs of Nalidixic Acid Through Human Skin

Compound	IPM		H₂O		
	$C_v{}^a$	J^b	$C_v{}^a$	J^b	log K^c
179	0.11	0.74	0.024	0.74	1.51
180	0.73	2.32	0.46	2.25	1.23
181	0.13	3.02	8.61	0.13	1.43
182	0.34	2.32	0.76	0.53	1.21
183	0.90	1.16	0.34	0.72	1.70
184	2.69	3.71	0.26	3.71	2.20
185	2.49	4.18	0.22	1.51	2.17

[a]Solubility in equivalent mg of nalidixic acid/ml of vehicle at 21 ± 1°C.
[b]Flux in mg/cm²/h × 10³ from suspensions in IPM or H₂O with a receptor phase at 37°C.
[c]Partition coefficients between 1-octanol and H₂O at 21°C.
Source: From Ref. 94.

human skin in diffusion cell experiments. This is in direct contrast with the results for the simple methyl ester **180** where 65 ± 15% of the intact ester was detected in the receptor phase at various sampling times. Thus, the acyloxymethyl type of prodrug does function as a prodrug and is effective in overcoming the stability problem of simple esters in the case of nalidixic acid.

The rates of delivery of nalidixic acid by the series of prodrugs through human skin from either IPM or water generally follow the same trend. The greater the lipid solubility of the prodrug by either the log K or IPM solubility criterion, the greater the rate of delivery..The only outlier to the trend is the delivery of nalidixic acid by the propionyloxymethyl derivative, **183**, from IPM; its rate of delivery is too low.

This trend is consistent with the previous results obtained for Drug-SH and Drug-NH acyloxymethyl derivatives. For a series of more lipid-soluble prodrugs, the more water-soluble members are more effective at delivering the parent drug through skin. For the 6-MP derivatives, all of the Drug-SH derivatives that are more soluble in water than 6-MP are among the more effective derivatives at delivering 6-MP from IPM. There is apparently a maximum in performance realized with the S⁶-butyryloxymethyl derivative, **138**. The S⁶-butyryloxymethyl derivative is the last member of the series (**136-137-138**) which is more soluble in water than 6-MP and is more soluble in IPM than the preceding members of the series (**136** and **137**). However, the differences between its performance and that of the valeryloxymethyl, **139**, and propionyloxymethyl derivatives, **137**, on either side are not significant. The situation is similar for the nalidixic acid series of acyloxymethyl derivatives, except that all the prodrugs that were evaluated are over an order of magnitude more soluble in water than the parent drug. The series has not been extended far enough to reach the point where the water solubility of the prodrug is less than that of nalidixic acid itself and the rate of delivery of nalidixic acid decreases. In fact, the series is not even close to that point. Thus, even better performances at delivering nalidixic acid through skin should be achieved before there is a decrease in performance by using acyloxyalkyl derivatives with even longer alkyl chains in the acyl portion of the promoiety. Whether the usual relationship between alkyl chain length in the acyl portion of the prodrug and the rate of delivery of the parent drug is observed for this series of prodrugs awaits the synthesis and evaluation of prodrugs containing longer alkyl chains.

Cromoglycic Acid

Cromoglycic acid, or cromolyn, is a very polar drug that has been used primarily in the treatment of bronchial asthma. However, it has been observed that topically applied sodium cromolyn has been effective in the treatment of atopic eczema in children (95). If a molecule as polar as sodium cromolyn was effective topically, it was anticipated that even better results could be obtained using prodrugs of cromolyn that exhibited lower melting points and were more soluble in lipids. To this end, Bodor and coworkers synthesized and evaluated a series of α-acyloxyalkyl esters on both carboxylic acid groups in cromolyn (Table 46) (96). No solubility data are available, but the melting points are useful indicators of relative solubilities as has been shown elsewhere in this chapter. Thus, of the bispivaloyloxymethyl (**187** and **190**) and bishexanoyloxymethyl (**188** and **191**) pairs, the hexanoyloxymethyl derivatives **188** and **191** are probably the more

Table 46 Physicochemical Properties of Cromoglycic Acid Prodrugs and Their Abilities to Deliver Cromoglycic Acid Through Skin

Compound	MP°C	% Diffused[a]
186, R = R' = Na	241–242(d)	0.50
187, R = H, R' = CH$_2$O(C=O)-C(CH$_3$)$_3$	133–135	—
188, R = H, R' = CH$_2$O(C=O)-C$_5$H$_{11}$	124–126	2.74
189, R = H, R' = CH(CH$_3$)O(C=O)-C$_5$H$_{11}$	Glass	3.07
190, R = NO$_2$, R' = CH$_2$O(C=O)-C(CH$_3$)$_3$	156–166	2.88
191, R = NO$_2$, R' = CH$_2$O(C=O)-C$_5$H$_{11}$	93–95	1.63
192, R = H, R' = CH$_2$(C=O)N(C$_2$H$_5$)$_2$	160–170(d)	1.86

[a]Applied 0.03 M suspensions in IPM.
Source: From Ref. 96.

lipid-soluble derivatives compared to the pivaloyloxymethyl derivatives on the basis of melting points. Although the bispivaloyloxymethyl ester, **187**, was not evaluated in a diffusion cell experiment, the combination of bispivaloyloxymethyl and nitrate esters, **190**, was evaluated and it performed better than the combination of bishexanoyloxymethyl and nitrate esters, **191**. This result suggests that **187** may outperform **188**, and hence may be the best member of this series at delivering cromolyn through skin.

The bis-α-(hexanoyloxy)ethyl derivative, **189**, is apparently the best example of this type of prodrug at enhancing delivery of cromolyn through skin. It also exhibits the lowest melting point of any of the prodrugs that were evaluated. However, the low melting point of **189** is probably due to the fact that two new optical centers are introduced into the molecules when the (C=O)-OCH(CH$_3$)-O(C=O) groups are incorporated into the promoiety. Since each optical center is a mixture of R and S, a low melting point is expected for such a racemic modification. On the other hand, **191** exhibits the next lowest melting point and it is the worst example of this type of prodrug at enhancing the delivery of cromolyn through the skin. Finally, the combination prodrug approach using the nitrate and α-(acyloxy)alkyl esters appears to be less effective than the α-(acyloxy)alkyl derivatives when used alone.

Aspirin

One of the problems associated with the design of prodrugs of aspirin is the rate at which the promoiety cleaves to regenerate aspirin. The acetyl group in aspirin undergoes hydrolysis to give salicylic acid with a half-life in human plasma of about 2 h, but when the carboxylic acid group is masked—so that it is no longer ionized under those conditions—the half-life for hydrolysis of the acetyl group is only 1–3 min (97). Thus, the promoiety on the carboxylic acid group must cleave faster than the acetyl group if the prodrug is to function as a prodrug of aspirin and not of salicylic acid. Although no α-(acyloxy)alkyl derivatives of aspirin have been evaluated in diffusion cell experiments, the data in Table 47 suggest that the acetyloxymethyl derivative, **194**, may be useful for enhancing the topical delivery of aspirin. Prodrug **194** is an oil which is much more lipophilic than aspirin, yet it retains significant water solubility and actually hydrolyses in 10% human plasma to give 29% aspirin. On the other hand, **195** gives only salicylic acid upon hydrolysis in plasma. For comparison purposes, the methyl ester of aspirin, **203**, also hydrolyses to give only salicylic acid.

Dialkylaminocarbonylmethyl Derivatives of Drug-(C=O)-OH: Drug-(C=O)-OCH$_2$(C=O)-NR$_2'$

As previously mentioned, one of the problems with simple alkyl ester prodrugs of carboxylic acids is that they are not sufficiently labile. One simple solution to the

Table 47   Physicochemical Properties of Prodrugs of Aspirin

$$\text{(C=O)OR}$$
$$\text{O(C=O)CH}_3$$

Compound	MP°C	$C_v{}^a$	log K^b
193, R = H (Aspirin)	128–129	3.84	0.22
194, R = CH$_2$O(C=O)-CH$_3$	oil	2.43	1.42
195, R = CH$_2$O(C=O)-C$_3$H$_7$	oil	0.35	2.50
196, R = CH$_2$(C=O)-N(CH$_3$)$_2$	75–76	7.50	0.38
197, R = CH$_2$(C=O)-N(C$_2$H$_5$)$_2$	76–77	2.28	1.16
198, R = CH$_2$(C=O)-N(C$_3$H$_7$)$_2$	50–51	0.72	2.09
199, R = CH$_2$(C=O)-N[CH(CH$_3$)$_2$]$_2$	108–109	0.18	2.03
200, R = CH$_2$(C=O)-N(CH$_3$)(CH$_2$CH$_2$OH)	70–71	—	0.06
201, R = CH$_2$(C=O)-N(CH$_2$CH$_2$)$_2$O	97–98	4.84	0.30
202, R = CH(CH$_3$)(C=O)-N(C$_2$H$_5$)$_2$	40–41	7.68	0.67
203, R = CH$_3$	47–49	2.81	1.46
204, R = CH$_2$SCH$_3$	oil	0.55	1.94
205, R = CH$_2$(S=O)CH$_3$	80–81	4.23	0.11
206, R = CH$_2$(O=S=O)CH$_3$	149–151	0.11	0.57

^{a}Solubility in water at 21°C in mg/ml.
^{b}Partition coefficient between octanol and water at 21°C.
Source: From Ref. 97.

problem is to use α-(acyloxy)alkyl derivatives of the carboxylic acid. This has already been discussed above.

Another solution is to find substituted alkyl groups that are more highly suscep-tible to enzymatic hydrolysis. An example of this approach is the use of dialkyl-aminocarbonylmethyl derivatives of carboxylic acids. Bundgaard and coworkers have generated a significant amount of data delineating the parameters that contribute to the rate of hydrolysis of this type of ester (98–100). The fastest rate of enzymatic hydrolysis is realized for the dialkylaminocarbonylmethyl deriva-tives: The 2-(dialkylaminocarbonyl)ethyl and 3-(dialkylaminocarbonyl)propyl derivatives hydrolyze at a much slower rate (99). The dialkylaminocarbonyl-methyl derivatives generally hydrolyze faster than the alkylaminocarbonylmethyl derivatives (98). Finally, their buffer stabilities are four or five orders of mag-nitude greater than their stabilities in plasma. Thus, this type of ester derivative exhibits physicochemical and biological properties that make it a very attractive prodrug candidate for carboxylic acids.

Nalidixic Acid

Of all the ester-type prodrugs of nalidixic acid that were evaluated by Bundgaard and coworkers (94), the diethylaminocarbonylmethyl derivative of nalidixic acid, **181**, is the least soluble derivative in IPM and the most soluble in water (see Table 45), and delivers over 4 times as much nalidixic acid through the skin from IPM as does nalidixic acid. On the other hand, 6 times as much nalidixic acid is delivered through skin from water by nalidixic acid as by **181**. Clearly, **181** is too soluble in water and not soluble enough in lipids to enhance the transdermal delivery of nalidixic from water: It is only barely more soluble in IPM than nalidixic acid. Since only this one example of this type of ester was evaluated, it is not clear that the lipid solubility of the next example to be tested needs to be increased, or the water solubility needs to be decreased, or both to realize increased transdermal delivery of nalidixic acid from IPM. However, since 50% of the prodrug diffused through intact, this type of prodrug approach for nalidixic acid will probably not be pursued further.

Cromoglycic Acid

Very little information about the physicochemical properties of the diethylamino-carbonylmethyl derivative of cromolyn, **192**, is available (96). It exhibits the highest melting point and the next to the lowest percent delivery of cromolyn through skin (see Table 46). However, as opposed to the nalidixic acid derivative, **192** delivers only cromolyn through skin.

Aspirin

Although none of the dialkylaminomethyl derivatives of aspirin have been evaluated in diffusion cell experiments, a large number of this type of ester prodrug of aspirin have been synthesized and characterized under the same conditions that the acyloxymethyl and methylthiomethyl type esters have been characterized (see Table 47) (97). Of those dialkylaminocarbonylmethyl derivatives, only **196**, **201**, and **202** are more soluble in water than aspirin, but they are almost all more lipophilic based on their log K values. The greatest advantage that these derivatives have is their potential to actually function as prodrugs and to deliver aspirin instead of salicylic acid. Upon hydrolysis in 10% human plasma, **196** generates 50% aspirin, **197** generates 38% aspirin, whereas **201** and **202** do not generate any aspirin. The percent of aspirin generated in undiluted plasma is essentially identical with the values from the diluted solutions. Comparison of the physicochemical properties of aspirin with those of the dialkylaminocarbonyl-methyl derivatives **196–202** shows that **196** is more soluble in water and more lipophilic than aspirin. Hence, since **196** also hydrolyses to give 50% aspirin, it should function as a prodrug of aspirin and increase the transdermal delivery of aspirin and salicylic acid.

α(Alkylthio)alkyl, α-(Alkylsulfinyl)alkyl, and α-(Alkylsulfonyl)alkyl Derivatives of Drug-(C=O)-OH

α-(Alkylthio)alkyl derivatives of carboxylic acids have been used as protecting groups for carboxylic acids because they are stable under a variety of conditions (101,102). However, subsequent oxidation of the methylthiomethyl group to the sulfoxide or the sulfone stage leads to a much more labile derivative which can be easily cleaved under neutral or alkaline conditions to the carboxylic acid. In addition, dimethylsulfoxide (DMSO) has been shown by numerous investigators to function as a penetration enhancer under certain conditions (103,104). It has been suggested that the biphasic solubility properties of DMSO contribute to its ability to function as a penetration enhancer. Hence, it was anticipated that the incorporation of a similar sulfoxide functional group or a sulfone functional group into a promoiety would increase the biphasic solubility of the prodrug and enhances its ability to deliver the parent drug through a biological membrane. This assumes that the prodrug reverts to the parent drug in vivo.

Application of this approach to aspirin did not give encouraging results (105). The only derivative that is more soluble in water than aspirin is the sulfoxide, **205**, but it is less lipophilic than aspirin (see Table 47) (97). The results from the diffusion cell experiments in which aspirin, **204** and **205**, were applied to hairless mouse skins show that neither of the prodrugs deliver aspirin. The sulfone, **206**, was not tested because of solubility problems. Under the conditions of the experiment only aspirin delivered aspirin through skin. The sulfoxide, **205**, performed no better than aspirin at delivering total salicylates through skin and the sulfide, **204**, is only about twice as effective as aspirin. None of the prodrugs exhibit the kind of biphasic solubility properties exhibited by prodrugs that are successful at enhancing the topical delivery of their parent drugs (97).

N,N-Dialkylhydroxylamine Derivatives of Drug-(C=O)-OH:

Drug-(C=O)-O-NR$_2'$

Acyl derivatives of dialkylhydroxylamines belong to a potentially attractive type of prodrug for drugs containing a carboxylic acid functional group. Although dialkylhydroxylamines are basic molecules, they are much less basic than the corresponding dialkylamines and are less toxic as well. For example, the basic pK_a of N,N-dimethylhydroxylamine is only 5.2 (106) and probably becomes even lower when the hydroxyl portion is acylated. Diethylhydroxylamine exhibits a topical LD_{LOW} of 2000 mg/kg in rabbits, whereas diethylamine exhibits a topical LD_{50} of 820 mg/kg in rabbits (107). The use of basic amines in transdermal delivery as penetration enhances or incorporated into prodrugs as the promoiety has already been discussed. However, the low pK_a of dialkylhydroxylamines compared to dialkylamines means that at physiological pH or the pH of the skin (≈4.5) less of the protonated form of the amine will be present at the vehicle-skin interface. Since partitioning into the skin is generally easier for uncharged species, the prodrugs derived from dialkylhydroxylamine should partition into the skin better than prodrugs containing higher pK_a basic functional groups as part of the promoiety. In addition, O-acyldialkylhydroxylamines have been used as activated esters of acyl compounds in amination reactions (108), so it was anticipated that dialkylhydroxylamine derivatives of carboxylic acids would hydrolyze quickly enough to function as prodrugs.

In order to evaluate this prodrug approach, several dialkylhydroxylamine derivatives of aspirin and indomethacin were synthesized and characterized (52). However, only the diethylhydroxylamine derivative of indomethacin, **207**, was evaluated in diffusion cell experiments and in various animal and human topical activity studies (109). In those experiments, **207** is twice as effective as indomethacin at delivering indomethacin through mouse skin from a polyethylene ointment or petrolatum formulation, but **207** in IPM is almost 10 times as effective. In all cases only indomethacin is detected in the receptor phases. In the animal model, **207** in IPM or propylene glycol is twice as effective as indomethacin in IPM or propylene glycol at inhibiting thermal edema. However, in a sunburn test with human volunteers, **207** and indomethacin in petrolatum or polyethylene glycol are only equally effective at inhibiting redness.

CH_3O $CH_2(C=O)ON(C_2H_5)_2$

207

Thus, dialkylhydroxylamine derivatives of drugs containing carboxylic acid functional groups may be useful for increasing the transdermal delivery of the drug. But increased delivery of indomethacin and other NSAIDs may not improve their ability to inhibit UV-B erythema. Instead, these prodrugs and the other types of prodrugs of NSAIDs discussed in this section might be used in efforts to improve the topical treatment of conditions such as allergic eczematous contact dermatitis where prostaglandins have been implicated as causative factors (110).

DRUG-OH

Drugs containing hydroxy functional groups are ubiquitous. However, for the purposes of this discussion the focus will be primarily on two types of drugs: steroids and nucleosides. Generally, the greater the number of hydroxy groups a molecule contains, the more polar the molecule is and the poorer its permeation through skin. For example, Chien and coworkers (111) have evaluated the effect of the sequential introduction of hydroxy groups and their substitution pattern in a lipophilic steroid molecule (progesterone, 208) on the rates of transdermal delivery of the substituted progesterones from their suspensions in 40% aqueous polyethylene glycol (PEG) 400. In Table 48 are listed the structures, melting points, and solubilities of the steroids in the 40% aqueous vehicle. Within a series of steroids with the same number of hydroxy groups (e.g., 209 through 211), the lower the melting point is, the higher the solubility. Also, the solubility in the polar vehicle generally goes up as more hydroxy groups are introduced (compare 209 to 212 to 214).

In Table 49 the effect of the hydroxy groups on rates of permeation are readily apparent. Within a series of steroids with the same number of hydroxy groups, the lower the melting point is and the higher the solubility is in the 40% aqueous PEG 400 vehicle, the higher the fluxes through both intact and stripped skin. Also, as more hydroxy groups are introduced into 208, the flux goes down as the solubility in the vehicle goes up (compare 209 to 212 to 214).

In terms of delivery through intact or whole skin, a major factor is solubility in the stratum corneum, since the unsubstituted molecule 208, which exhibits the highest stratum corneum solubility, also exhibits the second highest rate of delivery through intact skin. However, solubility of the molecule in the viable skin, which is much more aqueous in nature, is also important because 209, which exhibits 75% of the solubility of 208 in the stratum corneum and twice the solubility of 208 in the viable skin, permeates intact skin at twice the rate of 208. On the other hand, 214, which contains three hydroxy groups, is the most soluble of all the derivative in 40% aqueous PEG 400, yet it is less soluble in viable skin

Table 48   Physicochemical Properties of Progesterone Derivatives

Compound	MP°C[a]	C_v^b
208, R = R′ = R″ = H	127–131	208
209, R = OH, R′ = R″ = H	141–142	1380
210, R = H, R′ = OH, R″ = H	187–189	653
211, R = R′ = H, R″ = OH	222–223	121
212, R = R′ = OH, R″ = H	180–182	1840
213, R = OH, R′ = H, R″ = OH	212.8–216.8	457
214, R = R′ = R″ = OH	217–220	2590

[a]From the *Merck Index*, M. Windholz, ed., 10th Ed., Merck and Co., Inc., Rahway, N.J., 1983.
[b]Solubility in µg/ml in 40% (v/v) aqueous PEG 400 solution.
Source: From Ref. 111.

Table 49 Steady-State Rates of Permeation of Progesterone Derivatives Across, and Their Solubilities in Hairless Mouse Skin

Compound	J^a		$C_v{}^b$	
	Intact skin	Stripped skin	Stratum corneum	Viable skin
208	2.37	3.62	47.7	0.87
209	4.73	12.1	32.4	2.26
210	0.57	5.13	12.5	0.79
211	0.29	1.92	2.82	0.32
212	0.97	8.27	7.97	1.94
213	0.31	2.44	2.46	0.39
214	0.15	7.26	1.09	1.69

[a]Permeation in $\mu g/cm^2/h$ from 40% aqueous PEG 400 suspensions.
[b]Solubility in mg/ml calculated from permeation rates through intact and stripped skin. The viable skin is that part of the skin left after the stratum corneum is removed.
Source: From Ref. 111.

that either **209** with one hydroxy group or **212** with two hydroxy groups. Steroid **214** is also the least soluble of all the derivatives in the stratum corneum, so it is not surprising that **214** permeates the skin at a lower rate than any of the other derivatives and only 0.03 times that of **209**. Thus, both lipid solubility (solubility in the stratum corneum) and aqueous solubility (solubility in the viable skin) are important in optimizing transdermal delivery, and the introduction of too many hydroxy groups (e.g., **214**) has a detrimental effect on the rate of transdermal delivery of the drug through intact skin.

The effect of the solubility of the steroid in the viable skin, i.e., stripped skin, on permeation is especially evident in the data for the flux of the steroids through stripped skin. Steroid **209** permeates stripped skin almost 4 times better than **208**, whereas the even more polar steroids **212** and **214** permeate the stripped skin only about 2 times better than **208**. There is almost a perfect correlation between solubility in the viable skin and flux through the stripped skin.

It should also be noted that data for permeation of the same series of steroids through a silicone elastomer has been obtained under essentially the same conditions (112). As might be expected, **208** and **209** exhibit the highest solubility in the silicone membrane and permeated the membrane 20 and 10 times, respectively, better than the next best steroid. Moreover, other than the reversal of the relative rates of permeation of **208** and **209** in silicone compared to mouse skin membranes, the relative rates of permeation through the silicone membrane by the other steroids remained the same. This general correlation between the permeability of mouse skin and that of silicone suggests that silicone elastomer may be a reasonable substitute for skin in certain situations.

Acyl Derivatives of Drug-OH Groups: Drug-O-(C=O)-R'

One way to overcome the effect of a polar hydroxy group is to mask it with an acyl functional group to give an ester functional group. A prodrug containing an ester functional group in place of a hydroxy functional group is almost always more soluble in lipids than the parent drug, yet the first few members of the series frequently exhibit comparable if not superior water solubility compared to the parent drug as well. The effect of masking hydroxy groups with acyl groups on the transdermal delivery of a purine nucleoside has already been discussed. In that case, no solubility data were available and only a modest increase in the transdermal delivery of the purine by the acylated nucleoside was observed compared to the transdermal delivery by the nonacylated nucleoside.

Glucocorticoid steroids, which usually contain several hydroxy groups, have also been converted to their ester derivatives in attempts to improve their topical efficacies. Esters of the 21-OH group apparently function as prodrugs, since they bind to glucocorticoid receptors less tightly than the parent drug, yet exhibit enhanced topical biological potency compared to the nonacylated parent drug (113). On the other hand, esters of the 17-OH group bind more tightly to the receptors than the parent drug and hydrolyze much more slowly than the 21-esters. They also exhibit enhanced topical biological potency compared to the parent drug (113). Although the 17-esters are apparently not prodrugs, they do permeate skin more efficiently than the nonacylated parent drug (52).

Arabinofuranosyladenine

Arabinofuranosyladenine (Ara-A) has been found to be very effective in the systemic treatment of herpesvirus infections, but it has been found to be ineffective in the topical treatment of either oral or genital herpesvirus infections in humans (114). The lack of topical effectiveness has been attributed to its inability to permeate skin. Ara-A exhibits low aqueous solubility and a low partition coefficient value (Table 50), which suggest that it is not very soluble in lipids either (115). Thus, it lacks the biphasic solubility properties necessary to permeate skin. In addition, ara-A is very sensitive to adenosine deaminase, which degrades ara-A to its hypoxanthine analogue (115). The hypoxanthine analogue is much less potent an antiviral agent, so any prodrug of ara-A has two problems to overcome: delivery and premature metabolism (116).

In order to overcome these problems, a number of acyl derivatives of ara-A have been synthesized, characterized, and evaluated—primarily topically in an in vivo animal model. A list of the three series of derivatives from which the more potent compounds have come is given in Table 50. In the 2'-acyl series (216–219), the first member of the series, 216, is over 200 times more soluble in water than ara-A and is apparently more lipid soluble as well in spite of its more negative log partition coefficient value (log K). Assuming that the log K values can be extrapolated to the ratio of the saturated solubilities of 216 in octanol and water, and

Table 50 Physicochemical Properties of Acyl Derivatives of Ara-A

Compound	MP°C	$C_v{}^a$	log K^b
215, R = R′ = R″ = OH	257–257.5	0.4	–0.48
216, R = O(C=O)CH$_3$, R′ = R″ = OH	195–197^c	93.6^c	–0.89^c
217, R = O(C=O)C$_2$H$_5$, R′ = R″ = OH	207–210^c	11.7^c	–0.48^c
218, R = O(C=O)C$_3$H$_7$, R′ = R″ = OH	209–210^c	3.41^c	–0.02^c
219, R = O(C=O)C$_4$H$_9$, R′ = R″ = OH	164–166^c	10.4^c	0.41^c
220, R = R′ = OH, R″ = O(C=O)CH$_3$	197.5–198.5^d	6.6^d	0.12^d
221, R = R′ = OH, R″ = O(C=O)C$_2$H$_5$	201–203^d	9.2^d	0.58^d
222, R = R′ = OH, R″ = O(C=O)C$_3$H$_7$	184^d	16.1^d	0.90^d
223, R = R′ = OH, R″ = O(C=O)C$_4$H$_9$	glass^d	8.4^d	1.33^d
224, R = R′ = OH, R″ = O(C=O)C$_5$H$_{11}$	glass^d	2.5^d	1.78^d
225, R = R′ = OH, R″ = O(C=O)C$_7$H$_{15}$	glass^d	0.23^d	2.00^d
226, R = R′ = OH, R″ = O(C=O)C(CH$_3$)$_3$	glass^d	7.0^d	1.63^d
227, R = R′ = O(C=O)CH$_3$, R″ = OH	138–139^e	33.0^e	0.20^e
228, R = R′ = O(C=O)C$_2$H$_5$, R″ = OH	172–173^e	4.5^e	1.10^e
229, R = R′ = O(C=O)C$_3$H$_7$, R″ = OH	—	2.6^e	1.49^e

^{a}Solubility in mg/ml of pH 7.3 buffer at 37°C.
^{b}Partition coefficient between octanol and water at 37°C.
^{c}From Ref. 116.
^{d}From Ref. 115. Partition coefficient between pentanol and water at 37°C.
^{e}From Ref. 118. Partition coefficient between pentanol and water at 37°C.

knowing the saturated solubility in water, then it can be estimated that **216** is almost 100 times more soluble in octanol than ara-A (12 mg/ml compared to 0.13 mg/ml). In the 2′-acyl series (116), only the valerate, **219**, is more soluble in octanol (26.7 mg/ml) than **216**, yet **219** is inactive in the topical animal model and the more water-soluble acetate, **216**, is the only active member of the 2′-acyl series. In fact, **216** is arguably the most effective member of any of the series tested, and it is also more soluble in water than any of the other derivatives in either of the other two series.

In the 5′-acyl series the butyrate, **222**, is the most water-soluble member of the series, and it is the only member of the series that exhibits any topical activity (117). However, **222** is much less effective at reducing herpesvirus lesions than

216. Most of the members of the 5'-acyl series are much more soluble in pentanol than the members of 2'-acyl series were in octanol. For instance, **222** is over 10 times more soluble in pentanol than **216** is in octanol (127.9 mg/ml compared to 12 mg/ml) using the previously described method of estimating alcohol solubilities from measured partition coefficients and water solubilities. However, **216** is about 5 times more soluble in water and is more effective than **222**.

In the 2'-3'-diacyl series, the diacetyl derivative, **227**, is more soluble in water than the other members of the series and it is the only one of the series that exhibits any topical activity (117,118). Again, lipophilicity is not a critical criterion, since **227** and **228** exhibit comparable pentanol solubility, but **227** is about 7 times more soluble in water and it is the more effective prodrug.

Thus, for the acyl derivatives of ara-A, enhanced water solubility is the crucial criterion for improved topical delivery. Within every series the more water-soluble derivative is the more effective derivative. Among the three series, the most water-soluble derivative is the most effective and the least water-soluble derivative is the least effective. However, two points should not be lost sight of. First, all of the effective derivatives are at least 10 times more soluble in octanol or pentanol than ara-A, so lipid solubility is important. Second, the importance of the rate of hydrolysis of the derivatives should not be overlooked. The timing of the enzymatic hydrolysis to the parent drug is essential to deliver the parent drug to the site of action. All of the acyl derivatives are resistant to adenosine deaminase, but as soon as the acyl group is removed metabolism to the less active hypoxanthine become a competing event. Obviously, the timing of the hydrolysis to the parent active compound, the enhanced biphasic solubility, and the resistance of the prodrugs to deaminase are all factors that combine to modulate their in vivo efficacy in treating genital herpesvirus infection in guinea pigs.

Levonorgestrel

Levonorgestrel (LN) is a very lipophilic contraceptive drug which is very poorly soluble in water (1 µg/ml at 25°C), and does not permeate through skin at a sufficient rate to deliver an effective dose. In addition, various penetration enhancers are ineffective at enhancing the delivery of LN through skin to the desired rate (119). However, LN is also extremely potent, and hence still a candidate for transdermal delivery if a method of improving its physicochemical properties were available.

Two types of acyl derivatives of LN were synthesized, characterized, and evaluated in diffusion cell experiments to determine which direction to take in changing the physicochemical properties of LN (120). One type of acyl derivative consisted merely of medium alkyl chain esters of the 17-OH group to decrease the melting point of LN. The rationale was that the lower the melting point, the greater the transdermal flux. These derivatives indeed are lower melting, but they are also even more hydrophobic than LN (Table 51), since their partition coefficients

Table 51   Physicochemical Properties and Rates of Delivery of Levonorgestrel by Prodrugs of Levonorgestrel

Compound	MP°C	$C_v{}^a$	$\log K^b$	J^c
230, R = H	240	6.0 (100)	3.70	0.06
231, R = (C=O)OCH₂CH(OH)CH₂OH	147–148	13.0 (40)	3.22	1.95
232, R = (C=O)O(CH₂)₄CH(OH)CH₂OH	49–53	187 (40)	3.75	0.95
233, R = (C=O)C₅H₁₁	84–86	248 (95)	—^{d}	—
		53. (62)		0.35
234, R = (C=O)C₄H₉	170	11.2 (95)	—^{d}	0.10

^{a}Solubility in mg/ml in ethanol or ethanol-water mixtures at 32°C. The value in parentheses is % ethanol.
^{b}Octanol–pH 7.4 buffer partition coefficients at 24°C.
^{c}Flux in μg/cm²/h from suspensions in the ethanol-water mixtures from the C_v column.
^{d}Partition coefficients could not be determined because of the low water solubility of the prodrugs.
Source: From Ref. 120.

could not be determined owing to lack of detectable prodrug in the buffer phase. The valerate ester, **234**, is not much more effective at delivering LN from a suspension in 95% ethanol than LN itself from its suspension in 100% ethanol, whereas the hexanoate ester, **233**, in 62% ethanol is about 6 times more effective. Neither of the esters (**233** or **234**) are as effective as the better penetration enhancers at delivering LN through skin. Both prodrugs deliver only LN through mouse skin. The value for the rate of delivery of LN by LN from suspensions in various ethanol-water mixtures (40–100% ethanol) remained fairly constant at 0.06–0.07 μg/cm²/h, so the performance of the prodrugs relative to LN could be easily compared regardless of the percent ethanol in the vehicle.

The second type of acyl derivative contained hydrophilic instead of hydrophobic functional groups in the promoiety. The rationale was that if the viable epidermis rather than the stratum corneum were the rate-limiting membrane in the transdermal flux of LN, then a more water-soluble prodrug was in order. Increased water solubility should lead to increased partitioning into the viable epidermis, which is more aqueous in nature, and finally should lead to increased transdermal delivery. Two acyl derivatives (carbonates) containing hydroxy functional groups in the alkyl portion of the promoiety were synthesized, characterized, and evaluated in diffusion cell experiments. Although the prodrugs are more soluble in aqueous ethanol than LN, their log K values are still approximately the same as that of LN, so they are also more soluble in octanol than LN. Thus, the carbonate prodrugs, **231** and **232**, exhibit greater biphasic solubility than LN. They also enhance the transdermal delivery of total LN species by 30 and 15 times, respectively. However, because the prodrugs are carbonates, they are much more stable than the ester prodrugs **233** and **234**. Prodrug **231** delivers 80% intact prodrug, whereas **232** delivers 96% intact prodrug into the receptor phases. Although this lack of delivery of LN into the receptor phase shows that this type of prodrug would not be acceptable for dermal delivery, it is perfectly acceptable for transdermal delivery. These results emphasize the importance of increased aqueous as well as lipid solubilities in optimizing the transdermal delivery of a drug by the prodrug approach.

Testosterone

Testosterone is another lipophilic steroid which is not very soluble in water, but for which there has been some interest in developing a transdermal delivery device. Also like levonorgestrel, the rate of delivery of testosterone from typical topical formulations through skin is not high enough to deliver the targeted amount of testosterone. So implementation of a prodrug or a formulation approach using penetration enhancers is necessary to reach the targeted amount. However, in order to use prodrugs to deliver testosterone from a controlled-release delivery device, it was first necessary to examine the effect of prodrug structure on its delivery to the skin through a silicone elastomer. Medium chain length alkyl esters of testosterone were selected as the prodrug candidates. They were evaluated for their abilities to deliver intact prodrug through a silicone elastomer from their suspensions in 40% aqueous PEG 400 (121). The results are given in Table 52.

There are four conclusions that can be drawn from the relationships between flux and solubilities. First, the best correlation between flux and solubilities is between the flux and solubilities of the esters in silicone fluid, which is representative of the solubility of the esters in the membrane. Second, partition coefficients between the applied phase and the membrane (not given, but calculated from the solubilities in silicone divided by the solubilities in 40% aqueous PEG 400) are not good indicators of the rates of transmembrane delivery. If that were the case, **239**, which exhibits the highest partition coefficient, would be the most effective prodrug at delivering the esters through the membrane; **239** is not. Third, although solubility in the silicone membrane is a good predictor of relative transmembrane delivery by an homologous series of prodrugs, this is not the only predictor of absolute delivery. Prodrug **239** is almost 3 times as soluble in silicone fluid as testosterone, **235**, yet it permeates the membrane only half as fast. On the other hand, **235** is 10 times as soluble in the donor phase and over 13 times as soluble in water. So for prodrugs, solubility in a polar phase is important to transmembrane delivery even if the membrane is a silicone elastomer. Fourth,

Table 52 Solubilities and Rates of Delivery of Prodrugs of Testosterone Across a Silicone Elastomer

		$C_v{}^b$			
Compound	MP°C[a]	water	40% PEG	silicone	J[c]
235, R = H	155	40.3	508	156	8
236, R = (C=O)-CH₃	140–141	5.8	137	511	90
237, R = (C=O)-C₂H₅	118–122	3.7	115	590	750
238, R = (C=O)-C₄H₉	—	3.6	54	471	—[d]
239, R = (C=O)-C₆H₁₃	36–37.5	3.1	47	443	4

[a]*The Merck Index*, M. Windholz, ed., 10th Ed., Merck and Co., Inc., Rahway, N.J., 1983.
[b]Solubility in μg/ml at 37°C.
[c]Flux in μg/cm²/h from suspensions in 40% aqueous PEG 400 estimated from graphic data.
[d]Flux could not be accurately estimated, but it was less than that of **236** or **237** but more than that of **239**.
Source: From Ref. 121.

enhanced solubility of the prodrug in the donor phase is not a good indicator of enhanced transmembrane delivery by the prodrug. Although in this case, the second most soluble prodrug is the most effective prodrug.

Generally, the rate of delivery of an homologous series of prodrugs through a very lipophilic homogeneous membrane such as a silicone elastomer is not predictive of their relative rates of delivery of the parent drug through a heterogeneous membrane such as skin where lipid and water solubilities are important and enzymatic forces are at work. However, the previously observed general correlation of the permeation of progesterone and its hydroxy analogues through silicone elastomer with their permeation through skin suggests that the former data can be useful. Also, the clear dependence of transmembrane delivery by a series of prodrugs on their solubilities in the silicone membrane reinforces the previous conclusions about dependence of transdermal delivery on solubility in the skin.

Estradiol

The need for estrogen replacement therapy in postmenopausal women is well documented. However, oral administration, especially of the naturally occurring estrogens such as estradiol, leads to extensive loss of the oral dose through conjugation during absorption and metabolism in the liver. In order to overcome the liabilities associated with the oral administration of estradiol, Chien and coworkers investigated the use of esters of estradiol to enhance its transdermal delivery (122). The results of that investigation are shown in Table 53.

The first observation that is apparent from the data in Table 53 is the trend in the solubilities of the prodrugs in an aqueouslike solvent (40% aqueous PEG 400) and a lipidlike solvent (silicone fluid). As expected, the solubility in the aqueous solvent decreases with increasing alkyl chain length of the acyl promoiety and increases in the silicone fluid. However, the diacetate, **244**, is much more soluble in lipids than expected based only on added carbons, and it is also more soluble in water than expected based on added carbons. The large increase in lipid solubility has to be due to the fact that both polar hydroxy groups are masked in **244**; the same may be true for its water solubility.

Among the 17-esters, the valerate, **242**, gives the highest rate of delivery of estradiol, and it is neither the most lipid soluble nor the most soluble in water (40% aqueous PEG 400) of the members of the series. It exhibits the best biphasic solubility. Both the valerate and the heptanoate deliver only estradiol. The 17-acetate initially delivers only estradiol, but after about 12 h intact 17-acetate begins to appear in the receptor phase and the rate of delivery of the acetate approximates that of estradiol itself. The analysis of the relative performance of the 3,17-diacetate, **244**, is very similar to that of **242**. Prodrug **244** is more soluble in lipids and in water than the most effective member of the 17-ester series, **242**,

Table 53   Physicochemical Properties of 17-Esters and a 3,17-Diester of Estradiol and Their Abilities to Permeate Mouse Skin

Compound	$C_v{}^a$		J^b
	40% PEG 400	silicone fluid	
240, R = R' = H	220	3.08	7.87
241, R = H, R' = (C=O)-CH$_3$	26.1	23.4	4.79
242, R = H, R' = (C=O)-C$_4$H$_9$	9.33	131	22.9^c
243, R = H, R' = (C=O)-C$_6$H$_{13}$	3.07	322	13.3^c
244, R = R' = (C=O)-CH$_3$	18.1	1567	81.9

[a]Solubility in μg/ml at 37°C.
[b]Flux in μmol/cm^2/s × 10^8 through hairless mouse skin from suspensions in silicone fluid as the donor phase and using 40% PEG 400 in the receptor phase.
[c]Only estradiol detected in the receptor phase.
Source: From Ref. 122.

and it is much more effective at delivering estradiol: **244** exhibits better biphasic solubility characteristics. Like the 17-acetate, the 3,17-diacetate initially delivers only estradiol through the skin, but after about 12 h significant levels of the 17-acetate (the more stable ester) begin to appear in the receptor phase, and the rate of delivery of the 17-acetate by the 3,17-diacetate eventually approximates that of estradiol. The authors conclude that the delivery of estradiol depends on the concentration of the ester on the stratum corneum surface, but the results for the heptanoate, **243**, and the cypionate (data not given) do not fit. Prodrug **243** is almost 3 times as soluble in silicone fluid as **242**, but it gives a little over half the rate of permeation. On the other hand, the relatively poorer performance by **243** (and the cypionate) fits the biphasic solubility theory, since **243** is only 0.3 times as soluble in 40% aqueous PEG 400 as **242** (and the cypionate is only 0.1 times as soluble and delivers only 0.2 times as much estradiol).

Hydrocortisone

The target for topical delivery of hydrocortisone is not transdermal delivery but dermal delivery. Thus, most of the evaluations of esters of hydrocortisone and similar esters of other glucocorticoid steroids involve in vivo biological testing. However, in many cases steroid esters targeted for dermal delivery are still evaluated in diffusion cell experiments where only transdermal delivery is measured. In this section we will discuss examples of both methods of evaluation, and see the effect of using ester prodrugs containing a functional group in the promoiety in addition to the ester functional group.

Drug-O(C=O)-R′.   Although a very large number of esters of hydrocortisone and hydrocortisonelike steroids have been reported, in most cases the primary focus has been on their synthesis and the evaluation of their activities. Seldom are systematic evaluations of the physicochemical properties of the esters—their lipid and aqueous solubilities, their stabilities—presented along with the reports of their synthesis and activity. Thus, it is difficult to predict the effect of varying the alkyl chain length of the acyl promoiety on the solubility of the steroid prodrug, or, knowing the solubility, the effect of solubility on delivery into the skin and through the skin.

One of the few reports on the effect of steroid ester prodrug structure on delivery of the steroid through skin is the thesis of Smith (123). Some of the results that were generated from that work are given in Table 54. The water solubilities of all the 21-esters are much lower than that of hydrocortisone itself. There are two outliers to the trend of decreasing water solubility with increasing acyl chain length: the propionate, **247**, and the hexanoate, **250**. Each is 2–3 times more soluble in water than the preceding member of the series. Thus, it is interesting that these same two esters are also the esters that are among the more effective members of the series at delivering total hydrocortisone through hairless mouse skin regardless of whether or not an esterase inhibitor was present.

Table 54   Physicochemical Properties of 21-Ester Derivatives of Hydrocortisone and Their Abilities to Permeate Mouse Skin

Compound	$C_v{}^a$	J^b no inhibitor	inhibitor^c	J^d
245, R = H	0.44	0.686	1.15	27.8
246, R = (C=O)-CH₃	0.00848	0.147	0.316	1.34
247, R = (C=O)-C₂H₅	0.0176	1.72	1.22	3.74
248, R = (C=O)-C₃H₇	0.00590	2.54	0.719	0.82
249, R = (C=O)-C₄H₉	0.00123	0.873	0.480	0.52
250, R = (C=O)-C₅H₁₁	0.00374	7.40	0.785	0.89
251, R = (C=O)-C₆H₁₃	0.000683	2.29	0.082	0.38

^{a}Solubility in water in mg/ml at 37°C.
^{b}Flux in mg/cm^2/h × 10^4 from steroid suspensions in water calculated from the product of the given permeability coefficients and the solubilities in water. Lag times were on the order of 1–11 h.
^{c}A known inhibitor of esterase activity (0.01% p-nitrophenyl acetate) added to donor phase.
^{d}Late flux in mg/cm^2/h × 10^4 in presence of inhibitor. Lag times were on the order of 30–40 h.
Source: From Ref. 123.

The importance of the water solubility of prodrugs to their abilities to permeate skin is especially evident in the trend in flux values of the intact prodrug through hairless mouse skin in the presence of an esterase inhibitor. In those experiments only intact esters are detected in the receptor phase, and the relatively more water-soluble esters, **247** and **250**, and are the more effective delivery forms. In the absence of an esterase inhibitor, significant amounts of hydrocortisone are detected in the receptor from the application of suspensions of the acetate, **246**, and propionate, **247**, whereas the remaining esters deliver only hydrocortisone. The rates of delivery of total hydrocortisone by the esters are also much higher in the absence of the enzyme inhibitor except by the acetate. Hydrocortisone is also less effective in the absence of the enzyme inhibitor. Apparently "short circuiting of the aqueous tissue resistance (to the longer chain ester) by metabolism is more than a possibility but a phenomenon which is occurring to considerable extent" (123).

The rates of delivery of hydrocortisone by its simple medium chain length alkyl esters is somewhat predictive of their in vivo anti-inflammatory activity (124). In those in vivo experiments the hexanoate is the most potent (2.4), the butyrate (2.3) is the next most potent, and the acetate (2.0) is more potent than hydrocortisone (1.6). The fact that hydrocortisone itself delivers more hydrocortisone than the acetate under all experimental conditions, yet the acetate is more potent in vivo, suggests that there may be a depot effect with the acetate.

Drug-O-(C=O)-CH₂CH₂(C=O)-NR₂. Almost all of the ester derivatives of hydrocortisone (and similar steroids) that have been developed to enhance the topical anti-inflammatory potency of such steroids have been simple alkyl acyl esters. However, there is one report on the extensive investigation of the effect of incorporating an amide functional group into the promoiety in addition to the ester enabling functional group (125). The hypothesis was that since dimethylformamide was a known penetration enhancer (126), the incorporation of an amide group into the promoiety would enhance the penetration of the prodrug.

An abbreviated list of the prodrugs that were synthesized and evaluated in one of several in vivo biological models is given in Table 55. Most of the derivatives were prodrugs of hydrocortisone, although there were several prodrugs of 17-esters of hydrocortisone as well. Almost all of the derivatives were succinamate esters, but there were several esters derived from pyrrolidone-6-carboxylic acid and thiazolidine-4-carboxylic acid (results not shown).

The evaluation of the prodrugs of hydrocortisone, **252–259**, either in the blanching in human volunteers model or in the reduction in mouse ear edema model, identified the diethylsuccinamate ester, **253**, as the most potent prodrug. Prodrug **253** is more potent than **254** or any of the other prodrugs in the series in the blanching model, and **254** is the most potent of the prodrugs in the series that were tested in the mouse ear edema model. There is very little solubility data available for the series, and only **253** was evaluated in diffusion cell experiments. In the diffusion cell experiments, **253** delivers 3 times as much hydrocortisone as hydrocortisone itself and twice as much as hydrocortisone acetate from a finite dose of 0.03 M steroid in acetone:IPM (90:10). In addition, **253** is comparable to hydrocortisone and hydrocortisone 21-acetate in its systemic toxicity and is much less toxic locally as determined from its propensity to cause skin thinning. Thus, the succinamate esters of hydrocortisone are more potent and less toxic than hydrocortisone itself which is sold over the counter.

As mentioned before, the 17-esters of glucocorticoid steroids are not prodrugs per se, although they permeate skin better than hydrocortisone or hydrocortisone 21-acetate. The 17-esters are much more potent than hydrocortisone or generally any of the 21-esters. Therefore, once the diethylsuccinamate promoiety was identified as the optimum promoiety in the 21-ester series, it was an obvious extension to determine its effect in combination with the 17-esters of hydrocortisone. The members of that series, **260–262**, were generally less potent than their parent 17-esters in both in vivo activity models. However, in the toxicity tests the diethylsuccinamate of the 17-valerate, **262**, causes less systemic toxicity than the 17-valerate ester, which in turn is less toxic than the other 17-esters tested and even hydrocortisone itself. So, although the 21-succinamate esters of the 17-esters

Table 55 Anti-Inflammatory Activities of 21-Succinamate Esters of Hydrocortisone

$$\text{—O(C=O)CH}_2\text{CH}_2\text{(C=O)NR}_2'$$

Compound	MP°C	ED$_{50}$(M)^a score	Blanching^b
245, Hydrocortisone		0.011	1.7
246, Hydrocortisone 21-acetate		0.020	2.0–1.4
252, R = H, NR$_2'$ = N(CH$_3$)$_2$	228–233	0.0143	—
253, R = H, NR$_2'$ = N(C$_2$H$_5$)$_2$	100–105	—	2.0–2.5
254, R = H, NR$_2'$ = N(C$_3$H$_7$)$_2$	157–162	0.0013	2.0–1.5
255, R = H, NR$_2'$ = N(C$_4$H$_9$)$_2$	173–174	—	inactive
256, R = H, NR$_2'$ = N(C$_6$H$_{13}$)$_2$	148–149	—	inactive
257, R = H, NR$_2'$ = N(CH$_2$)$_4$	152–155	0.379	—
258, R = H, NR$_2'$ = N(CH$_2$CH$_2$)$_2$NCH$_3$	159–162	0.013	—
259, R = H, NR$_2'$ = N(CH$_2$CH$_2$)$_2$O	223–225	0.0176	—
260, R = (C=O)C$_2$H$_5$, NR$_2'$ = N(C$_2$H$_5$)$_2$	96–103	0.0011	3.0–3.5
261, R = (C=O)C$_3$H$_7$, NR$_2'$ = N(C$_2$H$_5$)$_2$	81–83	0.0008	3.0–3.5
262, R = (C=O)C$_4$H$_9$, NR$_2'$ = N(C$_2$H$_5$)$_2$	126–128	0.0019	3.0–3.5

^{a}Dose (3 × 10^{-5}, 3 × 10^{-4}, 3 × 10^{-3}, and 3 × 10^{-2} M) necessary to cause 50% reduction of swelling in mouse ear caused by topical application of croton oil (2% in acetone).
^{b}Blanching in human volunteers caused by topical application of 0.03 M steroids in acetone: IPM (90:10).
Source: From Ref. 125.

of hydrocortisone are less potent than the parent 17-esters, at least one of them is less toxic. This suggests that some separation of toxicity from increased potency using prodrugs is possible.

Betamethasone

Most of the available literature comparing derivatives of a glucocorticoid steroid does so using in vivo tests. One of the most popular tests is the blanching or vasoconstrictor test in human volunteers. This test can be used to evaluate the effectiveness of the formulation as well as the potency of the steroid in the formulation, and is still used extensively today. Originally introduced by McKenzie and Stoughton in 1962 (127), the vasoconstrictor test was used in 1964 to evaluate a whole series of different types of derivatives of betamethasone, not all of which were prodrugs (128). The partial results of that extensive evaluation are given in Table 56.

Generally the 17α-esters, **272–275**, are more potent than the 21-esters, **264–269**, and the 17α,21-ortho esters, **277–280**, are apparently even more potent than the 17α-esters. The lone 17α,21-orthocarbonate derivative, **281**, is comparable in potency to a 17α-ester, while the lone 21-carbonate ester, **271**, is less potent than the corresponding 21-ester. Prodrug **276** and the lone 21-carbamate, **270**, were only as potent as betamethasone itself. 17α,21-Diesters were not examined in the

Table 56 Relative Potencies of Betamethasone Derivatives

Compound	Relative potency
263, R = R' = H	0.8
264, R = (C=O)-CH₃, R' = H	18
265, R = (C=O)-C₃H₇, R' = H	85
266, R = (C=O)-C₄H₉, R' = H	26
267, R = (C=O)-C₅H₁₁, R' = H	123
268, R = (C=O)-C₈H₁₇, R' = H	2
269, R = (C=O)-C₁₅H₃₁, R' = H	0.1
270, R = (C=O)-N(C₂H₅)₂, R' = H	<1
271, R = (C=O)-OC₂H₅, R' = H	25
272, R = H, R' = (C=O)-CH₃	114
273, R = H, R' = (C=O)-C₂H₅	190
274, R = H, R' = (C=O)-C₃H₇	168
275, R = H, R' = (C=O)-C₄H₉	360
276, R,R' = CH(OC₂H₅)	1
277, R,R' = CCH₃(OC₂H₅)	67
278, R,R' = CC₂H₅(OC₂H₅)	402
279, R,R' = CC₃H₇(OCH₃)	402
280, R,R' = CC₄H₉(OCH₃)	150
281, R,R' = C(OC₂H₅)₂	166

Source: From Ref. 128.

work of McKenzie and Atkinson, but they are generally somewhat more potent than the 17α-esters. The 17α,21-ortho esters are not very stable and are readily hydrolyzed under acidic conditions, primarily to the 17α-esters. Since the skin is acidic, it is quite possible that some measure of the potency of the 17α,21-ortho esters is due to the activity of the 17α-esters formed upon hydrolysis of the ortho ester in vivo. However, that does not explain why the ortho ester is more potent than the corresponding 17α-ester in some comparisons. Either the ortho esters are more efficient at delivering the 17α-ester into the skin than the 17α-ester itself, or the 17α,21-ortho esters are also functioning as distinctly different drug entities compared to the 21-esters, which are merely functioning as prodrugs.

Metronidazole

Metronidazole was one of the first drugs for which a prodrug approach to enhance topical delivery was systematically evaluated (129). Before then, although there were numerous reports of different prodrug approaches to enhancing topical delivery, few reports had characterized the physicochemical properties of an homologous series of prodrugs (in this case esters), and had evaluated them in diffusion cell experiments to determine how effective they were in delivering the parent drug through skin. The choice of metronidazole was perhaps unfortunate, since all the esters (Table 57) except the acetate, which melted at 73–77°C, were

Table 57 Physicochemical Properties of Ester Derivatives of Metronidazole and Their Abilities to Deliver Metronidazole Through Skin

$$CH_3$$
$$N{-}N\,CH_2CH_2OR$$
$$NO_2$$

| | Half-lives[a] | | | |
Compound	buffer	plasma	log K[b]	% Permeated[b]
282, R = H			–0.05	64
283, R = (C=O)-CH₃	400	32	0.31	77
284, R = (C=O)-C₂H₅	507	3.2	0.92	98
285, R = (C=O)-C₃H₇	890	0.45	1.28	96
286, R = (C=O)-C₄H₉	802	0.21	1.94	72
287, R = (C=O)-C₅H₁₁	862	0.24	2.44	69

[a]Half-lives in hours at 37°C where the buffer was pH 7.4 phosphate and the plasma was 2.5% human plasma.
[b]Estimated from a graphic representation of partition coefficient between octanol and a pH 7.4 buffer versus % permeated.
Source: From Ref. 129.

oils. Thus, no water or lipid solubilities were measured and the only available criterion of relative solubilities are the log K values. As expected, the log K values increase incrementally as longer chain alkyl groups are introduced into the promoiety.

Because most of the derivatives were oils, it was not possible to use saturated solutions in the diffusion cell experiments. Instead, equimolar amounts of the esters in ethanol:PG (82:18) were applied to the skins. The ethanol evaporated, leaving behind a thin film of prodrug in PG. Only metronidazole was detected in the receptor phase under conditions where intact prodrug could have been detected. Since a constant drug concentration at the skin surface was not maintained, a steady-state rate of delivery was never achieved and the total percent permeated leveled off after about 80 h. Only percent permeated for each prodrug is listed in Table 57. There is not much difference in the performances of any of the prodrugs by this criterion. Moreover, if the plot of percent permeated versus hours is examined, the rate of delivery by each of the prodrugs shown is about the same as by metronidazole itself.

Possibly a better way to have evaluated the prodrugs of metronidazole, and for that matter any series of prodrugs that are oils, would have been to apply them neat. The oils can be dissolved in acetone or ethanol, etc., applied, and the acetone or ethanol allowed to evaporate to leave a thin film of the oil on the skin. In that way all the prodrugs could have been tested at unit thermodynamic activity.

DRUG-(C=O)

Drugs containing only a carbonyl functional group are usually not considered as candidates for prodrug modification. The carbonyl group usually does not impart much polarity to the drug molecule and does not contain an exchangeable heteroatom-H group capable of forming hydrogen bonds. However, carbonyl functional groups are usually quite reactive toward a wide range of nucleophiles and such premature reactions can inactivate the drug molecule before it reaches its site of action. In this section, two examples of prodrugs will be discussed where a carbonyl functional group is involved in the formation of the promoiety. In the first example, the carbonyl group is part of the drug molecule, and a thiazolidine type prodrug of the carbonyl group is examined for its ability to enhance the delivery of the carbonyl-containing drug through skin. In the second example, the enabling functional group is a procarbonyl group (an oxazolidine), and the drug contains a 2-aminoalcohol functional group. The oxazolidine prodrug is evaluated for its ability to deliver the drug—a 2-aminoalcohol—through skin.

Thiazolidine Derivatives of Drug-(C=O): Drug-C$\overset{S}{\underset{N}{\big\langle}}$

Hydrocortisone is an endogenous steroid which is rapidly metabolized in vivo to nontoxic, inactive molecules by reduction of the 3-ketone and by other routes as well. Hydrocortisone and other endogenous steroids such as progesterone and testosterone can be looked at as naturally designed, naturally occurring soft drugs (130). That is, they exhibit activity themselves but are metabolized in a controlled and predictable manner to inactive nontoxic molecules. On the other hand, prodrugs are usually designed to be inactive initially, but to be metabolized in a controlled and predictable manner to give the parent, active drug. Making a prodrug of a naturally occurring soft drug could protect the soft drug from premature metabolism and enhance its delivery to its site of action. In the case of hydrocortisone or testosterone, there are hydroxy functional groups present to which a promoiety can be attached. However, for progesterone only carbonyl groups are available for modification. In addition, ester prodrugs of hydrocortisone have no reported effect on preventing the reduction of the 3-ketone.

Thiazolidines derived primarily from cysteine ethyl ester or 2-aminoethanethiol were synthesized from a large number of hydrocortisone 17α-esters and hydrocortisone 21-acetate. In addition, a large series of thiazolidines derived from different esters of cysteine and hydrocortisone 21-acetate were synthesized (130). All of the thiazolidines functioned as prodrugs of hydrocortisone or the hydrocortisone 17-esters. Although all of the thiazolidines based on the different esters of cysteine and hydrocortisone 21-acetate are more potent than hydrocortisone 21-acetate or hydrocortisone in the mouse edema model, none of the thiazolidines are as potent as hydrocortisone 17α-butyrate. However, only the thiazolidine derived from 2-aminoethanethiol and hydrocortisone 21-acetate is more potent than hydrocortisone or its 21-acetate ester in the blanching model. It causes less systemic toxicity than the other thiazolidines, or its parent steroid, but it also causes more local toxicity than most of the other thiazolidines.

Only the thiazolidine derived from hydrocortisone 21-acetate and cysteine ethyl ester was evaluated in a diffusion cell experiment. The thiazolidine only delivers about 0.4 times as much hydrocortisone as hydrocortisone or 0.25 times as much as hydrocortisone 21-acetate through hairless mouse skin from the application of 0.03 M acetone:IPM (90:10) solutions. It was suggested that this result was due to the thiazolidine delivering more steroid into the skin and maintaining it there through a nonspecific reaction between the ring-opened thiazolidine thiol group and other thiols in the skin. This rationale is supported by the fact that when the thiazolidine derived from cysteine ethyl ester and progesterone was applied to hairless mice it delivered less progesterone through the skin (0.25 times), yet delivered a little over twice as much into the skin (131). Thus, a decreased rate of delivery through skin may not always correlate with decreased delivery into the skin and to the target epidermal cells. Conversely, increased delivery through skin may not correlate with increased delivery into the skin.

Oxazolidine Derivatives of Drug-(C=O): Drug-C$\left. \!\!\!\!\underset{N}{\overset{O}{<}} \right]$

In this section, the promoiety of the prodrug is derived from a carbonyl group instead of the carbonyl group being part of the drug molecule. The drug molecule in this case contains a 2-aminoethanol group. It is not clear that an approach that would work to enhance the topical delivery of a drug molecule containing a 2-aminoethanol group would necessarily work to enhance the topical delivery of a drug molecule containing a carbonyl functional group. The rationale for transiently converting the relatively basic 2-aminoethanol group to an oxazolidine is that the basic pK_a of the amine portion is lowered (132). Thus, the oxazolidine should present a lower concentration of its protonated form to the skin-vehicle interface than the parent 2-aminoethanol, and hence should partition into the skin better. That rationale would not necessarily apply to a drug molecule containing a carbonyl group. However, reference has already been made to the use of tertiary amines as penetration enhancers, and examples of the effect of incorporating amines into the promoiety on the ability of a prodrug to delivery the parent drug through skin have already been discussed. Thus, incorporation of an amino group into a promoiety of a drug containing a carbonyl group may be effective in enhancing its topical delivery, and one convenient way to incorporate the amine into a molecule containing a carbonyl group is in the form of an oxazolidine.

Bundgaard and coworkers (133,134) have characterized a number of examples of oxazolidines where substitution on the 2-aminoethanol or on the carbonyl group was varied to determine the effect of substitution on stability and partition coefficient. Generally, the oxazolidines are more stable when there are alkyl substituents α- to the amine portion of the 2-aminoethanol group and when there is increased alkyl or aryl substitution on the carbonyl carbon. All of the oxazolidines studied are less basic than the parent 2-aminoethanol and exhibit significantly higher log K values at pH 7.4.

Pitman and coworkers evaluated the oxazolidine formed from ephedrine and formaldehyde in diffusion cell experiments using human skin (135). The oxazolidine is more effective than ephedrine at delivering ephedrine from pH 7.0 to 10.88 aqueous buffers, but is less effective at delivering ephedrine from a liquid paraffin solution. However, the oxazolidine of ephedrine and ephedrine are equally ineffective at delivering ephedrine from a PG solution. In all the cases where the oxazolidine was applied in buffer, the solutions contained mixtures of ephedrine, formaldehyde, and oxazolidine because of the instability of the oxazolidine in water. Separate experiments showed that formaldehyde in the buffers causes no significant increase in the permeability of tritiated water compared to the buffers alone, so the increased delivery of ephedrine by its oxazolidine is not caused by formaldehyde damage to the skin. The oxazolidine is more effective at delivering ephedrine from the buffers (polar vehicle) and less effective from liquid paraffin (nonpolar vehicle) because of the increased lipophilicity of the oxazolidine compared to ephedrine: The calculated partition coefficients between water and liquid paraffin are 5.6 and 1.0, respectively. The oxazolidine is more soluble in liquid paraffin than ephedrine, and hence exhibits a "smaller tendency to escape" (135), whereas the opposite is true in water.

One general concept that resulted from the oxazolidine experiments is that the prodrug does not have to be completely stable in its vehicle to be effective. Although buffer solution which initially contained oxazolidines rapidly became mixtures of oxazolidine, ephedrine, and formaldehyde, the delivery of ephedrine was still enhanced. The equilibrium concentration of intact oxazolidine can be changed by adjusting the pH, the concentration of formaldehyde, and the initial concentration of oxazolidine. Thus, reproducible performances can be obtained even with an unstable prodrug under the appropriate circumstances.

CONCLUSIONS

In this chapter, we have described potential prodrug approaches and prodrug approaches that actually have been used to enhance the delivery of drugs through the skin (transdermal delivery) and into the skin (dermal delivery). Examples have been given of prodrug approaches that can be used to transiently mask amide, imide, amine, thionamide (thiol), carboxylic acid, hydroxy, and carbonyl functional groups. The functional groups that have been incorporated into the promoieties that form the prodrug have been shown to be capable of not only increasing the lipid solubilities of the prodrugs, but of also increasing their water solubilities. The balance between the lipid and water solubilities depends on the incorporated functional groups.

Two general types of prodrugs have been identified. They can be categorized as being either acyl or soft alkyl-type prodrugs depending on whether the enabling functional group is attached directly to the functional group that is to be masked in the drug, or it is separated from the functional group in the drug by a methylene or vinylogous methylene group. A greater degree of flexibility in the design of a prodrug approach to mask a particular functional group is possible using the soft alkyl type of prodrug. This is because the form of the enabling functional group in the prodrug is not limited by the existing heteroatom in the functional group that is to be masked in the drug.

Only a small number of the possible prodrug approaches to enhancing topical delivery have been evaluated, but significant improvement in the transdermal delivery of specific drugs has been achieved with some of those that have been evaluated. The greatest success was obtained from attempts to enhance the transdermal delivery of 6-MP. The combination of S^6-acyloxymethyl and 9-dialkylaminomethyl promoieties gave up to a 240 times increase in the transdermal delivery of 6-MP (see Table 40). The individual promoieties from the combination were effective as well. S^6-Acyloxymethyl derivatives of 6-MP gave up to a 66 times increase in transdermal delivery (see Table 34), whereas the 7-dialkylaminomethyl derivatives gave up to a 180 times increase (see Table 16).

The fact that the largest increases in transdermal delivery are observed for prodrugs of 6-MP may be due to the fact that the 6-MP itself is so polar and permeates skin so poorly. However, simple N-acyl derivatives of 5-FU gave up to a 40 times increase in transdermal delivery of 5-FU (see Table 25) and dihydroxyalkoxycarbonyl derivatives of levonorgestrel gave up to a 30 times increase in the transdermal delivery of levonorgestrel (see Table 51). Thus, the transdermal delivery of (a) a polar drug that can permeate skin reasonably well to begin with (5-FU), or (b) a drug that is very lipophilic (levonorgestrel) and does not permeate skin well can be enhanced significantly with prodrug approaches that transiently impart increased biphasic solubility to the drug.

The trends in the results from the use of the different prodrug approaches have several common features. First, the optimum member in an homologous series of more lipid-soluble prodrugs is the one which exhibits increased biphasic solubility. For prodrugs of very polar drugs such as 6-MP, 5-FU, theophylline, etc., the more efficient members of the series are the ones that exhibit the greater water solubility. The most effective member may not be the most water-soluble member but it is usually at least as water soluble as the parent drug. For prodrugs of very lipophilic drugs such as levonorgestrel, more water-soluble prodrugs performed better than prodrugs which were merely more lipid soluble.

Second, the members of an homologous series of prodrugs that exhibit higher solubilities in the donor phase are not the members that deliver the highest amounts of parent drug through skin. Generally, the more soluble a prodrug is in the donor phase the lower its activity coefficient or tendency to escape from that phase. However, if a member of the series is also more soluble in the skin as well as in the donor phase, the increased solubility in the skin appears to be the dominant feature.

Third, there is a good correlation between increased delivery through the skin (transdermal delivery) and increased delivery into the skin (dermal delivery). Two examples have been given where increased inhibition of epidermal DNA synthesis was observed from the topical application of prodrugs that were very effective at enhancing transdermal delivery (see Tables 7 and 15). In addition, numerous examples have been given where higher rates of transdermal delivery correlate with higher levels of accumulation of the parent drug in the skin (see Tables 21, 25, 28, 34, 36, 40, and 43).

Fourth, although the size of the permeant is certainly an important criterion in the selection of a particular prodrug approach, it does not appear to be a dominant factor within the members of a series of prodrugs. Instead, solubility is the dominant factor. An example has been given where the prodrugs were relatively similar in size and exhibited similar melting points, yet exhibited significantly different aqueous solubilities and were significantly different in their abilities to enhance topical delivery (see Tables 42 and 43).

Fifth, although it is difficult to measure, the solubility of the prodrug in the skin is an important factor in the ability of the prodrug to enhance the topical delivery of the parent drug. Solubility in skin does not merely mean solubility in the stratum corneum. Solubility in the viable skin, or the skin that remains after the skin is stripped of the stratum corneum, is also important, especially for drugs that are rather lipophilic to begin with. Obviously, the potential ability of the prodrug approach to increase the effective solubility of the parent drug in the skin gives it a significant advantage over any formulation approach in an attempt to increase the dermal or even the transdermal delivery of the parent drug. Primarily, a formulation approach affects the solubility of the parent drug in the vehicle and only secondarily affects its solubility in the skin as it permeates the skin along with the prodrug. Of course, the best strategy to optimize topical delivery would be to utilize both approaches.

It is clear that there are numerous types of prodrug approaches that can be used with each type of functional group that needs to be transiently masked in the parent drug. It is not clear which functional groups should be incorporated into a promoiety that is to be used for a particular drug if optimized topical delivery is to be achieved. That will be the subject of subsequent chapters. A case has been made in this chapter for using a functional group in the promoiety which, within a series of more lipid soluble prodrugs, imparts the greatest water solubility to the prodrug. However, it is not clear if that functional group will be the same for every type of prodrug or every type of drug.

REFERENCES

1. A. Albert, *Nature*, 182, 421 (1958).
2. S.M. Kupchan, A.F. Casy, and J.V. Swintosky, *J. Pharm. Sci.*, 54, 514 (1965).
3. V. Stella, in *Prodrugs as Novel Drug Delivery Systems* (T. Higuchi and V. Stella, eds.). American Chemical Society, Washington, D.C., 1975, pp. 1–115.
4. H. Bundgaard, in *Designs of Prodrugs* (H. Bundgaard, ed.). Elsevier, New York, 1985, pp. 1–92.
5. B. Barry, *Dermatological Formulations: Percutaneous Absorption*, Marcel Dekker, New York, 1983.
6. J. Hadgraft, in *Design of Prodrugs* (H. Bundgaard, ed.). Elsevier, New York, 1985, pp. 271–289.
7. W.I. Higuchi and C. D. Yu, in *Transdermal Delivery of Drugs* (A.F. Kydonieus and B. Berner, eds.). Vol. III. CRC Press, Boca Raton, Florida, 1987, pp. 43–83.
8. K.B. Sloan, *Adv. Drug Delivery Rev.*, 3, 67 (1989).
9. S.Y. Chan and A.L.W. Po, *Int. J. Pharm.*, 55, 1 (1989).
10. K.B. Sloan, S.A.M. Koch, K.G. Siver, and F.P. Flowers, *J. Invest. Dermatol.*, 87, 244 (1986).
11. K.B. Sloan, K.G. Siver, and S.A.M. Koch, *J. Pharm. Sci.*, 75, 744 (1986).
12. E.F. Sherertz, K.B. Sloan, and R.G. McTiernan, *J. Invest. Dermatol.*, 89, 147 (1987).
13. R.P. Waranis, K.G. Siver, and K.B. Sloan, *Int. J. Pharm.*, 36, 211 (1987).
14. K.B. Sloan, in *Prodrugs: Topical and Ocular Drug Delivery* (K.B. Sloan, ed.). Marcel Dekker, New York, 1992.

15. R.F. Fedors, *Polym. Eng. Sci.*, 14, 147 (1974).
16. A. Martin, P.L. Wu, and T. Velasquez, *J. Pharm. Sci.*, 74, 277 (1985).
17. A. Martin, P.L. Wu, Z. Liron, and S. Cohen, *J. Pharm. Sci.*, 74, 638 (1985).
18. K.B. Sloan and N. Bodor, *Int. J. Pharm.*, 12, 299 (1982).
19. K.B. Sloan, E.F. Sherertz, and R.G. McTiernan, *Arch. Dermatol. Res.*, 282, 484 (1990).
20. V.J. Stella and K.J. Himmelstein, *J. Med. Chem.*, 23, 1275 (1980).
21. K.B. Sloan, M. Hashida, J. Alexander, N. Bodor, and T. Higuchi, *J. Pharm. Sci.*, 72, 372 (1983).
22. J. Hadgraft, K.A. Walters, and P.K. Wotton, *Int. J. Pharm.*, 32, 257 (1986).
23. O. Wong, J. Huntington, T. Nishihata, and J.H. Rytting, *Pharm. Res.*, 6, 286 (1989).
24. B.J. Aungst, J.A. Blake, and M.A. Hussain, *Pharm. Res.*, 7, 712 (1990).
25. K.B. Sloan, S.A.M. Koch, and K.G. Siver, *Int. J. Pharm.*, 21, 251 (1984).
26. S.A.M. Koch and K.B. Sloan, *Int. J. Pharm.*, 35, 243 (1987).
27. K.G. Siver and K.B. Sloan, *Int. J. Pharm.*, 48, 195 (1988).
28. D. Ross, P.B. Farmer, A. Gescher, J.A. Hickman, M.D. Threadgill, *Life Sci.*, 32, 597 (1983).
29. C.F. Spencer and J.G. Michels, *J. Org. Chem.*, 29, 3416 (1964).
30. A.B.A. Jansen and T.J. Russell, *J. Chem. Soc.* 2127 (1965).
31. N. Bodor and K.B. Sloan, *Chem. Abstr.*, 87, P152278 (1977).
32. J.J. Voorhees and E.A. Duell, *Arch. Dermatol.*, 104, 352 (1971).
33. P.C. Bansal, I.H. Pitman, N.S.J. Tam, M. Mertes, and J.J. Kaminski, *J. Pharm. Sci.*, 70, 850 (1981).
34. H. Bundgaard and M. Johansen, *Int. J. Pharm.*, 5, 67 (1980).
35. A. DuVivier, R. Bible, R.K. Mikuriya, and R.B. Stoughton, *Br. J. Dermatol.*, 93, 1 (1975).
36. D.K. Goette, *J. Am. Acad. Dermatol.*, 4, 633 (1981).
37. T.A.Robinson and A.M. Kligman, *Br. J. Dermatol.*, 92, 703 (1975).
38. S. Ozaki, Y. Watanabe, T. Hoshiko, H. Mizuno, K. Ishikawa, and H. Mori, *Chem. Pharm. Bull.*, 32, 733 (1984).
39. A. Buur, H. Bundgaard, and E. Falch, *Int. J. Pharm.*, 24, 43 (1985).
40. B. Mollgaard, A. Hoelgaard, and H. Bundgaard, *Int. J. Pharm.*, 12, 153 (1982).
41. A. Buur, H. Bundgaard, and E. Falch, *Acta Pharm. Suec.*, 23, 205 (1986).
42. K.B. Sloan, M. Hashida, J. Alexander, N. Bodor, and T. Higuchi, *J. Pharm. Sci.*, 72, 372 (1983).
43. R.P. Waranis and K.B. Sloan, *J. Pharm. Sci.*, 76, 587 (1987).
44. R.P. Waranis and K.B. Sloan, *J. Pharm. Sci.*, 77, 210 (1988).
45. G.D. Weinstein, J.L. McCullough, W.H. Eaglstein, A. Golub, R.C. Cornell, R.B. Stoughton, W. Clendenning, H. Zackheim, H. Maiback, K.R. Kulp, L. King, H.P. Baden, J.S. Taylor, and D.D. Deneau, *Arch. Dermatol.*, 117, 388 (1981).
46. J.D. McGhee and P.H. von Hippel, *Biochemistry*, 14, 1281 (1975).
47. J. Alexander, *J. Org. Chem.*, 49, 1453 (1983).
48. H. Sasaki, E. Mukai, M. Hashida, T. Kimura, and H. Sezaki, *Int. J. Pharm.*, 15, 49 (1983).
49. K.B. Sloan and S.A.M. Koch, *J. Org. Chem.*, 48, 635 (1983).
50. D.D. Wheeler, D.C. Young, and D.S. Erley, *J. Org. Chem.*, 22, 547 (1957).

51. K.B. Sloan and S.A.M. Koch, *J. Heterocyclic Chem.*, 22, 429 (1985).
52. K.B. Sloan, unpublished results.
53. F. Sakamoto, S. Ikeda, H. Kondo, and G. Tsukamoto, *Chem. Pharm. Bull.*, 33, 4870 (1985).
54. H. Bundgaard and M. Johansen, *Arch. Pharm. Chemi. Sci. Ed.*, 8, 29 (1980).
55. H. Bundgaard and M. Johansen, *J. Pharm. Sci.*, 69, 44 (1980).
56. G.M. Loudon, M.R. Almond, and J.N. Jacob, *J. Am. Chem. Soc.*, 103, 4508 (1981).
57. H. Bundgaard and E. Falch, *Int. J. Pharm.*, 25, 27 (1985).
58. K.B. Sloan, E.F. Sherertz, and R.G. McTiernan, *Int. J. Pharm.*, 44, 87 (1988).
59. M. Johansen and H. Bundgaard, *Arch. Pharm. Chemi. Sci. Ed.*, 8, 141 (1980).
60. E.F. Sherertz, K.B. Sloan, and R.G. McTiernan, *Arch. Dermatol. Res.*, 282, 463 (1990).
61. S.A.M. Koch and K.B. Sloan, *Pharm. Res.*, 4, 317 (1987).
62. K.B. Sloan and K.G. Siver, *Tetrahedron*, 40, 3997 (1984).
63. A. Buur and H. Bundgaard, *Int. J. Pharm.*, 21, 349 (1984).
64. A. Buur and H. Bundgaard, *Arch. Pharm. Chemi. Sci. Ed.*, 12, 37 (1984).
65. A. Buur and H. Bundgaard, *J. Pharm. Sci.*, 75, 522 (1986).
66. A. Buur and H. Bundgaard, *Int. J . Pharm.*, 23, 209 (1985).
67. H.A. Staab, *Angew. Chem. Internat. Edit.*, 1, 351 (1962).
68. S. Ozaki, Y. Ike, H. Mizuno, K. Ishikawa and H. Mori, *Bull. Chem. Soc. (Jpn.)*, 50, 2406 (1977).
69. H. Sasaki, T. Takahashi, Y. Mori, J. Nakamura, and J. Shibasaki, *Int. J. Pharm.*, 60, 1 (1990).
70. H.D. Beall, research toward Ph.D. thesis, University of Florida.
71. T. Kametani, K. Kigasawa, M. Hiiragi, K. Wakisaka, S. Haga, Y. Nagamatsu, H. Sugi, K. Fukawa, O. Irino, T. Yamamoto, N. Nishimura, A. Taguchi, T. Okada, and M. Nakayama, *J. Med. Chem.*, 23, 1324 (1980).
72. A. Buur and H. Bundgaard, *Int. J. Pharm.*, 36, 41 (1987).
73. Y. Ishido, A. Hosono, S. Isome, A. Maruyama, T. Sato, *Bull. Chem. Soc. (Jpn.)*, 37, 1389 (1964).
74. N. Bodor, K. B. Sloan, Yu-Neng Kuo, and T. Higuchi, *J. Pharm. Sci.*, 67, 1045 (1978).
75. M. Giani and L. Molteni, *Chem. Abstr.*, 52, 12874h (1958).
76. H.K. Lee, H. Lambert, V.J. Stella, D. Wang, and T. Higuchi, *J. Pharm. Sci.*, 68, 288 (1979).
77. H. Sasaki, E. Mukai, M. Hashida, T. Kimura, and H. Sezaki, *Int. J. Pharm.*, 15, 61 (1983).
78. E. Mukai, K. Arase, M. Hashida, H. Sezaki, *Int. J. Pharm.*, 25, 95 (1985).
79. J. Alexander, R. Cargill, S.R. Michelson, and H. Schwam, *J. Med. Chem.*, 31, 318 (1988).
80. U.S. Gogate, A.J. Repta, and J. Alexander, *Int. J. Pharm.*, 40, 235 (1987).
81. R.D. Schoenwald and H.S. Huang, *J. Pharm. Sci.*, 72, 1266 (1983).
82. K.G. Siver, K.B. Sloan, R.P. Waranis, and A. Saab, *J. Heterocyclic Chem.*, 25, 1077 (1988).
83. R.P. Waranis and K.B. Sloan, *J. Pharm. Sci.*, 77, 210 (1988).
84. M. Johansen, H. Bundgaard, and E. Falch, *Int. J. Pharm.*, 13, 89 (1983).
85. R.P. Waranis and K.B. Sloan, *J. Pharm. Sci.*, 76, 587 (1987).

86. A.N. Saab and K.B. Sloan, *Int. J. Pharm.*, 57, 253 (1989).

87. A.N. Saab, K.B. Sloan, H.D. Beall, and R. Villanueva, *J. Pharm. Sci.*, 79, 1099 (1990).

88. K.G. Siver and K.B. Sloan, *J. Pharm. Sci.*, 79, 66 (1990).

89. J. Swarbrick, G. Lee, J. Brom, and N.P. Gensmantel, *J. Pharm. Sci.*, 73, 1352 (1984).

90. G.E. Parry, A.L. Bunge, G.D. Silcox, L.K. Pershing, and D.W. Pershing, *Pharm. Res.*, 7, 230 (1990).

91. E.T. Bororows and J.M. Johnson, *Br. Patent*, 1, 220, 447 (1971).

92. I. Barasoain, J.M. Rojo, C. Sunkel, and P. Portoles, *Int. J. Clin. Pharmacol.*, 16, 235 (1978).

93. V. Bohr, E.A. Abel, E.M. Farber, and P. Hanawalt, *Arch. Dermatol. Res.*, 279, 147 (1987).

94. H. Bundgaard, N. Mork, and A. Hoelgaard, *Int. J. Pharm.*, 55, 91 (1989).

95. S.A. Haider, *Br. Med. J.*, 1, 1570 (1977).

96. N. Bodor, J. Zupan, and S. Selk, *Int. J. Pharm.*, 7, 63 (1980).

97. N.M. Nielsen and H. Bundgaard, *J. Med. Chem.*, 32, 727 (1989).

98. H. Bundgaard and N.M. Nielsen, *J. Med. Chem.*, 30, 451 (1987).

99. N.M. Nielsen and H. Bundgaard, *J. Pharm. Sci.*, 77, 285 (1988).

100. H. Bundgaard and N.M. Nielsen, *Int. J. Pharm.*, 43, 101 (1988).

101. T.L. Ho and C.M. Wong, *J. Chem. Soc. Chem. Commun.*, 224 (1973).

102. P.M. Hardy, H.N. Rydon, and R.C. Thompson, *Tetrahedron Lett.*, 2525 (1968).

103. S.W. Jacobs, M. Bishel, and R.J. Herschler, *Curr. Ther. Res.*, 6, 193 (1964).

104. T.H. Sweeny, A.M. Downs and G. Matoltsy, *J. Invest. Dermatol.*, 46, 300 (1966).

105. T. Loftsson and N. Bodor, *J. Pharm. Sci.*, 70, 756 (1981).

106. W.P. Jencks and J. Carriuolo, *J. Am. Chem. Soc.*, 82, 1778 (1960).

107. Registry of Toxic Effects of Chemical Substances, R.J. Lewis and R.L. Tatken, eds., U.S. Department of Health and Human Services, NIOSH, 1980.

108. B.O. Handford, J.H. Jones, G.T. Young, and T.F.N. Jones, *J. Chem. Soc.*, 6814 (1965).

109. K.B. Sloan, S. Selk, J. Haslam, L. Caldwell, and R. Shaffer, *J. Pharm. Sci.*, 73, 1734 (1984).

110. M.W. Greaves and J. Sondergaard, *Arch. Dermatol.*, 101, 659 (1970).

111. K. Tojo, C.C. Chiang, and Y.W. Chien, *J. Pharm. Sci.*, 76, 123 (1987).

112. M.M. Ghannam, K. Tojo, Y.W. Chien, *Drug Dev. Ind. Pharm.*, 12, 303 (1986).

113. M. Ponec, *Int. J. Dermatol.*, 23, 11 (1984).

114. E.L. Goodman, J.P. Luby, and M.T. Johnson, *Antimicrob. Agents Chemother.*, 8, 693 (1975).

115. D.C. Baker, T.H. Haskell, S.R. Putt, *J. Med. Chem.*, 21, 1218 (1978).

116. D.C. Baker, S.D. Kumar, W.J. Waites, G. Arnett, W.M. Shannon, W.T. Higuchi, and W.J. Lambert, *J. Med. Chem.*, 27, 270 (1984).

117. W.M. Shannon, G. Arnett, D.C. Baker, S.D. Kumar, W.I. Higuchi, *Antimicrob. Agents Chemother.*, 24, 706 (1983).

118. D.C. Baker, T.H. Haskell, S.R. Putt, and B.J. Sloan, *J. Med. Chem.*, 22, 273 (1979).

119. D. Friend, P. Catz, J. Heller, J. Reid, and R. Baker, *J. Controlled Release*, 7, 243 (1988).

120. D. Friend, P. Catz, J. Heller, J. Reid, and R. Baker, *J. Controlled Release*, 7, 251 (1988).
121. Y. Sun, K. Tojo, and Y.W. Chien, *Drug Dev. Ind. Pharm.*, 12, 327 (1986).
122. K.H. Valia, K. Tojo, and Y.W. Chien, *Drug Dev. Ind. Pharm.*, 11, 1133 (1985).
123. W.M. Smith. An Inquiry into the Mechanism of Percutaneous Absorption of Hydrocortisone and Its 21-n-Alkyl Esters. Ph.D. Thesis, University of Michigan, Ann Arbor, 1982.
124. C.A. Schlagel, *Adv. Biol. Skin*, 12, 337 (1972).
125. N. Bodor and K.B. Sloan, *Int. J. Pharm.*, 15, 235 (1983).
126. D.D. Munro, *Br. J. Dermatol.*, 81(Suppl. 4), 92 (1969).
127. A.W. McKenzie and R.B. Stoughton, *Arch. Dermatol.*, 86, 608 (1962).
128. A.W. McKenzie and R.M. Atkinson, *Arch. Dermatol.*, 89, 741 (1964).
129. M. Johansen, B. Mollgaard, P.K. Wotton, C. Larsen, A. Hoelgaard, *Int. J. Pharm.*, 32, 199 (1986).
130. N. Bodor, K.B. Sloan, R.J. Little, S.H. Selk, and L. Caldwell, *Int. J. Pharm.*, 10, 307 (1982).
131. N. Bodor and K.B. Sloan, *J. Pharm. Sci.*, 71, 514 (1982).
132. H. Bundgaard and M. Johansen, *Int. J. Pharm.*, 10, 165 (1982).
133. M. Johansen and H. Bundgaard, *J. Pharm. Sci.*, 72, 1294 (1983).
134. A. Buur and H. Bundgaard, *Int. J. Pharm.*, 78, 325 (1984).
135. J.A. Young-Harvey, I.D. Rae, and I.H. Pitman, *Int. J. Pharm.*, 30, 151 (1986).

3

Prodrugs for Dermal Delivery: Solubility, Molecular Size, and Functional Group Effects

Gerald B. Kasting and Ronald L. Smith
The Procter & Gamble Company, Cincinnati, Ohio

Bradley D. Anderson
The University of Utah College of Pharmacy, Salt Lake City, Utah

INTRODUCTION

The development of prodrugs for topical or transdermal applications involves several key considerations—delivery through skin, chemical and enzymatic stability, and dermal irritancy and sensitization. This chapter is primarily concerned with the first of these considerations. In the first section, we review a theory which provides a rationale for the design of compounds with optimal topical delivery properties and outline extensions which provide it with broader applicability. The second section presents experimental evidence in support of the theory. The last section describes the results of a program in which these ideas were applied to the development of nonsteroidal anti-inflammatory drugs (NSAIDs) via a prodrug approach. On the basis of increased skin penetration rates plus favorable results from anti-inflammatory, skin irritation, and bioconversion studies, several of the new compounds are believed to hold potential as improved topical anti-inflammatory agents.

Most of the chapter deals with the topical delivery of drugs in general rather than focusing on prodrugs per se. This reflects our belief that a common set of principles governs the absorption of these agents. The emphasis is on concepts that are useful in a predictive sense; that is, they allow one to make quantitative predictions of percutaneous absorption rates prior to beginning experimentation. We have found these ideas to be particularly useful in the selection of compounds for study as either transdermal or topical drugs. A second area of applicability is the estimation of systemic exposure resulting from the contact of noxious chemicals with the skin.

THEORY OF SKIN PERMEABILITY

Nomenclature and Units

The following symbols and abbreviations are used throughout the chapter:

Symbol	Units	Identity
J	$\mu g/cm^2/h$	flux
J_m	$\mu g/cm^2/h$	maximum flux
P	cm/h	permeability coefficient
ΔC	$\mu g/ml$	concentration gradient
S_w	$\mu g/ml$	aqueous solubility
S_{oct}	$\mu g/ml$	octanol solubility
K_{oct}	–	octanol/water or octanol/buffer partition coefficient

Other symbols are defined as they are introduced. All logarithms are base 10. The units are chosen to be internally consistent, i.e., $P = J/\Delta C$, and as consistent as possible with published work. An alternative set of units having merit for prodrugs would have flux and concentrations expressed in molar quantities.

The permeability coefficient, P, is sometimes expressed as a function of its constituent components P_{lip}, P_{pol} and P_{aq}. In this notation the subscript "lip" refers to the stratum corneum lipid pathway, "pol" to the polar pathway, and "aq" to the aqueous layers in series with the stratum corneum lipids. The latter term includes both the viable skin layers and the aqueous (or proteinaceous) layers within the stratum corneum, should the diffusion path be transcellular. The diffusion coefficient, D, partition coefficient, K, and thickness, h, of each pathway or layer are defined as required. Partition coefficients are expressed with respect to water unless otherwise indicated.

A Membrane Permeation Model Incorporating Partition Coefficient, Lipid Solubility, and Molecular Size

Most researchers in transdermal delivery today would agree that the stratum corneum is a heterogeneous membrane comprised of morphologically distinct lipid and protein domains. The lipid domain consists of lipid bilayer forming lipids which reside largely in highly structured lamellae within the intercellular space of stratum corneum (1,2). The protein domain consists primarily of cross-linked keratin residing in the intracellular region (3). These domains are, to a certain extent, physically separable by solvent extraction, allowing their independent contributions to properties such as solute partitioning into the stratum corneum to be assessed (4).

In contrast to the overwhelming physicochemical and morphological evidence that the stratum corneum is heterogeneous, models which are typically applied to the transport of moderately lipophilic permeants through the skin assume that the stratum corneum, which governs the rate of transport of such solutes, is a homogeneous, isotropic membrane having lipidlike properties. Therefore, the flux of a permeant across the skin from an arbitrary vehicle is generally written as:

$$J = (D/h)*K_{m/v}*\Delta C \tag{1}$$

where h is the stratum corneum thickness, D is the diffusion coefficient of the permeant, and $K_{m/v}$ is the stratum corneum membrane/vehicle partition coefficient.

Certainly more complex models of skin transport are necessary and are frequently applied when the range of permeants under investigation extends in either direction beyond those moderately lipophilic permeants for which equation 1 applies. Thus, highly polar or ionic solutes may traverse the skin via proteinaceous or water-filled "pore" pathways which exhibit little selectivity to lipophilicity (5). On the other hand, the transport of highly lipophilic permeants may be rate limited by aqueous layers either within the stratum corneum or in the epidermis or dermis. Subsequent sections of this chapter address these more complex models.

For permeants which undergo apparent transport via a lipid pathway within the stratum corneum, an important issue which must be addressed is: How does the well-documented heterogeneity of the stratum corneum limit the utility of equation 1, which assumes the stratum corneum to be homogeneous? Recent studies by one of us have shown that a linear relationship between flux and the stratum corneum/vehicle partition coefficient, as expressed by equation 1, should not be expected to hold because the domain probed in equilibrium partitioning studies may not be the transport barrier domain (6). Moreover, human skin studies (7) and studies using reaggregated stratum corneum (8) suggest that there is no relationship between flux and the thickness of stratum corneum or the number of cell layers. Thus, the evidence available indicates that neither h nor $K_{m/v}$ as defined in equation 1 correlate with flux. Equation 1 is therefore incorrect.

Nevertheless, it is likely that the correlation frequently observed between skin permeability and permeant lipophilicity as measured by one of a number of possible lipophilicity scales may in fact reflect the tendency of the permeant to partition into the membrane barrier microenvironment from the vehicle, even though this particular partition coefficient cannot be directly measured. It is also reasonable that the flux of a permeant across the skin should be directly proportional to its effective diffusion coefficient and the length of the pathway it traverses, even though neither of these parameters can be measured directly at present. We, therefore, propose the following simple model for transport of moderately lipophilic solutes through the skin:

$$J = (D_{lip}/h_{lip})*K_{lip/v}*\Delta C \tag{2}$$

where h_{lip} is the effective thickness of the stratum corneum lipid barrier, D_{lip} is the diffusion coefficient of the permeant in this barrier, and $K_{lip/v}$ is the lipid barrier/vehicle partition coefficient. Under sink conditions, ΔC is simply the drug concentration in the vehicle, C_v. (The above relationship also assumes that the vehicle does not alter the barrier properties.)

Whereas equation 2 has the same form as equation 1, the parameters in equation 2 cannot at present be independently determined. Much is known, however, about the relationship between flux and molecular structure—particularly molecular size—of the permeant. Subsequent sections of this chapter and recent publications by the authors (9,10) and others (11) rationalize molecular size effects on flux by assuming that the effective diffusion coefficient may be taken to be an inverse power function of molecular weight as described in equation 3:

$$D_{lip} = D_0^*(MW)^{-b} \tag{3}$$

with a value of b in the range 3–5. (Recall that diffusion coefficients in liquids obey equation 3 with b of one-third to one-half (12,13), whereas values of b > 3 have been observed for diffusion in polymer membranes, lipid bilayers, and other biomembranes (13–18).)

Alternatively, the form of D arising from free volume theory for diffusion may be used (9,19,20).

$$D_{lip} = D_0^*\exp(-\beta v) \tag{4}$$

where v is the molecular volume of the permeant. For most purposes, molecular weight may be substituted for volume in equation 4, since, for organic compounds, these two properties are highly correlated. For the skin penetration datasets we have examined either equations 3 or 4 may be used and MW may be substituted for v with no loss of accuracy.

In addition to D_{lip}, a means of determining relative values of $K_{lip/v}$ with varying molecular structure is needed before equation 2 can be used in predicting relative permeabilities. Given the fact that stratum corneum/vehicle partition coefficients are often not reliable predictors of relative permeabilities, is there a more appropriate lipophilicity parameter for relating permeant flux to molecular structure? Biomembrane selectivities are generally related to bulk solvent/water partition coefficients through linear free energy relationships (21) as depicted in equation 5 for the lipid/water partition coefficient, K_{lip}. (K_{lip} and $K_{lip/v}$ are related by $K_{lip/v} = K_{lip}/K_v$, where K_v is the vehicle/water partition coefficient.)

$$\log K_{lip} = A^*\log K_{solvent/water} + B \tag{5}$$

According to equation 5, the most suitable model solvent for predicting skin penetration would be that system for which A = 1. Such a bulk solvent would exactly resemble in its selectivity the rate-limiting microenvironment of the stratum corneum barrier. Unfortunately, it is unlikely that such a bulk solvent system can be identified because the transport pathway in question probably comprises lipid bilayers which are highly ordered and anisotropic, whereas bulk solvents are homogeneous and isotropic. (An indication that the stratum corneum barrier microenvironment is much more highly ordered than bulk solvents is evident in the much greater sensitivity of skin transport to molecular size when compared to diffusion through bulk solvents.) Nevertheless, for both practical and theoretical reasons, it would be worthwhile to identify a model solvent system which most closely approximates in its chemical nature the stratum corneum barrier microenvironment.

One may find a variety of correlations between permeability coefficients through the skin and various bulk solvent/water partition coefficients, including mineral oil/water (22), olive oil/water (23), ether/water (24), and octanol/water (6,9,10). Although linear free energy relationships between partitioning systems are frequently assumed (25), plots of log K in one system versus log K for another solvent/water system often deviate from linearity when the solute structural variations include a varying number of hydrogen-bonding functional groups and when the organic solvents being compared differ in their hydrogen-bond donating or accepting abilities (25,26). Thus, the solvent systems listed above are not equivalent.

From an examination of a variety of data sets in previous publications (6,9,10) and additional data in this chapter, we have concluded that when molecular size effects are properly taken into account octanol/water partition coefficients most closely correlate with skin penetration data. Group contribution data (discussed in a later section) more directly support this view. Therefore, K_{lip} may be related to the octanol/water partition coefficient by the linear free energy relationship shown below,

$$logK_{lip} = A*logK_{oct} + B \qquad (6)$$

where the slope, A, is close to unity.

Equation 2 provides an explicit form for the flux of a compound dissolved in an arbitrary vehicle with a concentration gradient, ΔC, across the membrane. Equation 2 may also be rewritten in terms of the permeability coefficient, $P = J/\Delta C$. However, ΔC is limited by the solubility of the compound in the vehicle. Furthermore, the value of P is vehicle dependent (through $K_{lip/v}$) and must be determined in each solvent system of interest. Hence, equation 2 does not suffice for predicting which compound in a group can be best delivered topically. However, a useful relationship can be developed by invoking the concept of maximum flux (9,22,27).

Consider what happens to equation 2 as ΔC is increased to the solubility limit of the compound, S_v, with sink conditions existing on the dermal side of the skin. In this case, ΔC may be replaced by S_v and the product $K_{lip/v}S_v$ may in turn be replaced by the solubility of the solute in the lipid barrier, S_{lip}. The latter substitution follows from the assumption of a single rate-limiting microphase plus rapid establishment of partition equilibrium at each interface. The chemical potential of the solute at all points exterior to the barrier must be constant, and the surface layer of the barrier lipids must, therefore, be saturated with solute. The flux arising under these conditions is known as maximum flux, and may be written as

$$J_m = (D_{lip}/h_{lip})^* S_{lip} \tag{7}$$

Maximum flux has no explicit dependence on the properties of the vehicle in which the solute is applied and in that sense is a quantity which is vehicle independent. It provides an upper limit for the penetration rate of a given permeant, which is often the parameter of interest in a drug development program. Of course every solvent interacts with the skin to some degree, so that in practice J_m is solvent dependent. The interaction may be direct (solvation or fluidization of the stratum corneum) or indirect (a vehicle-induced change in the hydration state of the stratum corneum). Despite this drawback, the concept is very useful in comparing the relative delivery rates of different compounds applied under similar conditions.

Let us now combine the preceding equations in order that the explicit dependence of P or J_m on physical properties of the permeant can be examined. Assuming the power law model (eq. 3) for the dependence of D_{lip} on molecular weight, we have

$$\log P_{lip} = A \log K_{oct} - b \log MW + \text{const} \tag{8}$$

$$\log J_m = A \log S_{oct} - b \log MW + \text{const} \tag{9}$$

where the value of the constant term is $\log D_0/h_{lip} + B$. Equation 8 follows by substituting equations 3 and 6 into equation 2 and dividing the result by ΔC. (For simplicity, the vehicle has been assumed to be aqueous.) Equation 9 results from substituting equation 3 into equation 7 and replacing S_{lip} with octanol solubility, S_{oct}, multiplied by a free energy relationship similar to equation 6. The latter substitution provides a parallel structure to the equations, making them equivalent in the low solubility limit (where the partition coefficient may be expressed as a ratio of solubilities).

The corresponding equations for the exponential model (eq. 4) are

$$\log P_{lip} = A \log K_{oct} - (b'/2.303) * MW + \text{const} \tag{10}$$

$$\log J_m = A \log S_{oct} - (b'/2.303) * MW + \text{const} \tag{11}$$

Here, molecular weight has been substituted for molecular volume and the coefficient β replaced with b'. The constant terms have a different numerical value than those in equations 8 and 9 because the values of D_0 in equations 3 and 4 are not equivalent. In the following section, we will show that the value of A in all four of the above equations is very close to unity.

One can see from these equations that the permeability coefficient is related to partition coefficient, whereas maximum flux is related to lipid solubility. Since A

$\simeq 1$, one can search for molecular weight effects in a penetration dataset by plotting either of the quantities $\log (P/K_{oct})$ or $\log (J_m/S_{oct})$ versus MW or $\log$ MW. Relationships of the type shown in equations 8–11 have been demonstrated in a variety of biological membranes and models thereof, including the gut, the cornea, erythrocytes, plant cell membranes, toad urinary bladder, liposomes, and black lipid films. These findings have been discussed by Lieb and Stein (12,13) and by Cooper and Kasting (28). Donovan and coworkers (29,30) have recently demonstrated a steep size dependence for the absorption of polyethylene glycols through rat intestinal and nasal mucosa over the molecular weight range 200–1000 Da. For some membranes, solvents other than octanol have been shown to provide a better correlation with permeability. For example, Lieb and Stein (13) found that hexadecane-water partition coefficient plus molecular size provided the best fit to human erythrocyte permeability data for 10 permeants in the range 18–102 Da. Using an exponential form for the diffusion coefficient (eq. 4), they furthermore demonstrated that molecular volume provided a better fit than did molecular weight for this dataset.

Extension to a Composite Membrane

Equations 8–11 are predicated on the assumption that diffusion across lipid barriers is the rate-limiting step for absorption through skin. While this appears to be valid for a wide variety of materials, there are three conditions under which this approximation no longer holds. These occur when the permeant is either (a) very large, (b) very hydrophilic, or (c) very lipophilic.

In the first two cases, the lipid barrier is indeed formidable, owing to either an extremely low diffusion coefficient (Case 1) or to a low lipid/water partition coefficient or lipid solubility (Case 2). In either case, the so-called "polar pathway" through the stratum corneum must be taken into account in order to properly calculate permeability (6,23). The existence of such a pathway may be inferred from permeation studies which show that for sufficiently hydrophilic permeants there is no longer a correlation between permeability and lipid/water partition coefficient (5,31). Furthermore, this pathway appears to be relatively insensitive to molecular weight for compounds ranging in size from glucose (MW 180) to neomycin B (MW 614), based on Flynn's data in hairless mouse skin.

Estimates of the magnitude of the polar pathway permeability coefficient, P_{pol}, for neutral molecules in human skin range from 1×10^{-6} cm/h (23) to about 10 times that value. Anderson et al. (6) found that permeability of sucrose in human skin to be in the range of 5×10^{-6} to 1×10^{-5} cm/h. In the hairless mouse, Flynn (31) estimated a limiting permeability of 1×10^{-5} cm/h for solutes including glucose, thiourea, and adenine arabinoside (ara-A).

Similar or slightly higher estimates have been obtained for ionic species. (Here one must remember that passive transport of anions and cations are coupled by the requirement of electroneutrality.) Tregear's data on $^{24}Na^+$ penetration through human skin in vitro and in vivo (32) lead to an estimate of NaCl permeability of about 3–6 × 10^{-5} cm/h. A similar result was obtained for NaBr (as $Na^{82}Br$). Using excised human skin, Kasting and Bowman (33,34) found the median permeability coefficient for ^{22}NaCl to be in the range 3–5 × 10^{-5} cm/h, and Kasting et al. (35) found the permeability of disodium etidronate, a highly charged anionic drug, to be about 5 × 10^{-6} cm/h. Srinivasan et al. (36) found the permeability of tetraethyl ammonium bromide (in the presence of excess chloride ion) in human skin to be about 7 × 10^{-5} cm/h. While Donnan exclusion may modulate the transport of ions in skin (37), it seems that permeabilities comparable to those of hydrophilic neutral molecules are obtained for common ionic species.

The range of values shown above, as well as our own work (33–35), shows that there is substantial variability in the penetration rates of highly polar compounds through skin. It may therefore be unwise to assign a specific permeability to the skin's polar pathway, as it will vary considerably between samples. However, it is also clear that one should consider the consequences of this pathway for compounds whose observed or calculated permeabilities are smaller than about 10^{-4} cm/h. In order to provide a working estimate for the polar pathway permeability of human skin, we propose the following range of values for P_{pol}:

$$P_{pol} \simeq \begin{cases} 1 \times 10^{-6} \, (300/MW)^{1/2} \, cm/h & \text{(lower estimate)} \\ 1 \times 10^{-5} \, (300/MW)^{1/2} \, cm/h & \text{(upper estimate)} \end{cases} \qquad (12)$$

The lower estimate should be used when one is attempting to predict in vivo delivery through healthy skin. This recommendation is based on our belief that handling-induced defects contribute to the polar pathway permeability in excised skin, especially skin that has been stored frozen.

The molecular weight dependence in equation 12 has been arbitrarily chosen as that expected for diffusion in a liquid; it may underestimate the true dependence if, for example, diffusion through a protein network is involved. Although it cannot be rigorously defended, equation 12 provides more reasonable lower bounds for the permeation of large or hydrophilic solutes than do equation 8–11 taken alone. Thus, it will comprise a piece of our final model.

In the case of very lipophilic compounds (Case 3 above), a second phenomenon comes into play. Under these circumstances, water solubility may be so low that transport across aqueous layers in the skin becomes rate limiting. The steady-state behavior of such a system may be modeled by treating the skin as a bilaminate membrane composed of a lipid layer in series with an aqueous layer (38). The reciprocal permeabilities of the lipid and aqueous layers are additive in this approach.

An upper limit to the aqueous layer permeability coefficient may be obtained by considering the thickness of this layer, h_{aq}, to be the distance from the stratum corneum to the top of the capillary bed, which is approximately 200 μm (38), and calculating the diffusion coefficient, D_{aq}, from Scheuplein's data on the diffusion of n-alkanols in the dermis. Using this approach one obtains $P_{aq} = D_{aq}/h_{aq} \simeq 0.30$ $(300/MW)^{1/2}$ cm/h. A somewhat smaller value of $P_{aq} = 0.127$ cm/h was obtained by Anderson et al. (6) by measuring the permeability of hydrocortisone esters (MW $\simeq$ 450) through delipidized human skin. The permeabilities of lipophilic n-alkanols, phenols, and hydrocortisone esters in both human skin and hairless mouse skin in vitro appear to plateau at about 0.1 cm/h, with some evidence of a weak inverse molecular weight dependence (31).

Based on these data, we estimate the aqueous layer permeability of both human and mouse skin as follows:

$$P_{aq} \simeq 0.15 \ (300/MW)^{1/2} \ \text{cm/h} \tag{13}$$

As for P_{pol}, the molecular weight dependence for P_{aq} has been assumed to be that of a liquid and may ultimately prove to be stronger than suggested by equation 13 if an appreciable fraction of the resistance resides within the keratinized cells of the stratum corneum.

There is an interesting dichotomy in the physical interpretation of what regions of the skin are actually represented by equations 12 and 13. Those holding that transport through skin is primarily paracellular consider the polar pathway to represent the small leakage current through nearly impermeable keratinized cells, in addition to that through the skin appendages (31). However, a transcellular transport model would have what we have called the lipid pathway to be the oil-water multilaminate structure of the stratum corneum, with the polar pathway being primarily appendageal. In this case, an appreciable fraction of the aqueous barrier resistance reflected by equation 13 may reside within the keratinized cells of the stratum corneum. This could explain why the measured permeability of delipidized stratum corneum was only 0.127 cm/h (6). Defects also contribute to the polar pathway permeability, as evidenced by the wide sample-to-sample variation in the penetration rate of poor skin permeants.

For the present purposes it does not matter whether the paracellular model or the transcellular model is closer to the truth. Equations 12 and 13 are simply tools for providing reasonable limits to the lipid membrane model represented by equations 8–11. By combining these equations, a composite membrane model consisting of two parallel pathways through the stratum corneum, lipid and polar, in series with an aqueous layer may be developed. Such a model does not have a simple, exact solution. However, the approximate solution of Grass et al. (39) is adequate for our purposes. In analogy to parallel and series electrical circuits, one has

$$P = \left[K_v \left(\frac{1}{P_{lip} + P_{pol}} + \frac{1}{P_{aq}} \right) \right]^{-1} \tag{14}$$

(The vehicle/water partition coefficient, K_v, has been inserted into equation 14 to generalize the result to nonaqueous systems). An equation analogous to equation

7 for the maximum flux through the composite membrane may also be derived by multiplying equation 14 by the solubility of the permeant in the vehicle, S_v, and equating the products $K_{lip}S_v/K_v$ with S_{lip} and S_v/K_v with S_w. The result is

$$J_m = \left[\frac{1}{(D_{lip}/h_{lip})\, S_{lip} + P_{pol}S_w} + \frac{1}{P_{aq}S_w} \right]^{-1}$$

(15)

Equation 15 shows explicitly the importance of adequate water solubility, S_w, in obtaining a high value of the maximum flux. The lipid pathway parameters in equation 15 can be replaced by functions of molecular weight and octanol solubility to produce an equation for the composite membrane analogous to either equation 9 or equation 11 for the simple lipid membrane.

Equations 14 and 15 represent refinements to equations 8–11 which are only required for compounds whose permeation is not rate limited by the stratum corneum lipids. The analysis in the following section will allow us to estimate the parameters of the lipid pathway.

Treatment of Ionic Equilibria

For compounds that are partially ionized, a correction must be applied in order to relate the observed permeability constant to physical properties. In light of pH-partition theory, which holds that the neutral form of a molecule is far more membrane permeable than the ionized form(s) (40), the appropriate correction is often to multiply the vehicle concentration by the fraction of nonionized drug, f, and disregard the permeation of the ionized species. This correction can be easily applied to equations 8, 10, or 14 by replacing P_{lip} with fP_{lip}. For a monoprotic acid f is given by

$$f = 1/(1 + 10^{pH-pKa})$$

(16)

and for a monoprotic base,

$$f = 1/(1 + 10^{pKa-pH})$$

(17)

In many cases, accurate predictions of flux or permeability may be made by considering only the concentration of the unionized species. (For maximum flux measurements one must ensure that the vehicle is saturated with respect to this species.) However, if the nonionized fraction is very small, the permeation of the ionic form may have to be considered (41–43).

Calculation of Lipid and Aqueous Solubilities

In the absence of experimental solubility data, the lipid solubility of many drugs may be estimated from ideal solution theory. An equation suitable for this purpose is

$$\log S_{oct} \simeq 5.91 - \log \left\{ 1 - \left[1 - \exp \left(\frac{\Delta S_f(mp - T)}{R*(273.15 + T)} \right) \right] \frac{130.22}{MW} \right\}$$

(18)

which provides an estimate of the octanol solubility (in $\mu g/ml$) at temperature, T, of a lipophilic compound of molecular weight, MW, melting point, mp, and entropy of fusion, ΔS_f (R is the gas constant, 1.987 cal/deg/mol). The density of the solution is assumed to be that of octanol, 822 g/L. This is a slightly different form from that given by Yalkowsky et al. (44). For rigid molecules, ΔS_f is approximately 13.5 cal/mol (45); for flexible molecules ΔS_f may be estimated from the number of carbon atoms and heteroatoms in the flexible chain, n, as follows (45,46).

$$\Delta S_f(cal/mol) = 13.5 + 2.5(n - 5)$$

(19)

Alternatively, S_{oct} may be estimated from the product of K_{oct} and water solubility, S_w, which may be calculated as follows:

$$\log S_w \simeq -1.00 * \log K_{oct} - 1.11 * \left[\frac{\Delta S_f(mp - T)}{R*(273.15 + T)} \right] + \log MW + 3.54$$

(20)

Equation 20 is a modification of the equation given by Yalkowsky and Valvani (45), expressing S_w in $\mu g/ml$ and allowing for temperatures other than 37°C. The important feature to note from either equations 18 or 20 is that solubility decreases with increasing melting point in an approximately exponential fashion for compounds which melt more than 10°C above the test temperature. Furthermore, attempts to lower the melting point of a compound by introduction of an alkyl chain (as in an ester prodrug) may be partially offset by an increase in fusion entropy, in addition to the penalty of added size.

EXPERIMENTAL SUPPORT OF THEORY

A number of recent studies have demonstrated the applicability of the models represented by equations 8–11 to the estimation of skin penetration rates. These results are discussed below. We also present a reanalysis of two other published datasets which lends further support to the present approach. One dataset which appears to be an outlier is also discussed.

The Solvent Nature of the Stratum Corneum Barrier—
Group Contribution Information

While it is well known that permeability coefficients of agents which cross the skin via the so-called lipid pathway depend on permeant lipophilicity, which solvent/water partitioning system should be employed to most closely predict the tendency of a permeant to partition from an aqueous vehicle to the stratum corneum barrier microenvironment? A comparison of functional group contributions to the free energy of transfer of various solutes from water to a given bulk solvent with free energy values obtained from functional group effects on permeability coefficients provides the most direct and most sensitive quantitative answer to this question.

In a series of papers, Anderson and coworkers (4,6,10) examined the effects of substituting various functional groups on the partitioning and penetration of a series of hydrocortisone esters and methyl-substituted p-cresols into human skin in vitro. The structures of these compounds are shown in Figs. 1 and 2. From permeability data, group contributions to the free energy of transfer of various functional groups from water to the rate-determining microenvironment of the stratum corneum barrier, $\Delta(\Delta G^{\ddagger})_{-x}$, were calculated according to the following relationship:

$$\Delta(\Delta G^{\ddagger})_{-x} = -2.303RT \log (P[RX]/P[RH]) \tag{21}$$

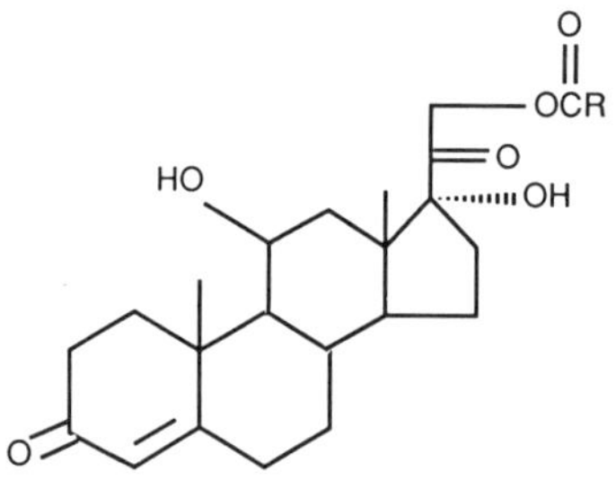

1a-k

Compound	R
a	-CH$_2$CH$_2$CONH$_2$
b	-CH$_2$CH$_2$CON(CH$_3$)$_2$
c	-CH$_2$CH$_2$COOCH$_3$
d	-CH$_2$CH$_2$COOH
e	-(CH$_2$)$_4$CH$_2$COOH
f	-(CH$_2$)$_4$CH$_2$CONH$_2$
g	-(CH$_2$)$_4$CH$_2$OH
h	-CH$_2$CH$_3$
i	-(CH$_2$)$_4$CH$_2$COOCH$_3$
j	-(CH$_2$)$_4$CH$_3$
k	-(CH$_2$)$_6$CH$_3$

Figure 1 Hydrocortisone esters studied by Anderson et al. (6).

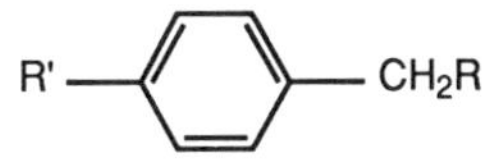

$$R' \text{—} \underset{\text{(benzene ring)}}{\bigcirc} \text{— } CH_2R$$

Compound	R'	R
a	-OH	-CONH$_2$
b	-OH	-OH
c	-OH	-COOH
d	-OH	-COOCH$_3$
e	-OH	-H
f		
g	-H	-CONH$_2$
h	-H	-OH
i	-H	-COOH
j	-H	-COOCH$_3$
k	-H	-H

Figure 2 Substituted p-cresols studied by Anderson and Raykar (10).

In a similar manner, group contributions to the standard free energy of transfer from water to various solvent environments (heptane, octanol, and stratum corneum protein domain) were obtained from equilibrium partition coefficients:

$$\Delta(\Delta G^0)_{-x} = -2.303RT \log (K^{RX}/K^{RH}) \tag{22}$$

Functional group contributions were found to be similar using both classes of compounds, suggesting that a group activity (contribution) approach for predicting permeability coefficients of closely related molecules is possible. The average group contributions obtained are shown in Table 1. Such data have important practical utility in predicting the effects of a given structural modification on a compound's permeability coefficient. For such practical purposes, a more convenient way of representing functional group effects is by means of enhancement factors (EF = P[RX]/P[RH]) as shown in Table 2. Thus, each additional methylene group incorporated into a parent compound increases its permeability coefficient by a factor of 2, whereas an additional -OH group decreases permeability coefficient by >50-fold. (These estimates do not consider molecular size effects, which would be relatively small for such changes.)

The group contribution data in Table 1 are shown graphically in Figure 3. From these "selectivity profiles," we can determine the degree to which a given solvent environment resembles the barrier microenvironment of the skin. Not surprisingly, the selectivity of the protein domain of human stratum corneum toward solutes varying in structure does not closely resemble that of the lipid barrier. Perhaps more surprising to some, however, may be the fact that the uptake of the

Table 1 Thermodynamic Group Contributions (cal/mol) to the Free Energy of Transfer of Various Functional Groups from Water to Hydrocarbon, Octanol, Stratum Corneum Protein Domain, or the Stratum Corneum Transport Barrier at 37°C

Functional group	Heptane	Octanol	Stratum Corneum	
			protein domain	transport barrier
-CH$_2$-	-800	-710	-210	-440
-CONH$_2$	6600	2800	660	3050
-CON(CH$_3$)$_2$	3500	1400	160	2600
-COOCH$_3$	1650	810	160	1250
-COOH	6050	1500	30	1950
-OH	5750	2350	580	2450

majority of solutes examined in these studies could be accounted for by partitioning into the protein domain alone. That is, partition coefficients into untreated stratum corneum were similar to those obtained using delipidized stratum corneum (4). These data, therefore, demonstrate conclusively that stratum corneum/water partition coefficients are not useful in a quantitative sense for predicting relative permeabilities.

Clearly, the transport selectivity profile more closely resembles the octanol/water profile than that of heptane/water. From this we conclude that the barrier microenvironment of the stratum corneum lipid pathway is capable of participating in hydrogen-bonding interactions and, thus, does not exhibit the properties expected if the barrier were the hydrocarbon interior of lipid bilayers.

A closer examination of the group contributions in Table 1 and Figure 3 reveals significant discrepancies, however, between the values obtained from transport data and those obtained from octanol/water partition coefficients. These differences suggest that octanol does not resemble the barrier domain *in detail*. Thus,

Table 2 Functional Group Enhancement Factors to the Permeability Coefficient from Aqueous Vehicles

Functional group	EF
-CH$_2$-	2
-CONH$_2$	1/143
-CON(CH$_3$)$_2$	1/67
-COOCH$_3$	1/8
-COOH	1/24
-OH	1/53

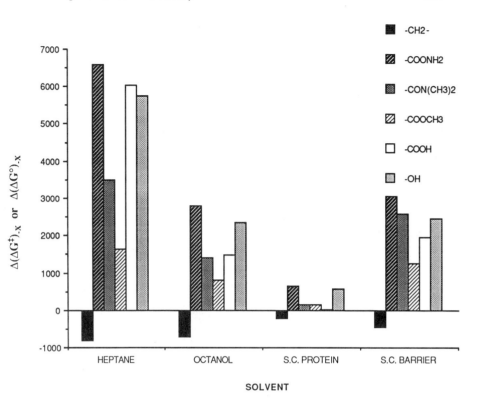

Figure 3 Solvent selectivity for functional groups based on the study of hydrocortisone esters and substituted p-cresols. The data are those from Table 1. (From Ref. 10.)

the methylene group contribution to transport (–440 cal/mol) is significantly less favorable than its contribution to transfer from water to octanol (–710 cal/mol). This difference may reflect a higher degree of order within the transport barrier, which would contribute to a less favorable entropy of permeant transfer (47). Also differing significantly are the free energies for the –COOCH$_3$ and –CON(CH$_3$)$_2$ groups calculated from permeability coefficients in comparison to the corresponding values obtained from octanol/water partitioning. As both groups are hydrogen acceptors, these discrepancies, if real, may indicate that the barrier microenvironment is a poor hydrogen bond donor relative to octanol. Nevertheless, in the absence of a superior model solvent system, the similarity in their selectivity profiles in Figure 3 suggests that octanol/water partition coefficients should be useful at least semiquantitatively in predicting permeability coefficients.

Correlations of Various Permeability Coefficient Data Sets
Using the Proposed Model

Consistent with the group contributions, the permeability coefficients obtained by Anderson and coworkers for hydrocortisone esters and substituted p-cresols in human skin (6,10) were highly correlated with octanol/water partition coefficients, yielding log-log plots with near unit slope in correspondence with equations 2 and 6. However, the line representing the hydrocortisone ester permeability data fell approximately two orders of magnitude below the line for the substituted p-cresols. In order to collapse these two relationships onto a single line, a strong molecular weight dependence was required. The coefficients of the fit to equation 8 and a plot of the relationship derived for permeability coefficient are shown in Fig. 4a. (Correlations were also obtained using heptane/water and stratum corneum/water partition coefficients, but the log-log slopes were far from unity and the log-log plots of hydrocortisone esters versus stratum corneum/water partition coefficients were distinctly nonlinear.)

Itoh and coworkers (11) studied the in vitro penetration of 13 compounds chosen from the steroid, NSAID, and paraben classes through shed snake skin. Permeability coefficients were calculated and the results analyzed according to penetration models of the form given in equations 8 and 10. The results (after conversion to our units) were A = 1.10, b = 3.72 and const = 3.46 (eq. 8) or A = 1.07, b' = 0.0145 and const = −3.71 (eq. 10) with $r^2 = 0.94$ in both cases. A plot of the former relationship is shown in Fig. 5.

Scheuplein and coworkers (48) reported the absorption of 14 corticosteroids through human skin in vitro in an oft-cited study. They found only weak correlation of permeability coefficient with either stratum corneum/water, amyl acetate/water, or hexadecane/water partition coefficient. On the basis of the observed permeability coefficients and some very long apparent lag times for the more polar steroids (e.g., $t_l = 220$ h for cortisone), they interpreted the results on the basis of diffusion coefficients which decreased markedly with increasing polarity of the molecules.

We find that either of equations 8 or 10 offers a more satisfactory explanation for these data. Table 3 gives the data from Scheuplein's study (48) along with the molecular weight and octanol/water partition coefficient for each compound. Fig. 6 shows a plot of the data according to equation 10, using an assumed value of unity for the coefficient A. Since the molecular weight range is narrow (270–362 Da), an adequate relationship could also be developed for this dataset without incorporating the molecular weight term; nevertheless, it is intriguing that a least squares fit to the data in Fig. 6 yields a molecular weight dependence which is comparable to that observed in the other penetration studies.

An outlier to this pattern of agreement with equations 8 or 10 may be found in the work of Michaels et al. (22). In this study, the human in vitro skin penetration rate of eleven drugs with widely varying properties from saturated aqueous

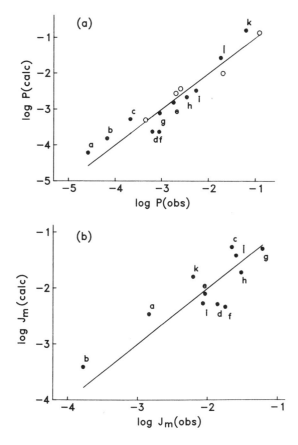

Figure 4 (a) Observed permeability coefficients versus those calculated from the equation $\log P = 0.87 \log K_{oct} - 4.6 \log MW + 6.80$ for the 16 compounds studied by Anderson and Raykar (10). ● — hydrocortisone esters; ○ — substituted p-cresols. (b) Hydrocortisone ester penetration data from Anderson and Raykar replotted in terms of maximum flux (calculations are shown in Table 6).

solutions was determined. The calculated permeability coefficients were well correlated with mineral oil/water partition coefficient. Substitution of octanol/water partition coefficient for mineral oil/water partition coefficient, with or without a molecular weight term, fails to provide as good a fit to these data as the original treatment.

A second dataset with a somewhat different physical properties dependence is Scheuplein's dilute, aqueous n-alkanol series (38). These data are shown in Table 4. The n-alkanol permeabilities follow equation 8 or 10 quite closely; however,

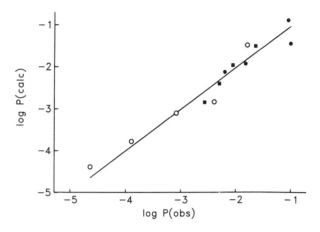

Figure 5 Observed permeability coefficients versus those calculated from the equation log P = 1.11 log K_{oct} - 3.72 log MW + 3.45 for 13 compounds from the steroid, NSAID and paraben families (11). Shed snake skin was the model membrane in this study. ● — NSAIDS; ○ — steroids; ■ — parabens.

Table 3 Percutaneous Absorption of Steroids

Compound	MW (Da)	mp (°C)	$K_{oct}{}^a$	P × 10⁵ cm/h
Estradiol	272	176	490	30
Estrone	270	260	575	360
Estriol	288	282	27	4
Hydrocortisone	362	215	34	0.3
Testosterone	288	155	2042	40
Progesterone	314	128	7410	150
17-α-Hydroxyprogesterone	330	222	1860[b]	60
Cortisone	360	222	30	1
Corticosterone	346	181	93	6
Cortexone	330	141	759	45
Pregnenolone	316	193	8130[c]	150
Hydroxypregnenolone	332	250	2040[c]	60
Cortexolone	346	215	288	7.5
Aldosterone	360	110	12[b]	0.3

[a]Values taken from Pomona College Medicinal Chemistry (MEDCHEM) database unless otherwise noted.
[b]Estimated value.
[c] Calculated according to MEDCHEM CLOGP program, Vers. 3.54.
Source: Data from Ref. 48.

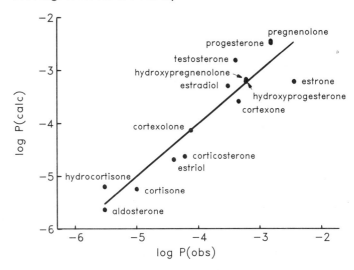

Figure 6 Observed permeability coefficients versus those calculated from the equation log P = log K_{oct} – (0.0223/2.303) MW – 2.26 for the 14 steroids studied by Scheuplein et al. (48). The data are given in Table 3.

Table 4 Percutaneous Absorption of n-Alkanols from Dilute Aqueous Solutions

Compound	MW (Da)	log K_{oct}[b]	P × 10^3 cm/h	P_{lip}[a] × 10^3 cm/h
Water	18	–1.38	0.5	0.5
Methanol	32	–0.77	0.5	0.5
Ethanol	46	–0.31	0.8	0.8
Propanol	60	0.25	1.2	1.2
Butanol	74	0.88	2.5	2.5
Pentanol	88	1.56	6	6
Hexanol	102	2.03	13	14
Heptanol	116	2.72	32	37
Octanol	130	2.97	52	67
Nonanol	144	4.26	60	83
Decanol	158	4.57	80	130

[a]Calculated from P by subtracting the effect of an aqueous boundary layer according to equations 13 and 14.
[b]Values taken from the Pomona College Medicinal Chemistry database.
Source: Data from Ref. 38.

the coefficients of optimum fit, A and b (or A and b′), are quite different from those already presented. Either a significantly higher value of b (or b′) or a lower value of A is required to model these data, even after correcting for boundary layer effects. This difference is examined in a later section.

Maximum Flux Estimates

The utility of the size and octanol solubility approach for estimating maximum flux through skin was demonstrated by Kasting et al. (9), using a human in vitro skin penetration model and 36 drug and druglike compounds. In this study, molecular size was taken to be the van der Waals volume of the molecule. The solubility factor alone explained about 53% of the variance in J_m values in this study and the volume term another 21%, giving an overall r^2 value for the fit of 0.74. A plot of the relationship developed between J_m, S_{oct} and molecular volume is shown in Fig. 7.

Roy and Flynn (43) studied the physical properties and in vitro human skin penetration rates of six narcotic analgesics from saturated aqueous solutions. Monotonic relationships were found between permeability coefficient and either solubility parameter or octanol/water partition coefficient, and the lower melting compounds were found to have higher values of P. We tested the present model on

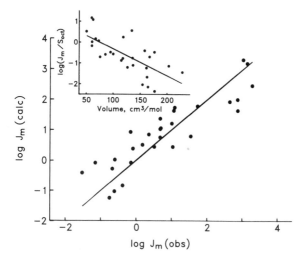

Figure 7 Observed versus calculated values of maximum flux for 29 compounds from Kasting et al. (9). The compounds tested as salts have been omitted (28). The calculated values were obtained from the regression equation $\log J_m = \log S_{oct} - (0.0295/2.303)*v - 2.04$, where v is molecular volume in cm^3/mol. The inset shows the volume dependence of normalized flux according to the model.

Table 5 Skin Penetration of Narcotic Analgesics

Compound	MW (Da)	mp (°C)	K_{oct}	S_w µg/ml	S_{oct}^a mg/ml	$P \times 10^5$ cm/h	J_m µg/cm²/h
Morphine	285	255	4.2	720	3	0.93	0.007
Hydromorphone	285	266	7.7	2250	17.3	1.41	0.032
Codeine	299	155	17.7	2140	38	4.91	0.105
Meperidine	247	35	529	6550	3460	336	22
Fentanyl	336	84	23390	51	1190	560	0.285
Sufentanil	388	97	38621	34	1310	1200	0.409

^{a}Calculated as $K_{oct}*S_w$.
Source: Data from Ref. 43.

this dataset, using equation 11 and the values in Table 5. The regression equation and a plot of the derived relationship are shown in Fig. 8. According to this model, meperidine had the highest flux because of its low molecular weight and high solubility in the barrier lipids (reflected by a large value of S_{oct}). Fentanyl and sufentanil were the next best owing to their high solubility. Note the inverse relationship between melting point and octanol solubility of these compounds.

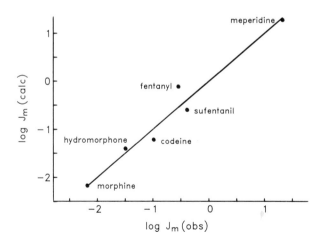

Figure 8 Observed values of maximum flux versus those calculated from the equation $\log J_m = S_{oct} - (0.0238/2.303)\ MW - 2.70$ for the six narcotic analgesics listed in Table 5. (The data were taken from the study by Roy and Flynn [43]).

In general, structural features which promote partitioning of a permeant from water into the stratum corneum barrier domain and thereby increase permeability coefficients (e.g., increasing lipophilicity) are not expected to have a parallel influence on maximum flux. This is because the maximum flux reflects the favorability of transfer of the permeant from its crystalline phase to the stratum corneum barrier microenvironment whereas permeability coefficients, at least from aqueous vehicles, reflect solute transfer from water to the stratum corneum barrier. Since the crystalline phase of any organic solute more closely resembles the stratum corneum lipid barrier than does water, the effects of changes in solute structure on maximum flux will be diminished in comparison to their effects on permeability coefficients. This represents a significant limitation to the degree of enhancement in maximum flux achievable using the prodrug approach.

To illustrate this point, the permeability coefficient description of hydrocortisone ester penetration summarized in Fig. 4a may be reexamined in terms of maximum flux. The relevant solubility data for these compounds (B. D. Anderson, unpublished) are shown in Table 6, along with permeability coefficients and calculated values of maximum flux. A plot of the maximum flux relationship is shown in Fig. 4b. Examining these data, we see that whereas the permeability coefficients spanned a range of 2400-fold, the maximum flux values (the product of the permeability coefficient and aqueous solubility) vary in magnitude by only 350-fold. There is furthermore a completely different rank ordering of compounds according to this criterion than was exhibited by the permeability coefficient. The more lipophilic compounds have the higher permeability coefficients, but the more octanol-soluble ones exhibit the higher maximum flux, provided that molecular size does not vary significantly.

The compounds in Table 6 were prepared to obtain group contribution information. They were not intended to be prodrugs of hydrocortisone for enhanced transport; hence their skin permeation rates were not compared directly with the parent compound under maximum flux conditions. However, indirect comparisons performed in one of our laboratories (BDA) suggest that it might be very difficult to develop a 21-ester of hydrocortisone with a dramatically higher maximum flux than hydrocortisone.

The naproxen derivatives discussed in a following section present a somewhat more optimistic picture for the prodrug approach to enhanced skin penetration. However, even in this more favorable case the maximum flux enhancements attained in vitro were no more than a factor of 10 (except for the unstable aldehyde derivative), and the flux enhancements under small-dose conditions in vitro and in vivo were smaller yet. The preferred derivatives were those which led to the maximum increase in lipid solubility with a minimal increase in size.

Table 6 Skin Penetration of Hydrocortisone Esters

ID Compound	MW (Da)	mp (°C)	K_{oct}	S_{oct}^a mg/ml	S_w μg/ml	$P \times 10^5$ cm/h	$J_m^b \times 10^3$ μg/cm²/h
a - $CH_2CH_2CONH_2$	461	227	27	1.5	56	2.6	1.5
b - $CH_2CH_2CON(CH_3)_2$	489	223	108	0.27	2.5	6.7	0.17
c - $CH_2CH_2COOCH_3$	476	143	380	39.5	104	21	21.8
d - CH_2CH_2COOH	462	171	130	2.9	22	63	13.9
e - $(CH_2)_4CH_2COOH$	506	112	1800	9.2	5.1	180	9.2
f - $(CH_2)_4CH_2CONH_2$	503	185	200	4	20	89	17.8
g - $(CH_2)_4CH_2OH$	478	144	610	40	66	91	60
h - CH_2CH_3	418	196	990	8.7	8.8	340	30
i - $(CH_2)_4CH_2COOCH_3$	518	142	5000	8	1.6	540	8.9
j - $(CH_2)_4CH_3$	460	152	30000	42	1.4	1800	25
k - $(CH_2)_6CH_3$	488	115	310000	31	0.10^c	6200	6.2

[a]Calculated as $K_{oct}*S_w$.
[b]Calculated as $P*S_w$.
[c]Calculated according to equations 19 and 20.
Source: Data from Ref. 6.

Systematic Analysis of Skin Penetration Datasets

In order to compare results from the several studies which have been discussed and to simplify the confusing variety of equations and exponents obtained, we reanalyzed each of the above datasets and the additional results in the section entitled Application to the Development of Topical NSAID Prodrugs on a common basis. The results are shown in Table 7. We used molecular weight or its logarithm (rather than molecular volume) for the size-dependent term in equations 8–11 and fixed the coefficient of the partition coefficient term at unity; i.e., A = 1. The former approximation was adequate for the present purposes based on the comparisons made by Kasting et al. (9) and additional tests with the data in the above mentioned section. The latter choice was arrived at by first fitting each of the datasets to these equations via multiple linear regression and examining the coefficient of the partition coefficient or solubility term. Two of the datasets (10,48) yielded A values slightly less than one, two (9,11) yielded A slightly greater than one, and one (43) yielded A almost identically one. (The naproxen, NSAID, and alkanol datasets were not tested in this fashion owing to collinearity between the molecular weight and log K_{oct} values.) However, in every case the value of A so obtained was not significantly different from one and forcing A = 1 did not appreciably degrade the fit.

Table 7 shows that strong molecular weight dependencies were calculated for all of the datasets and that, except for the alkanols (discussed below), either the power law or exponential form for molecular weight dependence could be used to describe them. The coefficient b in the power law fits (again excepting the alkanols) ranged from 3.6 to 7.9 and the corresponding parameter, b', in the exponential fits ranged from 0.014 to 0.024. Considering that the stronger molecular weight dependences were obtained on datasets which were limited in either molecular weight range or number of compounds, the agreement between the different studies was quite satisfactory.

The n-alkanol permeabilities clearly had a different physical properties dependence than the other datasets. To show this we first corrected the observed permeabilities according to equations 13 and 14 to obtain P_{lip}. (This corrected for the aqueous boundary layer effects evident with the longer chain alcohols.) A straight line was fit to the experimental octanol/water partition coefficient versus chain length data in Table 4 to obtain smoothed values of K_{oct}. (This eliminated the apparent anomalies in K_{oct} for octanol and nonanol.) We then fit equations 8 and 10 to the corrected data using several different values of A. With A = 1 a much stronger molecular weight dependence was required for the alkanols than for the other datasets (see Table 7). Furthermore, the exponential model (eq. 10) provided a significantly better fit to the data than did the power law model (eq. 8). We concluded that neither equation 8 nor equation 10 was completely correct over the full range of molecular weights provided by the alkanols in combination with the other datasets (18–518 Da).

Table 7 Regression Equations for Skin Penetration Datasets

Ref.	Eq. No.	Parameters[a]			n	s	r^2
		b	b'	Const			
10	8	5.04	—	7.57	16	0.36	0.92
	10	—	0.0185	−2.09	16	0.37	0.92
11	8	3.63	—	3.53	13	0.27	0.93
	10	—	0.0144	−3.54	13	0.28	0.92
48	8	6.17	—	9.08	14	0.38	0.84
	10	—	0.0193	−3.70	14	0.38	0.84
38	8	8.12	—	2.90	11	0.26	0.91
	10	—	0.0528	−1.67	11	0.15	0.97
9	9	3.56	—	4.78	29	0.63	0.78
	11	—	0.0156	−1.95	29	0.64	0.78
43	9	7.59	—	12.95	6	0.26	0.94
	11	—	0.0238	−2.70	6	0.27	0.94
Naproxen compounds (p. 150)	9	4.92	—	7.94	18	0.27	0.83
	11	—	0.0178	−1.92	18	0.28	0.82
NSAIDS (p. 148–150)	9	5.40	—	9.07	31	0.42	0.84
	11	—	0.0197	−1.71	31	0.42	0.84

[a] The value of A was set equal to one in these fits.
[b] Salts omitted as in Ref. 28

In spite of these difficulties, it seemed worthwhile to combine the results of the above analyses into an equation which would reflect a best estimate of human skin permeability to topically applied drugs, based on the available data. In order to arrive at an equation which would conservatively estimate permeabilities for compounds having physical properties within the range exhibited by most drug molecules and which would extrapolate reasonably outside of this range, we proceeded as follows: Using the value $A = 1$ for the dependence of P on partition coefficient (or J_m on solubility), we found that the exponential model with the value $b' = 0.018$ best represented the molecular weight dependence for all of the datasets. Using $A = 1$ and $b' = 0.018$, the best-fit constant in equation 10 or 11 was determined for each dataset. These values were then averaged to obtain the final equation. The result of this process is shown in equation 23:

$$\log P_{lip} = \log K_{oct} - (0.018/2.303) \; MW - 2.87 \tag{23}$$

When combined with equations 12–14, equation 23 completes the composite membrane model for skin already discussed. These equations provide a method for estimating the permeability coefficient in skin of a wide range of compounds from just the molecular weight and octanol/water partition coefficient of the compound. Given the octanol solubility of the compound and the value of one more parameter (B or D_0/h_{lip}, see eqs. 4–7) maximum flux for the composite membrane model can also be calculated by making the appropriate substitutions into equation 15. When the lipid barrier is rate limiting, this simplifies to equation 24, which is an explicit form of equation 11:

$$\log J_m = \log S_{oct} - (0.018/2.303) \; MW - 2.87 \tag{24}$$

Equations 23 and 24 represent our current best estimate of the permeability characteristics of the lipid pathway of human stratum corneum.

APPLICATION TO THE DEVELOPMENT OF TOPICAL NSAID PRODRUGS

Design of NSAID Database

Nonsteroidal anti-inflammatory drugs (NSAIDs) are widely used for the treatment of pain and inflammation. Given orally, they are effective systemic medications, the chief limitation to their use being the degree of gastrointestinal irritation produced by chronic exposure to anti-inflammatory doses of the drugs. In Europe, there is an appreciable, but fragmented, topical antirheumatic market, with ibuprofen being the most popular agent.

This section reviews the results of a research program aimed at developing topical NSAID therapy with improved safety and efficacy. The data have been presented previously (49–52). The approach taken was to chemically modify existing NSAIDs in a bioreversible fashion in order to enhance their skin penetration rates, and concurrently to monitor their potential for skin irritation. Two particularly promising compounds, the *sec*-butyl ester of naproxen and the 2-methylbutyrate ester of naproxol (the alcohol analog of naproxen), emerged from this program. The theory described in the previous two sections suggested the following strategy for the design of prodrugs with improved skin penetration properties: Prepare bioreversible derivatives which maximize lipid solubility with a minimal increment in molecular size. In practice, this can be achieved by converting polar functionalities in the parent molecule to less polar forms or by adding flexible chains which disrupt crystallinity. The most successful compounds described below incorporate both of these features.

Experimental Section

Materials

S(+)-Naproxen, aspirin, ketoprofen, and indomethacin were purchased from the Sigma Chemical Co. Ibuprofen, sulindac, and piroxicam were extracted from Motrin (Upjohn), Clinoril (Merck), and Feldene (Pfizer) tablets, respectively. The structures of these compounds are shown in Fig. 9. Derivatives of the drugs were designed and synthesized at Miami Valley Laboratories by L. G. Mueller. Much of the derivatization was conducted with naproxen, yielding the structures shown in Fig. 10. The derivatives were characterized by [^{1}H]-NMR (nuclear magnetic resonance) spectroscopy and gave spectra consistent with the assigned structures. The purity of each compound was established by HPLC, thin layer or gas chromatographic analysis (>95%) and by elemental analysis. Optical purity was also confirmed for selected naproxen derivatives to determine that the synthetic conditions did not induce racemization of the S(+)-naproxen.

Physical Properties and Skin Penetration Results

Steady-state penetration rates through excised human skin, solubilities in propylene glycol, octanol, and isopropyl myristate, molecular volumes, and octanol/water partition coefficients were determined as described by Kasting et al. (9). Solvent solubility and in vitro skin penetration analyses were conducted using reversed-phase HPLC (Zorbax-ODS) combined with ultraviolet (UV) detection at 254 nm. The mobile phase was comprised of acetonitrile-water (with 0.1% acetic acid to suppress ionization) and, depending on the elution time of the solute, the composition varied from 50 to 80% acetonitrile. Under these conditions, detection limits ranged from 0.1–0.5 µg/ml. For the ester prodrugs, penetration was calculated as the sum of the prodrug and parent parent compound found in the receptor solutions.

The skin penetration experiments employed dermatomed skin (0.25 mm) from human cadavers mounted in glass diffusion cells maintained at 37°C. At least five replicates were performed for each compound studied. The stratum corneum was dosed with 1 ml/cm^2 of a saturated solution of drug in propylene glycol, providing

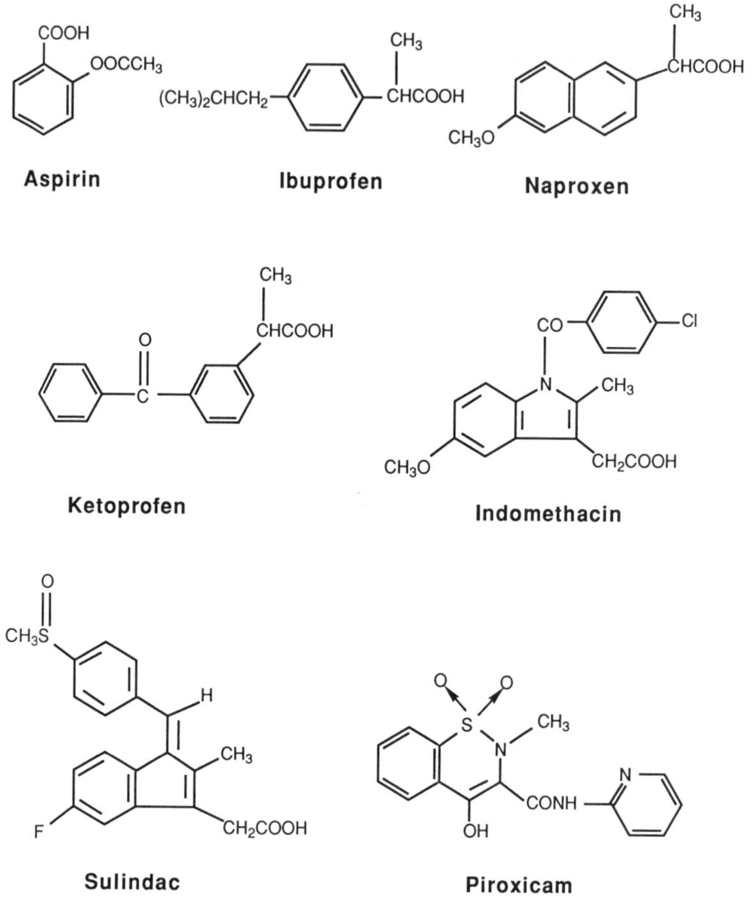

Figure 9 Parent structures for the NSAID prodrug studies.

an effectively infinite reservoir of drug for the 72-h duration of the experiment. The dermis was bathed with a 1:1 (v:v) solution of distilled water and ethanol containing 0.02% sodium azide to inhibit bacterial growth. This solution was replaced at 0, 6, 24, 48, and 72 h and assayed for the penetrant. After 24 h, the penetration rates were close to their final values, although they still increased gradually with time. The steady-state flux J_m was calculated from the amount of drug penetrated between 48 and 72 h.

Subsequent to these measurements we learned more about the effects of ethanol on skin through our own work and that of others (53–55). In these studies, high concentrations of ethanol were shown to provide a strong enhancing effect on the

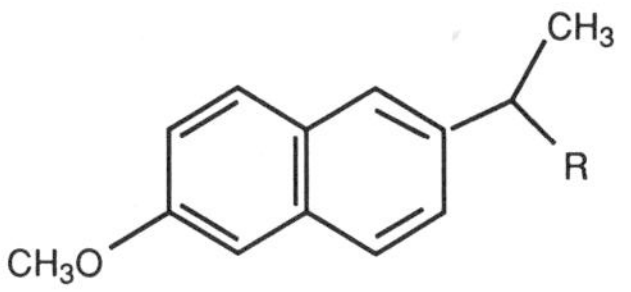

R

COOH (naproxen)

Esters

COO-ethyl
COO-isopropyl
COO-n-butyl
COO-(S,R)-sec-butyl *
COO-(S)-sec-butyl
COO-tert-butyl
COO-crotyl
COO-n-hexyl
COO-2-hexyl *
COO ⌐

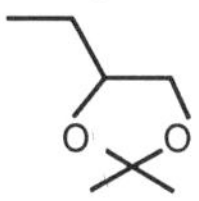

COO-1-glyceryl *
COOCH$_2$SCH$_3$
COOCH$_2$S(O)CH$_3$ *

Oxidation state analogs

CH$_2$OH
CHO

Reverse esters

CH$_2$O-acetate
CH$_2$O-2-methylbutyrate*

* 50:50 mixture of diastereomers

Figure 10 Naproxen derivatives prepared for skin penetration and metabolism studies.

permeation of lipophilic solutes through mouse or rat skin. Our own work (G. B. Kasting, unpublished) showed that the same was true for human skin for sufficiently lipophilic permeants. This may be due in part to the diminished effect of the aqueous skin layers (see eq. 13) in the presence of ethanol. Thus, the conditions employed in this study may have biased the results in favor of the more lipophilic compounds. However, since these compounds were already shown to be non-optimal under the study conditions, we believe that valid conclusions may still be drawn from the work.

In Vitro and In Vivo Bioconversion Measurements

In vitro bioconversion of selected naproxen esters was performed using a medium of reconstituted lyophilized human serum (Ortho Diagnostics) and a human skin-serum homogenate. Homogenates were prepared using one part frozen ($-70°C$) dermatomed human cadaver skin and nine parts reconstituted serum. A satisfactory skin-serum suspension was obtained using approximately 20 15-s bursts in a sonicating homogenizer. Samples were cooled in ice between sonic bursts to minimize heat denaturation.

Aliquots of cold serum or homogenate (0.9 ml) were combined with 0.1 ml ethanol containing 0.1 µmol naproxen prodrug and 0.5 µmol internal standard (ibuprofen) and incubated at 37°C for 0.25, 0.5, 1.0, 3.0, and 6.0 h. Liquid-liquid extraction of acidified samples into dichloromethane, followed by evaporation and subsequent reconstitution in mobile phase was done to prepare the samples for gradient elution HPLC analysis. This extraction procedure was found not to induce ester hydrolysis to the parent carboxylic acid.

A preliminary in vivo absorption and bioconversion study was conducted in male Wistar rats following topical application of ethanol-propylene glycol (1:1) solutions containing 5% (w/w) of either naproxen (3), its *sec*-butyl ester (20), naproxol (30), or its 2-methylbutyrate (33). Aliquots (0.2 ml) of each solution were topically applied to a shaven, depilated area (10 cm^2) of the back. The total applied dose was 30 mg compound/kg. One animal was used for each test solution and time point. Sacrifice times were 1, 3, 6, 12, and 24 h. Plasma samples were prepared for HPLC analysis the same as for the in vitro studies, with indomethacin (0.1 µmol) serving as the internal standard.

Variation in Data

Naproxen and its derivatives were tested in three separate skin penetration experiments, each one employing skin from a different donor. Within each experiment five to 10 penetrants were tested, with five to eight replicates per penetrant. Some of the compounds were tested in more than one experiment to allow a comparison between the different skin samples. The results showed that the three skin samples were of comparable permeability, so the results of the three experiments were combined.

The distribution of skin penetration data was found to be approximately lognormal. Therefore, results for each penetrant were calculated as geometric means and dispersions. The dispersions so obtained ranged (in base 10 logarithmic units) from 0.13 to 0.45 and had a pooled value of $s_{\log J} = 0.285$. This was similar to the value $s_{\log J} = 0.30$ obtained by the same method in an earlier study (9). Hence, the relative standard error of the reported flux values (for n = 5) is $10^{+0.285/\sqrt{5}}$, or about 30%.

In the course of obtaining the full 31 compound NSAID dataset, skin from four additional donors was employed. Limited reproducibility tests indicated that the permeability of these samples differed from those used in the naproxen work by as much as a factor of two. This factor contributed to greater departures from the theoretical model for the larger dataset.

Results of Physical Property and In Vitro Skin Penetration Measurements

Seven widely used NSAIds and a total of 26 derivatives thereof were evaluated. The derivatives consisted of esters and oxidation state analogues, all derivatization being conducted at the free carboxyl group. Six ethyl esters, three alcohol analogues, and one aldehyde were prepared. Seventeen of the derivatives were related to naproxen, which was selected for a detailed study because its small size and high melting point made it an ideal candidate for the prodrug approach. The compounds, along with their physical properties and steady-state penetration rates through human skin under maximum flux conditions are listed in Tables 8–10.

Parent NSAIDs, Ethyl Esters and Alcohol Analogues

The seven parent NSAIDs showed a range of flux through skin of nearly 10^4 (Table 8). The large and poorly octanol-soluble drugs sulindac and indomethacin penetrated most slowly, whereas the smaller, more soluble compounds (ibuprofen, ketoprofen, and aspirin) penetrated best. These findings agree qualitatively with the predictions of the model discussed in previous sections. With the exception of naproxol (30), the alcohol analogue of naproxen, simple ethyl ester derivatives or alcohol analogues of these drugs afforded the best marginal improvements in penetration rate (Tables 9 and 10).

The findings with the ethyl esters can be interpreted as resulting from offsetting effects of solubility and size. Although substantial decreases in melting points were obtained through esterification, the increases in octanol solubility were substantially less than those predicted by equation 18. The increase in molecular weight of 28 Da for each ethyl ester over its parent acid (corresponding to a molecular volume difference of about 21 cm^3/mol) may have been sufficient to counteract the increased solubility of the ester, resulting in little or no change in skin penetration rate.

The results with the alcohol analogs were surprising. In the case of naproxol, the increase in octanol solubility without an increase in molecular volume resulted in an approximately fourfold penetration enhancement, as expected. Ibuprofen alcohol (12) and ketoprofen alcohol (14) did not penetrate better than the parent drugs, even though the changes in their physical properties were similar to those seen for naproxol. In the case of ibuprofen, this inconsistency might well result from the fact that ibuprofen penetrated better than expected—with time its flux tended to deviate sharply upward from the steady state, indicative of possible

Table 8 Physical Properties and Steady State Skin Penetration Rates for Various NSAIDs

NSAID	MW (Da)	mp (°C)	log K_{oct}[a]	Solubility (mg/ml)			J_m $\mu g/cm^2/h$
				PG[b]	Octanol	
1. Aspirin	180	131	1.1	NM[c]	NM[c]		90[d]
2. Ibuprofen	206	76	3.51	220	250		350
3. Naproxen	230	155	3.26	18	30		5.8
4. Ketoprofen	254	93	3.00	125	200		24
5. Indomethacin	358	159	3.08	8.2	12		0.25
6. Sulindac	356	180	4.53	12	6.7		0.03
7. Piroxicam	331	198	0.05	1.7	4.1		0.73

[a]Octanol-water partition coefficient.
[b]Propylene glycol.
[c]Not measured.
[d]Tested with lower dose (20 μl at 0 and 24 h).

Table 9 Physical Properties and Steady-State Skin Penetration Rates for NSAID Derivatives

NSAID	MW (Da)	mp (°C)	log K_{oct}[a]	Solubility (mg/ml)		J_m μg/cm²/h
				PG[b]	Octanol	
8. Aspirin ethyl ester	208	oil	2.05	NM	NM	90[d]
9. Ibuprofen ethyl ester	234	oil	4.46	40	270	150
10. Ibuprofen 2-pyridylmethyl ester	297	oil	4.28	610	140	51
11. Ibuprofen 2-methoxyphenyl ester	312	oil	5.22	18	360	11
12. Ibuprofen alcohol	192	oil	3.60	M[e]	M[e]	71
13. Ketoprofen ethyl ester	282	oil	3.95	102	520	20
14. Ketoprofen alcohol	240	oil	3.09	75	M[e]	25
15. Indomethacin ethyl ester	386	96	3.96	0.7	5.3	0.02
16. Sulindac ethyl ester	384	128	5.48	5.3	7.3	0.05

[a-d]See Table 8.
[e]Miscible. Compound 12 was tested at 50% w/w.

Table 10 Physical Properties and Steady-State Skin Penetration Rates for Naproxen and Derivatives

Compound	MW (Da)	mp (°C)	log K_{oct}[a]	Solubility (mg/ml)			J_m µg/cm²/h
				PG[b]	Octanol		
Naproxen (3)[c]	230	155	3.26	19	30		5.8
Naproxen esters							
17. ethyl	258	75	4.21	4.6	52		3.1
18. isopropyl	272	64	4.62	10	95		9.9
19. n-butyl	286	67	5.27	2.1	38		2.2
20. dl-sec-butyl[d]	286	oil	5.15	28	650		49
21. d-sec-butyl[e]	286	45	5.15	15	150		18
22. tert-butyl	286	93	5.24	1.5	26		0.4
23. crotyl	284	60	4.94	4.4	51		4.0
24. n-hexyl	312	42	6.32	6.2	300		4.9
25. dl-2-hexyl	312	oil	6.20	42	M[f]		32
26. solketal	344	49	3.92	<46	37		3.2
27. glyceryl	304	61	1.85	330	120		6.6
28. methylthiomethyl	290	78	4.50	3.6	20		2.6
29. methylsulfinylmethyl	306	112	2.26	1.0	10		0.6
Oxidation state derivatives							
30. naproxol	216	87	3.35	26	63		21
31. naproxen aldehyde	214	62	3.02	76	350		160
32. naproxol acetate	258	61	4.21	14	88		14
33. naproxol 2-methylbutyrate	300	oil	5.68	28	M		53

[a-c]See Table 8.
[d]51:49 mixture of S,S and S,R diastereomers.
[e]90:10 mixture of S,S and S,R diastereomers.
[f]Miscible.

barrier damage under the conditions of the test. The finding for ketoprofen alcohol, however, was not well explained by the model.

Ibuprofen Derivatives

Table 9 summarizes the results for several ibuprofen derivatives. None of these materials penetrated the skin as well as ibuprofen, a finding which was consistent with the model and the atypical behavior of ibuprofen discussed above.

Naproxen and Derivatives

The results for naproxen and 17 derivatives are shown in Table 10. The penetration rates spanned a range of more than two orders of magnitude about that of the parent compound. Several of the compounds penetrated the skin markedly better than naproxen. These included the aldehyde analog (**31**; twenty-eight–fold), naproxol (**30**; fourfold), naproxol-2-methylbutyrate (**33**; ninefold), naproxen-*sec*-butyl ester (**20**; eightfold), and naproxen-2-hexyl ester (**25**; sixfold).

The better-penetrating compounds fell into two categories: oxidation state analogues of reduced polarity (**30** and **31**) and small, chiral esters (**20, 25, 33**). The aldehyde (**31**) was the best skin penetrant, but was too unstable to be of practical interest. The alcohol (**30**) was of greater interest, particularly since bioconversion studies showed that this compound reverted to naproxen in vivo. The esters, however, showed even more promise. Compound **20**, the *sec*-butyl ester, is the smallest possible chiral ester of naproxen, and compound **33**, the 2-methylbutyrate ester, is the smallest chiral ester of naproxol. These compounds, as well as the 2-hexyl ester (**25**), are mixtures of (S,S) and (S,R) diastereomers in approximately equal proportions. Compound **21**, a nearly pure (S,S) analog of **20**, was a good skin penetrant (threefold enhancement vs naproxen), although less so than **20**. Compound **20** penetrated at least twice as well as **21**, as would be expected if the two diastereomers diffused independently of one another.

Following the suggestion of Loftsson and Bodor (56) for aspirin prodrugs, the methylthiomethyl (**28**) and methylsulfinylmethyl (**29**) esters of naproxen were prepared; however, they offered no advantages in penetration. The glyceryl ester (**27**) penetrated as well as naproxen, although it was the most polar compound in the dataset. This result is consistent with equations 9 or 11, but would not be consistent with a model for maximum flux in which partition coefficient, rather than solubility, was the governing parameter.

Finite Dose Study with Naproxen and Derivatives

The experiments discussed in the preceding section demonstrated that under maximum flux conditions (infinite dose, saturated donor solutions), the skin penetration rate of certain derivatives of naproxen delivered from a propylene glycol vehicle could be 6–28 times that of the parent compound. The in vivo analogy of these conditions is to apply the drug from a patch containing propylene glycol and a larger reservoir of drug. Penetration studies were subsequently conducted with three of the naproxen compounds in order to determine whether or not similar enhancements could be obtained using finite doses of the drug on the skin. The conditions were chosen to simulate the effect of rubbing a small amount of each formulation onto the skin.

The results of this study are shown in Table 11. The rates of skin penetration through 8 h were in order.

naproxol (**30**) ≃ naproxen-*sec*-butyl ester (**20**) > naproxen (**3**)

with relative fluxes of approximately 2:2:1, respectively. After 4–8 h the ester, a liquid, penetrated more rapidly than the crystalline alcohol or parent acid. By 28 h, approximately 40% of the ester had been absorbed.

A separate experiment (data not shown) with naproxol-2-methylbutyrate, (**33**, another liquid derivative), yielded results similar to those with compound **20**.

Prodrug Bioconversion

An essential feature for a topical prodrug is that during or after skin transport, a reversion process occurs to liberate pharmacologically active drug. The prodrug linkage may be chemically or enzymatically labile, with the latter approach usually providing the greatest flexibility in prodrug design (57). The

Table 11   The Skin Penetration Rate of Small Doses of Naproxen and Two of Its Derivatives[a]

Compound	Concentration % (w/w)	Cumulative Amount Penetrated[b] ($\mu g/cm^2$)				
		0–2 h +36% −24%	0–4 h +26% −21%	0–8 h +25% −20%	0–28 h +19% −16%	% dose penetrated in 28 h
Naproxen (3)[c]	2.0	4	11	15	21	15%
Naproxol (30)[d]	2.5	9	18	23	28	16%
Naproxen dl-*sec*-butyl ester (20)[d]	2.0	8	17	27	56[e]	39%[e]

[a]The vehicle for these experiments consisted of propylene glycol (50% w/w) and isopropyl alcohol (balance of formulation). The dose was 5 μl per 0.7 cm^2 cell.
[b]Geometric mean. The percent error in each column is the pooled relative standard error of the geometric mean value.
[c]See Table 8.
[d]See Table 10.
[e]Significantly different from naproxen (> one 95% Least Significant Difference based on pooled variance).

viable epidermis and dermis are both relatively rich in non-specific esterase and other enzymatic activity (58). Hence, prodrugs are often designed to revert to parent drug during their transverse diffusion across these biophases. For topical prodrugs surviving enzymatic reversion during skin transport into the systemic circulation, other biophases, such as, bloodstream, muscle tissue, liver, kidney, etc., become important sites for the reversion process (59).

It was of interest to examine the bioconversion of several naproxen prodrugs whose skin penetration and physicochemical properties differed markedly from that of the parent drug. One series of in vitro experiments examined the rate of enzymatic hydrolysis of five aliphatic esters in human serum and serum skin homogenates. Another study involved the in vivo absorption and biotransformation of three liquid or low melting derivatives—the *sec*-butyl ester (**20**), the 2-methyl-butyrate (**33**), and naproxol (**30**)—following topical application to Wistar rats.

In Vitro Bioconversion: Human Serum and Skin-Serum Homogenates

The percent naproxen found in human serum and skin-serum homogenates following incubation of several ester derivatives is depicted in Figs. 11a and b, respectively. The hydrolytic rate of formation was approximated by first-order kinetics (Table 12) where, in serum, the order of hydrolytic susceptibility was glyceryl (**27**) > n-butyl (**19**) > > n-hexyl (**24**) > ethyl (**17**) > *sec*-butyl (**20**). Whereas the lysis of the alkyl ester bonds is expected to occur by a single Phase 1 biotransformation (via ester hydrolase), cleavage of the glyceryl ester can also occur by a separate hydrolytic reaction involving serum lipase (59). This

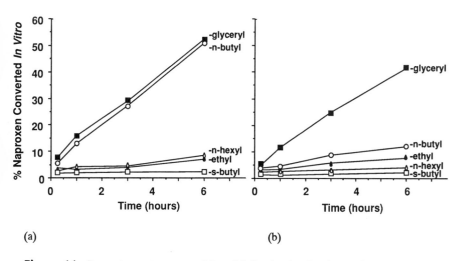

(a)   (b)

Figure 11 Percent parent compound found following in vitro incubation of naproxen prodrug derivatives in biological media. (a) Human serum; (b) serum-skin homogenate.

combined action may be the principal reason for its observed greater rate of hydrolysis than the alkyl esters.

The preferred enzymatic hydrolysis of the n-butyl (19) promoiety versus the other n-alkyl congeners, i.e., ethyl (17) and n-hexyl (24), is consistent with the results of Johansen et al. (60), who observed in a series of metronidazole n-alkyl prodrug esters a parabolic relationship (maximum = n-butyl) between the rate of ester hydrolysis in human plasma and ester carbon chain length. The lack of any measurable hydrolysis of the *sec*-butyl ester (20) underscores the significant role that a branching alkyl group can have on ester hydrolysis.

In the homogenate, all of the naproxen esters except the ethyl showed a substantial decline in the rate of hydrolysis. This decrease may reflect a competing adsorption/partition equilibrium between the lipoidal skin constituents and the highly lipophilic esters, resulting in longer apparent half-lives of hydrolysis.

In Vivo Bioconversion in Wistar Rat

The topical absorption and biotransformation of naproxen and naproxen-*sec*-butyl ester (20), naproxol (30), and naproxol 2-methylbutyrate (33) were examined in the Wistar rat. These derivatives were selected for study based on their enhanced in vitro human skin permeation and potential for development. Following topical application of 5% (w/w) solutions of the compounds in an ethanol-propylene glycol vehicle, the presence of parent and/or prodrug in rat plasma was determined using gradient elution HPLC. Only parent drug was detected in the plasma (detection limit 25 ng/ml), indicating efficient and complete biotransformation of prodrug to parent naproxen in vivo. Figure 12 depicts the naproxen plasma concentration–time profile. It is noteworthy that there was no evidence of prodrug

Table 12 $t_{1/2}$ Values for the Formation of Naproxen from Its Ester Derivatives in Human Serum and Skin-Serum Homogenates

Compound	$t_{1/2}^{a}$ (h) at 37°C	
	human serum[b]	skin-serum homogenate[b]
Naproxen esters		
ethyl[c]	63	58
n-butyl[c]	4.2	30
(d,l)-s-butyl[c]	>140	>140
n-hexyl[c]	53	>140
glyceryl[c]	3.5	7.9

[a]Half-time of formation of naproxen based on first-order kinetics.
[b]Average of two replicates.
[c]See Table 10.

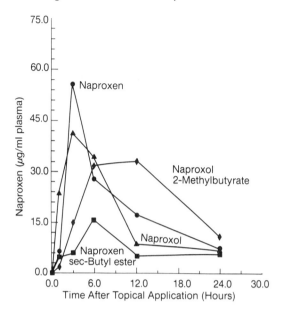

Figure 12 The naproxen plasma concentration-time profile following topical application of naproxen, naproxen-*sec*-butyl ester, naproxol and naproxol-2-methylbutyrate (5% in ethanol/propylene glycol) to rats.

in the plasma, yet very significant levels of parent drug were recoverable. This raises the possibility that conversion of these prodrugs to naproxen occurred in the peripheral tissues, e.g., skin, local blood compartment, or muscle, prior to systemic absorption. However, rapid hepatic metabolism of the prodrug could very likely yield the same result. It is worth noting that two biotransformation reactions, namely alcohol dehydrogenase followed by aldehyde oxidase, are required to convert naproxol **(30)** to naproxen in vivo.

As Figure 12 illustrates, naproxen applied topically was well absorbed and the low melting/liquid derivatives did not yield significantly higher systemic levels of parent drug. Based on the substantially higher in vitro human skin permeation for these derivatives, it was somewhat surprising that elevated parent blood levels were not observed. While there is always uncertainty in comparing animal skin (in this case Wistar rat) to human in terms of diffusion barriers and enzymatic activity, the results are suggestive of a rate-limiting diffusion step in the viable tissue. The uncharged, highly lipophilic naproxen prodrugs, while perhaps having the correct characteristics to efficiently penetrate the stratum corneum, would partition poorly into the aqueous skin layers. In terms of the composite membrane model for skin represented by equations 14 and 15, their flux would be limited by the aqueous barrier. This may be seen by considering the flux calculated from equation 15 for a permeant with a very large value of S_{lip} and a very small value of S_w.

Discussion

Implications for Prodrug Design

The fact that the permeability coefficients of polar materials can be increased by making lipophilic derivatives has been appreciated for some time (61–63). The increase in P has frequently been attributed to an increase in the diffusion coefficient of the permeant brought about by blocking polar functionalities (such as OH) which can hydrogen bond within the stratum corneum (48,64,65).

We believe the alternative interpretation provided by the model in the second section to be correct. According to this model, the major effect of converting a polar substituent to a less polar one is to increase the material's solubility, S_{lip}, in the barrier microenvironment of the stratum corneum, a lipophilic environment with discrimination properties similar to octanol. If the size of the molecule is not significantly changed by the derivatization, the skin permeation rate is increased in proportion to S_{lip}. If the derivatized molecule is larger than the parent, the diffusion coefficient is decreased by $\exp(-b'MW)$, partially or even totally offsetting the gain in penetration rate due to S_{lip}.

It is important to note that the quantity to be maximized for maximum drug delivery is the product of the molecular weight factor with S_{lip}, not the corresponding partition coefficient, K_{lip}. This follows directly from the structure of equations 8–11 when one recognizes that maximum flux, not permeability coefficient, is the governing parameter in most instances. The exception would be a situation in which the concentration of the compound in a topical vehicle was fixed by external requirements rather than by solubility; in that case, one would want to maximize partitioning at that concentration.

The study of naproxen derivatives showed that there are two effective ways to increase the percutaneous absorption of this compound through structural modification. The first is to lower the melting point by replacing the carboxyl group with a less polar group of comparable size. Naproxen alcohol (naproxol) and naproxen aldehyde exemplify this approach. While the aldehyde lacked the stability required for a product and may be a skin irritant as well, the alcohol showed considerable promise as a topical agent. Bioassay results (M. E. Loomans and H. H. Reller, unpublished data) showed that naproxol retained the anti-inflammatory activity of the parent acid against UV-induced erythema in the guinea pig and against croton oil–induced aural inflammation in the mouse. HPLC analysis of the blood of rats dosed with naproxol showed only naproxen in the plasma. The most likely location for oxidation to the acid form to occur is in the liver; hence, the topical activity of this compound suggests that naproxol itself is biologically active.

The second way to increase the absorption of naproxen is to esterify the parent acid with a small, chiral alcohol. Since the parent contains a chiral center at the α-propionic site, the use of a racemic alcohol results in a mixture of diastereomers. The sum of the mutual solubilities of these isomers is greater than that of a pure compound (cf. Table 10). In the case of naproxen, the parent compound is highly enriched in the S-isomer so that the racemic mixture contains one pair of diastereomers. Other α-propionic acids (e.g., ibuprofen) are available as racemates, so that the chiral ester approach would lead to two pairs of diastereomers.

The diastereomeric enhancement in total absorption appeared to work just as well when the alcohol and acid functionalities were interchanged, as shown by the high penetration rate of naproxol-2-methylbutyrate ester. Another possible way to increase total absorption, not yet confirmed, would be to mix two or more chemically distinct esters in the dosing formulation, e.g., *sec*-butyl and 2-methylpentyl. Again, one would expect the sum of the mutual solubilities of the compounds to exceed their individual solubilities. This technique has been shown to increase the in vitro release rate of steroids from a topical formulation (66).

Like naproxol, the improved-penetrating chiral esters were effective antiinflammatory agents and were hydrolyzed to naproxen in vitro and in vivo. The fact that these materials were liquids at room temperature was an additional advantage, allowing them to be formulated at higher concentrations and to penetrate the skin more efficiently after the vehicle in which they are dosed had dissipated.

Correspondence with Penetration Model

The skin penetration and physical properties data in Tables 8–10 were analyzed for correspondence with the diffusion models represented by equations 9 and 11. Two groups of compounds were considered—naproxen and its analogues and the full NSAID dataset.

The results of this analysis are shown in Table 7 and Figure 13. Although the correspondence was best when just the naproxen compounds were considered, the model provided an adequate description of both datasets. A detailed error analysis showed that the solubility term accounted for about 68% of the variation in log (J_m) values, and the molecular weight term for an additional 14–16%, giving overall r^2 values in the range 0.82–0.84. The maximum deviations between observed and calculated values of log J_m were 0.58 for the naproxen compounds and 0.95 for the NSAIDs, corresponding to multiplicative errors in predicted J_m values of 3.8 and 8.9, respectively.

CONCLUSIONS

For many compounds of pharmaceutical interest, including commonly prepared topical prodrugs, percutaneous absorption rates may be estimated by considering the skin to be a homogeneous, lipoidal barrier having solvent properties similar to

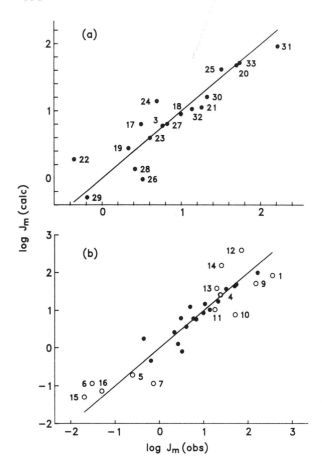

Figure 13 (a) Comparison of observed flux values for naproxen and its derivatives through excised human skin versus those calculated from the equation $\log J_m = \log S_{oct} - (0.0178/2.303) \, MW - 1.92$. The compounds are identified in Table 10. (b) Comparison of observed flux values for 31 of the 33 NSAIDs listed in Tables 8–10 with those calculated from the equation $\log J_m = \log S_{oct} - (0.0197/2.303) \, MW - 1.71$ (aspirin and its ester were omitted owing to missing solubility data). The numbers on the graph represent the compounds in Tables 8 and 9; the solid circles are the naproxen compounds.

those of the hydrogen-bonding solvent n-octanol. Diffusion coefficients of materials in the barrier microenvironment show a steep inverse dependence on molecular size (or molecular weight) similar to that seen in polymer membranes. For compounds which are either very large, very hydrophilic, or very lipophilic a composite membrane model which includes both a lipid pathway and a polar pathway through the stratum corneum in series with an aqueous layer is required in order to correctly predict absorption. When applied to the design of topical prodrugs, these principles suggest a strategy of preparing small, low-melting derivatives having increased oil (octanol) solubility with respect to the parent compound. A study of NSAID prodrugs highlighted two types of structures—oxidation state analogues and small, chiral esters—where this strategy appeared to be successful.

REFERENCES

1. P. M. Elias, *Arch. Dermatol. Res.*, 270, 95–117 (1981).
2. P. W. Wertz, D. C. Swartzendruber, K. C. Madison, and D. T. Downing. *J. Invest. Dermatol.*, 89, 419–425 (1987).
3. T.-S. Sun and H. Green, *J. Biol. Chem.*, 253, 2053–2060 (1978).
4. P. V. Raykar, M.-C. Fung, and B. D. Anderson, *Pharm. Res.*, 5, 140–150 (1988).
5. C. Ackermann and G. L. Flynn, *Int. J. Pharm.*, 36, 61–66 (1987).
6. B. D. Anderson, W. I. Higuchi, and P. V. Raykar, *Pharm. Res.*, 5, 566–573 (1988).
7. P. M. Elias, E. R. Cooper, A. Korc, and B. E. Brown, *J. Invest. Dermatol.*, 76, 297–301 (1981).
8. W. P. Smith, M. S. Christensen, S. Nacht, and E. H. Gans, *J. Invest. Dermatol.*, 78, 7–11 (1982).
9. G. B. Kasting, R. L. Smith, and E. R. Cooper, in *Pharmacology and the Skin*. Vol. 1 (B. Shroot and H. Schaefer, eds.). Karger, Basel, 1987, pp. 138–153.
10. B. D. Anderson and P. V. Raykar, *J. Invest. Dermatol.*, 93, 280–286 (1989).
11. T. Itoh, R. Magavi, R. L. Casady, T. Nishihata, and J. H. Rytting, *Pharm. Res.*, 7, 1302–1306 (1990).
12. W. R. Lieb and W. D. Stein, in *Transport and Diffusion Across Cell Membranes* (W. D. Stein, ed.). Academic Press, New York, 1986, pp. 69–112.
13. W. R. Lieb and W. D. Stein, *J. Membr. Biol.*, 92, 111–119 (1986).
14. W. R. Lieb and W. D. Stein, *Nature*, 224, 240–243 (1969).
15. W. D. Stein and S. Nir, *J. Membr. Biol.*, 5, 246 (1971).
16. B. E. Cohen and A. D. Bangham, Diffusion of small nonelectrolytes across liposome membranes. *Nature*, 236, 173–174 (1972).
17. B. E. Cohen, *J. Membr. Biol.*, 20, 235–268 (1975).
18. J. M. Wolosin and H. Ginsburg, *Biochim. Biophys. Acta*, 389, 20–33 (1975).
19. M. H. Cohen and D. Turnbull, *J. Chem. Phys.*, 31, 1164 (1959).
20. C. A. Kumins and T. K. Kwei, in *Diffusion in Polymers* (J. Crank and G. S. Park, eds.). Academic Press, New York, 1968, pp. 108–126.
21. S. S. Davis, T. Higuchi, and J. H. Rytting, in *Advances in Pharmaceutical Sciences*. Vol. 4. (H. S. Bean, A. H. Beckett, and J. E. Carless, eds.). Academic Press, New York, 1974, pp. 73–251.
22. A. S. Michaels, S. K. Chandrasekaran, and J. E. Shaw, *A.I.Ch.E.J.*, 21, 985–996 (1975).
23. R. J. Scheuplein and I. H. Blank, *Physiol. Rev.*, 51, 702–746 (1971).
24. C. Ackerman, G. L. Flynn, and W. M. Smith, *Int. J. Pharm.*, 36, 67–71 (1987).
25. A. Leo, C. Hansch and D. Elkins, *Chem. Rev.*, 71, 525–616 (1971).

26. B. D. Anderson, in *Physical Chemical Properties of Drugs* (S. H. Yalkowsky, A. A. Sinkula, and S. C. Valvani, eds.). Marcel Dekker, New York, 1980, pp. 252–253.
27. S. K. Chandrasekaran, in *Transdermal Delivery of Drugs*. Vol. III (A. F. Kydonieus and B. Berner, eds.). CRC Press, Boca Raton, Florida, 1987, pp. 23–42.
28. E. R. Cooper and G. B. Kasting, *J. Controlled Release*, 6, 23–35 (1987).
29. M. D. Donovan, G. L. Flynn, and G. L. Amidon, *Pharm. Res.*, 7, 808–815 (1990).
30. M. D. Donovan, G. L. Flynn, and G. L. Amidon, *Pharm. Res.*, 7, 863–866 (1990).
31. G. L. Flynn, in *Percutaneous Absorption* (R. L. Bronaugh and H. I. Maibach, eds.). Marcel Dekker, New York, 1985, pp. 27–51.
32. R. T. Tregear, *J. Invest. Dermatol.*, 46, 16–23 (1966).
33. G. B. Kasting and L. A. Bowman, *Pharm. Res.*, 7, 134–143 (1990).
34. G. B. Kasting and L. A. Bowman, *Pharm. Res.*, 7, 1141–1146 (1990).
35. G. B. Kasting, E. W. Merritt, and J. C. Keister, *J. Membr. Sci.*, 35, 137–159 (1988).
36. V. Srinivasan, M.-H. Su, W. I. Higuchi, and C. R. Behl, *J. Pharm. Sci.*, 79, 588–591 (1990).
37. R. R. Burnette and B. Ongpipattanakul, *J. Pharm. Sci.*, 76, 765–773 (1987).
38. R. J. Scheuplein, in *The Physiology and Pathophysiology of the Skin*. Vol. 5 (A. Jarrett, ed.). Academic Press, New York, 1978, pp. 1659–1752.
39. G. M. Grass, E. R. Cooper, and J. R. Robinson, *J. Pharm. Sci.*, 77, 24–26 (1988).
40. S. C. Harvey, Drug absorption, action and disposition. In *Remington's Pharmaceutical Sciences*, 17th ed. (A. R. Gennare, ed.). Mack Publishing Co., Easton, Pennsylvania, 1985, pp. 725–731.
41. C. Fleeker, O. Wong, and J. H. Rytting, *Pharm. Res.*, 6, 443–448 (1989).
42. J. Swarbrick, G. Lee, J. Brom, and N. P. Gesmantel, *J. Pharm. Sci.*, 73, 1352–1355 (1984).
43. S. D. Roy and G. L. Flynn, *Pharm. Res.*, 6, 825–832 (1989).
44. S. H. Yalkowski, S. C. Valvani, and T. J. Roseman, *J. Pharm. Sci.*, 72, 866–870 (1983).
45. S. H. Yalkowski and S. C. Valvani, *J. Pharm. Sci.*, 69, 912–922 (1980).
46. S. H. Yalkowski, *I&EC Fundam.*, 18, 108 (1979).
47. J. A. Marqusee and K. A. Dill, *J. Chem. Phys.*, 85, 434–444 (1986).
48. R. J. Scheuplein, I. H. Blank, G. J. Brauner, and D. J. MacFarlane, *J. Invest. Dermatol.*, 52, 63–70 (1969).
49. G. B. Kasting, E. W. Merritt, R. L. Smith, D. Walker, L. G. Mueller, and A. F. Estelle, *Pharm. Res.*, 4, S–59 (1987).
50. L. G. Mueller, A. F. Estelle, G. B. Kasting, E. W. Merritt, L. J. Tulich, R. L. Smith, D. D. Walker, and E. R. Cooper, *Pharm. Res.*, 4, S–71 (1987).
51. R. L. Smith, D. D. Walker, L. D. Ryan, J. A. Schaefer, L. G. Mueller, A. F. Estelle, M. E. Loomans, and R. E. Smyth, *Pharm. Res.*, 4, S–62 (1987).
52. L. G. Mueller, U.S. Patent No. 4,912,248 (Mar. 27, 1990).
53. R. L. Bronaugh and R. F. Stewart, *J. Pharm. Sci.*, 73, 1255–1258 (1984).
54. A. H. Ghanem, H. Mahmoud, W. I. Higuchi, U. D. Rohr, S. Borsadia, P. Liu, J. L. Fox, and W. R. Good, *J. Controlled Release*, 6, 75–83 (1987).

55. W. I. Higuchi, U. D. Rohr, S. A. Burton, P. Liu, J. L. Fox, A. H. Ghanem, H. Mahmoud, S. Borsadia, and W. R. Good, in *Controlled Release Technology, Pharmaceutical Applications*, ACS Symposium Series 348, American Chemical Society, Washington, D.C., 1987, pp. 232–240.

56. T. Loftsson and N. Bodor, *J. Pharm. Sci.*, 70, 756–761 (1981).

57. A. A. Sinkula and S. H. Yalkowski, *J. Pharm. Sci.*, 64, 111 (1975).

58. U. Tauber, in *Dermal and Transdermal Absorption* (R. Brandau and B. H. Lippold, eds.). Wissenschaftliche Verlagsgesellschaft, Stuttgart, 1982, pp. 133–151.

59. C. M. MacDonald and R. G. Turcan, in *Comprehensive Medicinal Chemistry* Vol. 5. (C. Hansch, P. G. Sammes and J. B. Taylor, eds.). Pergamon Press, New York, 1990, pp. 111–141.

60. M. Johansen, B. Mollgaard, P. K. Wotton, C. Larsen, and A. Hoelgaard, *Int. J. Pharm.*, 32, 199–206 (1986).

61. R. B. Stoughton, W. E. Clendenning, and D. Kruse, *J. Invest. Dermatol.*, 35, 337 (1960).

62. N. Bodor, J. Zupan, and S. Selk, *Int. J. Pharm.*, 7, 63–75 (1980).

63. W. M. Smith, Ph.D. Thesis, University of Michigan, Ann Arbor, 1982.

64. B. Idson and C. R. Behl, in *Transdermal Delivery of Drugs*. Vol. III (A. F. Kydonieus and B. Berner, eds.). CRC Press, Boca Raton, Florida, 1987, pp. 85–151.

65. R. H. Guy and J. Hadgraft, in *Transdermal Delivery of Drugs*. Vol. III (A. F. Kydonieus and B. Berner, eds.). CRC Press, Boca Raton, Florida, 1987, pp. 3–22.

66. A. D. Marcus, R. E. Dempski, T. Higuchi, and J. D. DeMarco, *J. Pharm. Sci.*, 54, 495–496 (1965).

4

A Computational Method for Predicting Optimization of Prodrugs or Analogues Designed for Percutaneous Delivery

David W. Osborne* and William J. Lambert[†]
The Upjohn Company, Kalamazoo, Michigan

INTRODUCTION

Four empirical models were evaluated to determine their ability to predict percutaneous absorption of drugs (1,2). Two of the predictive models evaluated were developed by Berner and Cooper (3), the third was taken from a publication by Michaels et al. (4), and the fourth was proposed by Albery and Hadgraft (5). In this previous study (2), 50 drugs having a wide range of physical properties were evaluated and their resulting predicted transdermal flux values compared to experimental values. It was found that these permeation equations are useful for predicting the flux of a drug through the skin barrier when values for the water solubility, an oil-water partition coefficient, and molecular weight of the drug are known, or can be calculated.

For the scientist concerned with the design of prodrugs to enhance skin absorption, these models provide useful insight into the relationship between prodrug lipophilicity and percutaneous transport. As noted by Sloan (6), increasing the lipid solubility of the promoieties almost always results in enhanced transdermal delivery of the parent drug; however, maximum transport additionally requires use of the more water-soluble members of these prodrug series. The α-acyloxyalkyl series was used as an example. As the acyl chain length increased, the water solubility decreased, whereas the lipid solubility, and consequently, the partition coefficient increased. No significant differences in the rate of transdermal delivery of the parent drug by the first few members of the series of

Current affiliations:
*Calgon Vestal Laboratories, St. Louis, Missouri
[†]Pfizer Central Research, Groton, Connecticut

prodrugs was observed, but then the rate decreased with increasing lipophilicity. Thus, merely increasing the lipophilicity of the drug by the transient masking of a polar functional group is not sufficient to maximize percutaneous transport of the parent drug. Rather, careful selection of the interrelated water solubility, partition coefficient, and molecular weight of the promoieties is required for successful development of dermal prodrugs.

The balance between water solubility and lipophilicity as a homologous series is ascended has been described for inert membranes (7). In this detailed analysis, the penetration rate of a series of p-aminobenzoate esters across dimethyl polysiloxane sheeting was determined as a function of alkyl chain length of the ester. A parabolic dependence between rate of penetration and alkyl chain length was found with the maximum rate occurring for the propyl and butyl esters. These results were successfully described by a diffusional model which incorporated diffusion layer involvement and solubility restrictions. While such rigorous descriptions are not the subject of this chapter, it is important to realize that mechanistic insight can be obtained following the application of established theory to carefully designed experiments.

DESCRIPTION OF THE MODELS

Since the models have been described in detail in both the original publications and in the previous technical update, only a brief description will be presented here. The two-parallel-pathway model for skin permeation proposed by Berner and Cooper (3) separates permeation through the skin's barrier function into two paths, a polar (aqueous) path and a nonpolar (lipophilic) path. The diffusion constants for the polar, D_P, and lipophilic, D_L, pathways are calculated using equations 1 and 2:

$$D_P = (3.8 \times 10^{-5})e^{-0.016M} \tag{1}$$

$$D_L = (1.7 \times 10^{-5})e^{-0.016M} \tag{2}$$

where M is the molecular weight of the drug, and the resulting diffusion constants are given in cm^2/h. Because the fluxes of the polar and lipophilic pathways are considered additive, the total flux (J) of the drug through the stratum corneum can be stated in terms of the diffusion coefficients from equations 1 and 2, as follows:

$$J = \frac{(A_P D_P + A_L K D_L)C_W}{L} \tag{3}$$

where A_P and A_L are the area fractions of the polar and lipophilic pathways, respectively; K is the partition coefficient of the nonpolar phase; C_W is the drug's water solubility (in mg/ml); and L is the thickness of the stratum corneum (in cm). Berner and Cooper suggest that $A_P = 0.1$ and $A_L = 0.9$. The octanol/water partition coefficient is used for K, and a value of 0.0015 cm is suggested for the thickness of the stratum corneum. Using these values for the parameters, J will have the units ng/cm^2·h. This represents the maximum flux from a saturated aqueous solution, assuming that the stratum corneum is unchanged by either the drug or vehicle over the period of application.

Berner and Cooper have also proposed a three-parallel-pathway model (3), which combines not only the polar and lipophilic pathways, but also an oil/water multilaminate pathway. Use of the same values for L, D_L, D_P, and A_P as for the two-parallel-path model, and decreasing the value for A_L from 0.9 to 0.5, the equations to calculate the upper (J^U_{max}) and lower (J^L_{max}) bounds of the maximum flux through the stratum corneum are given in equations 4 and 5. The values for J^U_{max} and J^L_{max} have been averaged in this evaluation to provide a single pathway for the three parallel path model.

$$J^U_{max} = \frac{2(C_W)e^{-0.016(M)}}{15} \left(\frac{(85(K) + 190)(38 + 153(K))}{(228 + 238(K))} \right) \tag{4}$$

$$J^L_{max} = \frac{(C_W)e^{-0.016(M)}}{15} \left(85(K) + 38 + \frac{5 \times 10^{-3}(K)}{380 + 170(K)} \right) \tag{5}$$

In the heterogeneous structural model described by Michaels et al. (4), the barrier function is treated as a dispersion of hydrophilic protein in a continuous lipid matrix through which the drug migrates by dissolution and Fickian diffusion. Based on this reasonable assumption concerning the structure of the stratum corneum, the simplified flux equation is given below, where K is the partition coefficient, which is set equal to the mineral oil/water partition coefficient in the original paper. The octanol/water partition coefficient has also been successfully used (1,2).

$$J = 0.27(K)(C_W) \left[\frac{1160 + 3.4 \times 10^{-3}(K)}{160 + 2(K)} \right] \tag{6}$$

The last model was adapted from a theoretical description of percutaneous absorption published by Albery and Hadgraft in 1979 (5). In steady-state applications, the total fluxes can be predicted using the following equation:

$$J = \frac{36C_W}{2.82 + 29.6/K} \tag{7}$$

COMPARISON OF PREDICTED EXPERIMENTAL FLUX VALUES

When compiling a list of experimental values, the most striking result is the huge value range that is found on the few occasions in which values are determined by more than one investigator. Partition coefficients and water solubilities can vary by two orders of magnitude, whereas experimentally determined transdermal flux values can vary by three to five orders of magnitude. In the case of transdermal flux measurements, such variability is usually the result of using significantly different experimental techniques. In many respects, the "ballpark" predictive nature of these empirical models is desirable over "quick and dirty" in vitro transdermal experiments, especially if the purity of radiolabel is questionable.

In total, 50 compounds have been evaluated using each of the four models listed above (2). While the experimental in vitro flux for some of these compounds were from saturated solvents other than water, reasonable correlations existed between experimental and calculated flux values for each of the 50 compounds. In order to compare the predictive ability of the models, the natural logarithm of the experimental value can be plotted against the natural logarithm of the predicted value. If the experimental and predictive values were in complete agreement, the plot would have an $r^2 = 1.00$, and a slope of unity. Coincidentally, both the two-parallel-pathway and three-parallel-pathway models of Berner and Cooper gave a correlation value (r^2) of 0.88, whereas the remaining two models had equivalent correlations of 0.73.

Perhaps a more enlightening comparison is the resulting slopes of the plots. The two-parallel- and three-parallel-path models resulted in slopes of 1.15 and 1.13, respectively, and crossed the ideal (slope equal to unity) correlation line at flux values of 60 and 1100 $\mu g/cm^2 \cdot h$, respectively. Thus, predicted flux values from these two models that are greater than 60 $\mu g/cm^2 \cdot h$, (or 1100 $\mu g/cm^2 \cdot h$ for the three-parallel-path model) will tend to be less than the experimental results. However, the slopes are sufficiently close to unity that this trend will be less than the scatter of the data, until low flux values are reached. The predictability of Berner and Cooper's models is superior to that of the other models that had slopes of 0.75 (4) and 0.70 (5) and that crossed the ideal flux line at 90 and 0.5 $\mu g/cm^2 \cdot h$, respectively.

APPLICATION OF MODELS TO PRODRUG SELECTION

Contour Plots

Without specifying any structural details of the prodrug, these models can be used to generate percutaneous flux contour plots that serve as qualitative guidelines that will aid the synthetic chemist in designing prodrugs to enhance transdermal delivery. In the past, vague guidelines existed indicating that increases in lipophilicity results in increased permeability, and that major changes in molecular weight were required to produce significant differences in diffusivity (8). While these generalities were very useful, more detailed insight into the relation between a drug's physical properties and percutaneous permeation can be obtained by use of contour plots of the predicted flux that are plotted as a function of the partition coefficient vs water solubility at a fixed molecular weight.

Contour plots based on equations 3–5 for molecular weights of 50, 100, 300, and 500 are given in Fig. 1. As seen for each molecular weight, the predicted flux values smoothly increase as both water solubility and partition coefficient increase. Generally speaking, the upper right corner of the contours plot is seldom attainable. Most notable on these plots are the shape of the contours and changes in this shape as molecular weight is increased. Changing the physical properties of a drug in a manner that results in movement parallel to a flux contour line will result in neither an increase nor a decrease in the predicted transdermal delivery of the drug. Conversely, changing the physical properties of a drug in a manner that results in movement perpendicular to a flux contour line will provide the greatest change in predicted delivery. For example, increasing the partition coefficient from 0.05 to 0.37 (ln partition coefficient = -3 to -1) while maintaining the water solubility at 2.72 mg/ml (ln water solubility = -1) results in a 5.3-fold increase in predicted flux for a drug of molecular weight 300, but only a 2.4-fold increase in the predicted flux for a drug molecular weight 100.

Calculation of Partition Coefficient and Water Solubility

The a priori prediction of maximum drug flux by any of the models requires knowledge of the water solubility and partition coefficient of the drug. The partition coefficient of the models actually represents the transfer of the solute from the aqueous environment to the lipophilic stratum corneum pathway. For a number of reasons, including convenience, the octanol/water partition coefficient is often used to estimate the stratum corneum/water partition coefficient. As will be discussed in a later section, the use of the octanol/water partition coefficient may represent a significant source of error in predicting drug flux.

The synthetic chemist has several methods available for the estimation of octanol/water partition coefficients. The most popular approach involves the use of substituent or fragment constants (9–11). Both methods assume that the partition coefficient is an additive-constituent property. Owing to this assumption, predicted partition coefficients may vary from experimental values due to interaction or proximity effects. Extensive listings of constants are available from several sources (12–14). In addition, a commercial computer program-based on the work of Hansch and Leo is available for estimating partition coefficients (CLOGP, Pomona College). This program also attempts to correct for various fragment interactions.

A method has been described for the a priori prediction of octanol/water partition coefficients based solely on geometrical and quantum chemical description (15). The molecular descriptors include surface area, volume, weight, and atomic charge density. This approach, while empirical, would appear to avoid the additivity assumption of the substituent or fragment approach.

It is often desirable to experimentally determine the partition coefficient of one compound in a series. The calculation of partition coefficients is much simpler if the partition coefficient of a related compound is known (10). Octanol/water partition coefficients are normally determined by the traditional shake-flask

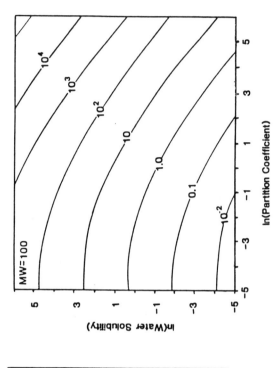

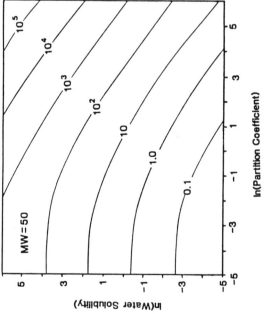

(a)

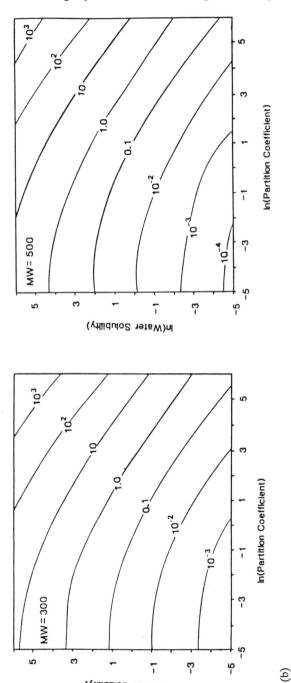

(b)

Figure 1 Plot for drugs of molecular weight 50, 100, 300, and 500. Contour lines are mean values from equations 3–5 of predicted transdermal flux in units of μg/cm²·h. The ordinate and abscissa are natural logarithm scales of water solubility (mg/ml) and octanol/water partition coefficients, respectively.

method (16,17). Owing to the laborious nature of the shake-flask method, a number of alternative methods are available. The centrifugal partition chromatograph (18) and the AKUFVE apparatus (19) both allow for the on-line determination of oil/water partition coefficients.

In addition to direct methods, reverse-phase chromatographic retention times can be used to estimate oil/water partition coefficients. This technique, made popular owing to its speed and need for only milligram quantities of compound, has been reviewed by several authors (20–25). In general, a good correlation is found between log octanol/water partition coefficients and log capacity factor using octadecyl silica (ODS) columns. However, specific interactions between solutes and the stationary phase (e.g., free silanol groups) have been suggested to differentiate between various classes of compounds (25). The use of polymer-based stationary phases provides an alternative to the ODS method which avoids silanol interactions and also allows the use of highly acidic or basic mobile phases (26–28). C-18 derivatized polystyrene-divinylbenzene phases have also been used to estimate alkane/water partition coefficients (26).

Owing to the importance of aqueous solubility in many fields, it is not surprising to find that many methods are available for the estimation of aqueous solubility (29). A common approach is to utilize octanol/water partition coefficients as an estimate of the activity coefficient of the drug in water (30). The underlying assumption for the use of the octanol/water partition coefficient is that the polarities of most drugs are similar to octanol, and thus, the activity coefficients of most drugs in octanol are near unity. The use of the octanol/water partition coefficients is fortunate, since this parameter is readily estimated, as described above. In fact, Hafkenscheid and Tomlinson (31) utilized chromatographic capacity factors to directly estimate aqueous solubility.

The ideal solubility (X) of a crystalline drug is also governed by lattice energies (32). Thus, estimation of the melting point (T_m), the heat of fusion (ΔH_f), and the heat capacity difference between the crystalline and liquid drug (ΔC_p) is required, as given by

$$\ln X = \frac{-\Delta H_f}{RT_m}\left(\frac{T_m - T}{T}\right) + \frac{\Delta C_p}{R}\left(\frac{(T_m - T)}{T} - \ln\frac{T_m}{T}\right)$$

(8)

where R is the gas constant and T is the temperature of interest. The right-hand term in the equation 8 is assumed to be negligible, and $\Delta H_f/T_m$ may be replaced by the entropy of fusion (ΔS_f), since the free energy of fusion equals zero at the melting point. ΔS_f may be approximated by 13.5 eu for rigid molecules, or 13.5 + 2.5(n-5) eu for flexible molecules, where n is the number of nonhydrogen atoms in a flexible chain (30). Unfortunately, an accurate method of predicting the melting point of a compound is not available. Thus, for crystalline drugs, it is necessary to experimentally determine the melting point in order to estimate the solubility and maximal drug flux. Specific equations for estimating a solubility are given in Table 1 (33).

Table 1 Equations for Prediction of Water Solubility (where $S_w = C_w$, PC = K, and MP = melting point)

Fundamental equations
Liquid solutes
   $\log S_w = -1.072 \log PC + 0.672$
Crystalline solutes—rigid non–electrolyte drug molecules
   $\log S^c_w \simeq -\log PC - 0.01 MP + 1.05$

Applied equations
Rigid polycyclic aromatic hydrocarbons (e.g., napthalene)
   $\log S^c_w = -0.88 \log PC - 0.01 MP - 0.012$
Mono- and multifunctional halobenzenes (e.g., 1,2-dichlorobenze)
   $\log S^c_w = -0.99 \log PC - 0.01 MP + 0.72$
Steroid hormones (e.g., progesterone)
   $\log S^c_w = -0.88 \log PC - 0.01 MP + 0.08$
Hexamethylmelamines (e.g., hexamethylmelamine)
   $\log S^c_w = -0.904 \log PC - 0.007 MP + 0.07$
Alkyl *para*-substituted benzoates (e.g., hexyl-p-aminobenzoate)
   $\log S^c_w = -1.14 \log PC - 0.005 MP + 0.633$
Alkylphenols
   $\log S^c_w = -0.0997 \log PC - 0.008 MP + 1.43$

Source: Ref. 33.

The above discussion assumes that the drug of interest is a nonelectrolyte. Solubilities and partition coefficients are dramatically affected by the ionization of basic or acidic functionalities. Thus, the pharmaceutical scientist should consider the acid dissociation constant(s) of the compound of interest. The estimation of dissociation constants can be performed by applying linear free relationships, as reviewed by Perrin et al. (34) and Harris and Hayes (35).

The Lipophilic Stratum Corneum Pathway

The intercellular volume of the stratum corneum is thought to comprise between 5 and 30% of the total volume (36,37). Lipids derived from the lamellar bodies of the underlying stratum granulosum fill the intercellular space, and are thought to be responsible for the barrier properties of the stratum corneum (38,39). These lipids, which are primarily neutral in nature, have been shown to form bilayer structures in the intercellular space (40–42).

The use of a bulk oil such as octanol to mimic the complex mixture of lipids in the stratum corneum is sure to have some shortcomings. First, the insertion of a solute into a structured lipid bilayer is thought to have an entropic cost that would not be associated with transfer into a bulk oil (43). In addition, the physical properties of the structured intercellular lipids should be anisotropic. The permeation of solutes in bilayers has been considered at length by Diamond and Katz (44). These authors suggest that the head-group region of bilayers may present the most resistance to the permeation of lipophilic solutes, whereas the interior alkanelike portion of the bilayer may limit the permeation of more polar solutes (Fig. 2). This has led several investigators to suggest that alkane/water partition coefficients may be more appropriate for assessing permeation through biomembranes, since most drugs contain multiple polar functionalities (26,45,46). Additional research is likely required in this area before the popular octanol/water system is replaced.

Examples from the Literature

The predictive ability of these models is well represented by the in vitro percutaneous transport study of a series of mitomycin C analogues. As seen in Table 2, both the ranking of the analogues and the absolute flux values were reasonably well predicted within the order of magnitude expected for the models. Since the experimental data were obtained after application of saturated isopropyl myristate solutions, the applicability of these models to even nonaqueous systems demonstrates the versatility of these calculations.

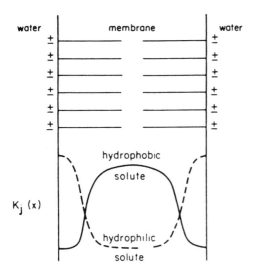

Figure 2   Expected dependence of nonelectrolyte partition coefficients [Kj(x)] on position within a lipid bilayer. (From Ref. 44.)

Table 2 Comparison of Predicted and Experimental Transdermal Flux Values

Compound	Molecular weight	Octanol/water partition coefficient	Water solubility (mg/ml)	Experi- mental flux	Calculated flux (eq. 3)
Mitomycin C (MMC)	334	0.41	0.94	0.32	0.030
Benzyl MMC	434	39	0.65	3.2	0.25
Benzoyl MMC	448	78	0.0045	0.0072	0.0028
Benzylcarbonyl MMC	462	34	1.0	0.3	0.22
Benzyloxycarbonyl MMC	478	110	0.285	2.5	0.14
Propyloxycarbonyl MMC	430	33	0.14	0.12	0.05
Pentyloxycarbonyl MMC	458	280	0.27	1.7	0.50
Nonyloxycarbonyl MMC	514	3700	0.00013	0.012	0.0013

Experimentally determined values for the octanol/water partition coefficient, water solubility, and transdermal flux ($\mu g/cm^2/h$) are from Mukai et al. (47).

A good example of moving along a contour line is seen in the experimental transdermal flux results for the mitomycin C (MMC) analogues (47). Note that the partition coefficient of pentyloxycarbonyl MMC is twofold greater than the partition coefficient for benzyloxycarbonyl MMC, while the water solubilities and molecular weights are approximately the same. The experimental results show that the in vitro percutaneous absorption of these substances are essentially the same, just as anticipated based upon the contour plot for molecular weight 500. Alternatively, benzyl MMC and propyloxycarbonyl MMC can be compared. Both compounds have essentially the same molecular weights and lipophilicity, but benzyl MMC has about fourfold greater water solubility than propyloxycarbonyl MMC. In this case, the increased water solubility of the analogue increases drug flux by greater than an order of magnitude. Again, this increase in flux of the drug would have been anticipated from noting the perpendicular crossing of the contour line in Fig. 3.

Liquid Prodrugs

While well-characterized crystalline drugs may be required for certain dosage forms, dermal delivery is often improved when the active species is a liquid at ambient conditions. If a topical cream or ointment is used as the vehicle, a liquid drug can readily be incorporated in the semisolid, without being concerned about slow crystallization from a supersaturated solution, or Oswalt rippening of a more stable polymorph. For transdermal delivery from a patch, dissolving/dispersing the drug in the adhesive or elastomer matrix may be greatly facilitated when the bulk drug is a lipophilic oil. Thus, unlike solid dosage forms, liquid prodrug esters of the parent species may be acceptable or even preferable for dermal delivery.

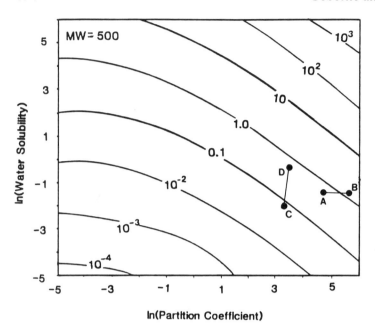

Figure 3 Benzyloxycarbonyl MMC is located on the contour plot at a water solubility of 0.28 mg/ml and a partition coefficient of 110 (labeled A) whereas pentyloxycarbonyl MMC has a water solubility of 0.27 mg/ml and a partition coefficient of 280 and is located at the position labeled B. The increase in partition coefficient does not correspond to a significant increase in the experimentally determined transdermal flux (47). This is expected since the change in physical properties of the prodrug results in movement on the contour plot that is approximately parallel to the 1 µg/cm^2/h contour line. This can be compared to propyloxycarbonyl MMC (water solubility = 0.14 mg/ml PC = 33) labeled C and benzyl MMC (water solubility = 0.65 mg/ml, PC = 39) labeled D. The increase in water solubility represents a change in prodrug physical properties that moves perpendicular to the 1 µg/cm^2·h contour line.

The prediction of percutaneous flux values is more widely applicable for liquid drugs than crystalline drugs, since the water solubility can be calculated directly from the partition coefficient (see Table 1). While most topically applied drugs are delivered from formulations that contain less than 10% of the active component, it is possible that a liquid drug could be applied neat.

Remember that each of the models assumes that the drug is being delivered from a saturated aqueous solution; therefore, water solubility is a factor in the equations. The use of saturated solutions is significant because this characteristic ensures that the driving force or chemical potential is equal for each system. When considering the penetration of solvents or liquid drugs, this means that percutaneous transport from a saturated aqueous solution should be the same as percutaneous transport of a neat liquid. However, this is to be expected only if the stratum corneum is unchanged by the vehicle or drug. Since water may serve as a percutaneous penetration enhancer (occlusion, for example), it is unlikely that an oil-saturated aqueous solution will provide the same level of transport as a neat oil applied to the skin.

Ocular Prodrugs

The chapter in this text on improved ocular delivery with prodrugs (see Chap. 7) prompts the question of whether the simple computational methods described in this chapter for stratum corneum transport could be utilized to predict corneal permeability of a series of promoieties. Occular drug delivery presents additional challenges compared to dermal drug delivery. First, absorption of topically applied opthalmics can occur via the cornea, the conjunctiva, and the nasal mucosa. As a result, factors such as vehicle viscosity and drug concentration can have a significant impact upon the amount of drug absorbed into the eye compared to systemic absorption (48,49). In a series of articles (50,51) Grass and Robinson described mechanisms of corneal drug penetration. The third paper in this series (52) considered modeling of molecular transport for the cornea. The model utilized apparent diffusion coefficients for the stroma, lipid epithelium, and the epithelial pores. The equation for the permeability coefficient was based on a dataset of approximately 50 molecules. For the 11 compounds described in the paper, a correlation coefficient of 0.74 was found for a log-log plot of the experimental permeability coefficient versus the calculated permeability coefficient.

ADDITIONAL CONSIDERATIONS

Although these contour plots are of obvious utility, it must be remembered that these computational methods provide predicted flux values that are generally within an order of magnitude of the experimental values determined using in vitro transdermal methods. It is fully expected that such computational methods may not be appropriate for topical drugs which uniquely interact with the bilayer-structured epidermal lipids or for drugs that alter the barrier properties of the skin. The second consideration can be seen when considering data for the keratolytic salicylic acid in which the predicted flux (~ 0.2 $\mu g/cm^2 \cdot h$) is 10,000 times less than the experimentally determined flux value. It must also be noted that each of these models assumes that diffusion is stratum corneum–controlled rather than dermally controlled.

Also important to remember is that the compounds initially investigated to establish the empirical parameters were nonelectrolytes. Thus, drug molecules that will dissociate should be evaluated with reservation. As seen in the previous study (2), these computation methods can be predictive for drugs that dissociate. However, predictions for compounds that fall outside the assumptions of the models must be considered suspect. Likewise, use of these techniques to predict the percutaneous delivery of polypeptides is likely unfounded. Octanol/water partition coefficients for polypeptides are often larger than would be expected compared with the non–hydrogen-bonding solvent/water partition coefficients.

Use of mineral oil/water or alkane/water partition coefficients may be more predictive of the actual percutaneous flux values. Finally, remember that only the two models by Berner and Cooper utilize the molecular weight of the compound. For compounds of molecular weight above 1000, the resulting flux values from these two models will likely be more predictive of experimental results.

REFERENCES

1. D. W. Osborne, *Pharmaceut. Manufact.*, 3(4), 41 (1986).
2. D. W. Osborne, in *Topical Drug Delivery Formulations* (D. W. Osborne and A. H. Amann, eds.). Marcel Dekker, New York, 1990, p. 109.
3. B. Berner and E. R. Cooper, in *Transdermal Delivery of Drugs*. Vol. II (A. F. Kydonieus and B. Berner, eds.). CRC Press, Boca Raton, Florida, 1987, p. 41.
4. A. S. Michaels, S. K. Chandrasekaran, and J. E. Shaw, *A.I.Ch.E. J.*, 21, 985 (1975).
5. W. J. Albery and J. Hadgraft, Percutaneous absorption: In vivo experiments. *J. Pharm. Pharmacol.*, 31, 140 (1979).
6. K. B. Sloan, *Adv. Drug Deliv. Rev.*, 3, 67 (1989).
7. G. L. Flynn and S. H. Yalkowsky, *J. Pharm. Sci.*, 61, 838 (1972).
8. J. L. Zatz, CTFA Scientific Monograph Series No. 2 CTFA, Washington, D.C., 1983, p. 29.
9. T. Fujita, J. Iwasa, and C. Hansch, *J. Am. Chem. Soc.*, 86, 5175 (1964).
10. A. Leo, P. Y. C. Jow, C. Silipo, and C. Hansch, *J. Med. Chem.*, 18, 865 (1975).
11. G. G. Nys and R. F. Rekker, *Chim. Ther.*, 8, 521 (1973).
12. W. J. Lyman, in *Handbook of Chemical Property Estimation Methods, Environmental Behavior of Organic Compounds* (W. J. Lyman, W. F. Reehl, and D. H. Rosenblatt, eds.). McGraw-Hill, New York, 1982, Chap. 1.
13. C. Hansch and A. Leo, *Substituent Constants for Correlation Analysis in Chemistry and Biology*, Wiley, New York, 1979.
14. M. S. Tute, *Adv. Drug Res.*, 6, 1 (1971).
15. N. Bodor, Z. Gabanyi, and C. K. Wong, *J. Am. Chem. Soc.*, 111, 3783 (1989).
16. J. C. Dearden and G. M. Bresnen, *Quant. Struct. Act. Relat.*, 7, 133 (1988).
17. A. Leo, C. Hansch, and D. Elkins, *Chem. Rev.*, 71, 525 (1971).
18. H. Terada, Y. Kosuge, W. Murayama, N. Nakaya, Y. Nunogaki, and K. I. Nunogaki, *J. Chromatogr.*, 400, 343 (1987).
19. H. Reinhardt and J. Rydberg, *Chem. and Indust.*, 488 (1970).
20. K. Valko, *Trends Anal. Chem.*, 6, 214 (1987).
21. W. Klein, W. Kordel, M. Weib, and H. J. Poremski, *Chemosphere*, 17, 361 (1988).

22. ECETOC Technical Report, *Assessment of Reverse-Phase Chromatographic Methods for Determining Partition Coefficients*. European Chemical Industry Ecology and Toxicology Centre, Brussels, 1983.

23. R. Kaliszan, *CRC Crit. Rev. Anal. Chem.*, 16, 323 (1986).

24. T. Braumnan, *J. Chromatogr.*, 373, 191 (1986).

25. H. Terada, *Quant. Struct.-Act. Relat.*, 5, 81 (1986).

26. W. J. Lambert, L. A. Wright, and J. K. Stevens, *Pharmacol. Res.*, 7, 577 (1990).

27. A. Bechalany, T. Rothlisberger, N. El Tayar, and B. Testa, *J. Chromatogr.*, 473, 115 (1989).

28. K. Miyake, F. Kitaura, N. Mizuno, and H. Terada, *Chem. Pharm. Bull.*, 35, 377 (1987).

29. W. J. Lyman, in *Handbook of Chemical Property Estimation Methods, Environmental Behavior of Organic Compounds* (W. J. Lyman, W. F. Reehl, and D. H. Rosenblatt, eds.). McGraw-Hill, New York, 1982, Chap. 2.

30. S. H. Yalkowsky and S. C. Valvani, *J. Pharm. Sci.*, 69, 912 (1980).

31. T. L. Hafkenscheid and E. Tomlinson, *J. Chromatogr.*, 218, 409–425 (1981).

32. J. H. Hildebrand and R. L. Scott, *Regular Solutions*. Prentice-Hall, Englewood Cliffs, New Jersey, 1962.

33. S. C. Valvani and S. H. Yalkowsky, in *Physical Chemical Properties of Drugs* (S. H. Yalkowsky, A. A. Sinkula, and S. C. Valvani, eds.). Marcel Dekker, New York, 1980, p. 201.

34. D. D. Perrin, B. Dempsey, and E. P. Serjeant, *pKa Prediction for Organic Acids and Bases*. Chapman and Hall, London, 1981.

35. J. C. Harris and M. J. Hayes, in *Handbook of Chemical Property Estimation Methods, Environmental Behavior of Oraganic Compounds* (W. J. Lyman, W. F. Reehl, and D. H. Rosenblatt, eds.). McGraw-Hill, New York, 1982, Chap. 6.

36. R. J. Scheuplein and I. H. Blank, *Physiol. Rev.*, 51, 702 (1971).

37. P. M. Elias and D. S. Friend, *J. Cell. Biol.*, 65, 180 (1975).

38. A. G. Matoltsky and P. F. Parakkal, *J. Cell. Biol.*, 24, 297 (1965).

39. L. Landman, *J. Invest. Dermatol.*, 87, 202 (1986).

40. P. M. Elias, *Arch. Dermatol. Res.*, 270, 95 (1981).

41. P. M. Elias, in *Topical Drug Delivery Formulations* (D. W. Osborne and A. H. Amann, eds.). Marcel Dekker, New York, 1990, p. 13.

42. S. E. Friberg, I. H. Kayali, M. Margosiak, D. W. Osborne, A. J. I. Ward, in *Topical Drug Delivery Formulations* (D. W. Osborne and A. H. Amann, eds.). Marcel Dekker, New York, 1990, p. 29.

43. J. A. Marqusee and K. A. Dill, *J. Chem. Phys.*, 85, 434 (1986).

44. J. M. Diamond and Y. Katz, *J. Membr. Biol.*, 17, 121 (1974).

45. B. D. Anderson, in *Physical and Chemical Properties of Drugs* (S. H. Yalkowsky, A. A. Sinkula, and S. C. Valvani, eds.). Marcel Dekker, New York, 1980.

46. J. H. Rytting, S. S. Davis, and T. Higuchi, *J. Pharm. Sci.*, 62, 816 (1972).

47. E. Mukai, Karase, M. Hashida, and H. Sezaki. *Int. J. Pharm.*, 25, 95 (1985).

48. S.-C. Chang, D.-S. Chien, H. Bundgaard, and V. H. L. Lee, *Exp. Eye Res.*, 46, 59 (1988).

49. S.-C. Chang and V. H. L. Lee, *J. Ocular Pharmacol.*, 3, 159 (1987).

50. G. M. Grass and J. R. Robinson, *J. Pharm. Sci.*, 77, 3 (1988).
51. G. M. Grass and J. R. Robinson, *J. Pharm. Sci.*, 77, 15 (1988).
52. G. M. Grass, E. R. Cooper, and J. R. Robinson, *J. Pharm. Sci.*, 77, 24 (1988).

5

Use of Solubility Parameters from Regular Solution Theory to Describe Partitioning-Driven Processes

Kenneth B. Sloan
University of Florida, Gainesville, Florida

INTRODUCTION

The solubility parameters of solute (δ_1) and solvent (δ_v) have been used for sometime by Hildebrand (1) and others (2–4) to attempt to quantitate the effect of solute-solvent interactions on the solubility of solutes in solvents. The mole fraction solubility of the solute, or in this case the drug, is represented by equation 1, where X_i is the mole fraction solubility of the drug (i) in the solvent or vehicle (v), ΔH_f is the heat of fusion of the drug at its melting point (T_i). T is the temperature at which the solubility is measured, and γ_1 is the activity coefficient of the drug in the vehicle. The first part of the right-hand side of the equation gives the ideal solubility, whereas the second part, γ_i, gives the contribution of solute-solvent interactions to the deviations of the measured solubility, X_i, from the ideal solubility. The activity coefficient of the drug in the vehicle can then be given by equation 2 from regular solution theory where δ_1 and δ_v have been defined above, ϕ_v is the fraction of the solution volume occupied by the vehicle, and V_i is the molar volume of the drug. Values for the terms in equations 1 and 2 can be determined experimentally or calculated from functional group contributions as described by Fedors (5) and illustrated by Martin (6) and others (7). The historical evolution of this approach to predicting solubility and, more important from the perspective of this chapter, to predicting the deviations from ideal solubility based on the theoretical considerations of the interaction between solute and solvent has been reviewed by Martin and Mauger (8).

$$-\log X_i = (\Delta H_f/2.3RT)\ [(T_i-T)/T_i] + \log \gamma_i \tag{1}$$

$$\log \gamma_i = (V_i\phi_v2/2.3RT)\ (\delta_i-\delta_v)^2 \tag{2}$$

Transdermal delivery of a drug is a diffusion process that depends on the development of a concentration gradient within the membrane to drive the process. The concentrations of the drug in that layer of the skin at the interface with the vehicle or donor phase (C_i) and at the interface with the plasma or receptor phase (C_2) are difficult to measure. On the other hand, the concentrations of the drug in the donor phase or vehicle (C_v) and in the receptor phase (C_R) are easy to measure, especially in the diffusion cell experiments. Thus, the equation for flux developed from Fick's first law for diffusion (eq. 3) is usually expanded to give equation 4, which contains terms that are more easily evaluated, or under certain controlled circumstances are assumed to be constants. In equation 4, J_i is the flux of the drug through the membrane, D_i is the diffusion coefficient of the drug in the skin, h_s is the thickness of the membrane, and K_i is the partition coefficient of the drug between the vehicle and the membrane. The term K_iC_v is substituted for C_1, and C_2 is assumed to represent sink conditions in equation 3, so $C_2 = 0$. Hence, equation 3 reduces to equation 4.

$$J_i = (D_i/h_s)\ (C_1-C_2) \tag{3}$$

$$J_i = (D_i/h_s)\ K_iC_v \tag{4}$$

If the vehicle does not significantly change or compromise the permeability of the membrane, it may be assumed that D_i and h_s are constants. The concentration of the drug in the vehicle, C_v, is easily measured, and the partition coefficient for the distribution of the drug between the vehicle and the membrane, K_i, can be measured in vitro. Alternatively, solvents with physicochemical properties similar to the membrane can be substituted for the membrane in the distribution experiments to give K_i for model systems. However, there are difficulties with either experimental approach, so a theoretical approach to evaluating K_i was developed.

The distribution of a drug between two phases to form saturated, nonideal solutions is given by equation 5. Since each activity coefficient in equation 5 can be calculated from equation 2, a theoretical partition coefficient can be calculated by substituting the values for the calculated activity coefficients into equation 5. The expanded form of equation 5 is equation 6, where $\gamma_{i,v}$ and $\gamma_{i,s}$ are the activity coefficients of the drug in the vehicle and in the membrane (skin), respectively; δ_i, δ_v, and δ_s are the solubility parameters of the drug, vehicle, and skin, respectively; V_i is the molar volume of the drug; and ϕ_s2 and ϕ_v2 approach 1, so equation 6 reduces to equation 7.

$$\log K_i = \log (\gamma_{i,v}/\gamma_{i,s}) \tag{5}$$

$$\log K_i = \frac{(\delta_i - \delta_v)^2 V_i \phi_v^2}{2.3RT} - \frac{(\delta_i - \delta_s)^2 V_i \phi_s^2}{2.3RT} \tag{6}$$

$$\log K_i = \frac{[(\delta_i - \delta_v)^2 - (\delta_i - \delta_s)^2] V_i}{2.3RT} \tag{7}$$

In the next sections we will illustrate the use of solubility parameters to describe biological processes other than transdermal delivery, and then their use to evaluate the effect of vehicles on the flux of drugs through skin. Finally, we will examine the use of solubility parameters to evaluate the effect of changes in the physicochemical properties of prodrugs on their ability to deliver their parent drugs through skin.

APPLICATIONS TO PARTITIONING-DRIVEN PROCESSES

Drugs: Nontransdermal

Examples of the use of solubility parameters to describe biological processes other than transdermal delivery is limited. Khalil and Martin (9) used solubility parameters in their analysis of the factors affecting the transfer of salicylic acid from one phase to another in a system designed to model absorption from the gastrointestinal tract. The rates of transfer of salicylic acid from pH 2 aqueous solutions (representing the stomach contents) through nonpolar immiscible liquids (representing the gastrointestinal membrane) exhibiting solubility parameter values of 7.1 to 10.7 $(cal/cm^3)^{1/2}$ and into pH 7.4 aqueous solutions (representing plasma) were measured. Their results from that model system show that the closer the δ value of the nonpolar liquid is to that of salicylic acid [$\delta_i = 10.8$ $(cal/cm^3)^{1/2}$], the faster the rate of disappearance of salicylic acid is from the pH 2.0 solution and the slower its rate of appearance is in the pH 7.4 solution. Generally, a solute exhibits its highest solubility in a solvent whose solubility parameter value is equal to that of the solute. Thus, partitioning into the model membrane is faster for those model membranes in which salicylic acid is most soluble.

On the other hand, partitioning of a solute from a solvent into a membrane will be slowest from those solvents in which the solute is most soluble; i.e., for solvents whose solubility parameter value is closest to that of the solute. Martin and coworkers (10) examined the effect of the composition of polyethylene glycol 400/water mixtures on the in vivo absorption of theophylline from the mixtures into rat intestinal membrane. They found that the closer the δ value of the polyethylene glycol 400/water mixture was to the δ value of theophylline, the slower the rate of disappearance of theophylline was from the mixture into the rat intestine. Thus, increasing the solubility of the solute in the solvent, if there is no concomitant increase in the solubility in the membrane, decreases the rate of partitioning driven processes.

Cohen and coworkers (11,12) have also used regular solution theory to explain how some molecules can be depressors (anesthetics) of the nervous system, whereas other quite similar molecules can be stimulants (convulsants). They explain the difference by extending the concept of Mullins (13), which is that the biological action of a chemical depended on the biophase in which the chemical acts. Thus, drug specificity is a consequence of its ability to preferentially partition into a subregion of the membrane exhibiting a bulk solubility parameter similar to that of the drug. In this case, drugs exhibiting lower δ values caused excitation, whereas those exhibiting higher δ values caused depression.

Similarly, Bustamante and Selles (14) have shown that the binding sites of drugs on protein correspond to amino acid sequences that exhibit solubility parameter values similar to that of the most tightly bound drug. For example, the δ value for the binding site of sulfonamides was determined to be 12.33 $(cal/cm^3)^{1/2}$, which closely corresponds to the average solubility parameter of the seven amino acid sequence in human serum albumin thought to be the primary binding site for sulfonamides.

Drugs: Transdermal

Two groups have investigated the use of regular solution theory to describe the partitioning process in topical delivery. Sloan and coworkers (7,15–17) and Cohen and coworkers (18–20) have used regular solution theory to explain the effect of vehicles on the rates at which a drug is delivered through skin. The experimental design used in the work reported by Sloan and coworkers contains three unique components. First, only saturated solutions of drug/vehicle are applied to the membranes in the diffusion cell experiments. Second, after each initial application period, a 24-h washout period—where there is no applied donor phase—is used to determine the effect of the drug/vehicle combination on accumulation of the drug in the membrane. Third, after the washout period, a "second" application of a standard solute/vehicle is made to determine the extent of any damage to the membrane that the initial drug/vehicle may have caused.

Saturated solutions of the drugs are used to ensure that they are being tested at their maximum thermodynamic activity. Also, when the drugs are tested as saturated solutions and a mole fraction concentration scale is used, the activities of the drug in the skin ($\alpha_{i,s}$) and in the vehicle ($\alpha_{i,v}$) are equal when equilibrium is established between the two phases. Thus, K_i from equation 5 can be calculated using the activity coefficients from equation 2 only if saturated solutions are being evaluated.

One advantage of being able to calculate K_i from activity coefficients derives from the relationship of K_i to the permeability coefficient P_i (eq. 8). If D_i and h_s are constants, then equation 8 reduces to equation 9, and the permeability coefficient is equal to the product of the partition coefficient and a constant. Then, since the form of equation 6 dictates that the relationship between calculated K_i and the solubility parameter values for the vehicles used (δ_v) takes the form of a parabola with a minimum where $\delta_v = \delta_i$, the relationship between experimental P_i and δ_v should take the same form. Hence, to determine if the differences in the rates of delivery of a drug by various vehicles can be explained by regular solution, it is only necessary to plot log calculated K_i against δ_v and determine if the plot of log experimental P_i against δ_v approximates the shape of the log K_i versus δ_v plot and is separated from it by a constant that corresponds to D_i/h_s.

$$P_i = K_i(D_i/h) = J_i/C_v \tag{8}$$

$$P_i = K_i \cdot \text{constant} \tag{9}$$

If the differences in the rates of delivery of a drug by various vehicles can be explained by regular solution theory, then it is possible to predict P_i for delivery of the drug from other vehicles based on calculated K_i for the partitioning of the drug from those vehicles into skin. It is then only necessary to measure the solubilities of the drug in those vehicles, C_v, and to calculate the flux, J_i, from those vehicles using equation 8.

The other advantage of being able to calculate K_i from activity coefficients is that it obviates the need of determining experimental K_i from partitioning of the drug between vehicles and membranes. Significant changes in the degree of hydration and other physicochemical properties of skin result if skin samples are equilibrated with vehicles for extended periods of time (21). Thus, such experimental K_i may not be as appropriate as they intuitively appear to be. On the other hand, it is possible to obtain very accurate K_i for the partitioning of a drug between a vehicle (water) and a solvent that serves as a model for the biological membrane. Frequently, octanol is used as the model solvent, but many other water-immiscible solvents have been used as well. It is also possible to calculate a theoretical K_i using fragment constants for the various functional groups in a drug which are derived from the previously determined experimental K_i values (22,23). However, this approach cannot be used to evaluate most of the vehicles that are potentially of interest as components of topical delivery formulations because the vehicles are either miscible or at least partially soluble in either octanol or water, or both. For example, it would be virtually impossible to measure K_i, and hence be able to calculate theoretical K_i, in systems where propanol, dimethyl sulfoxide, dimethylformamide, propylene glycol, formamide, glycerin, isopropyl myristate, or oleic acid are the vehicles of interest and 1-octanol is the model for the biological membrane.

The skin accumulation data obtained from the washout period in the diffusion cell experiments of Sloan and coworkers (see Chap. 2) are important to any approach to optimize dermal delivery. There must be a correlation between delivery of a drug through the skin or transdermal delivery (which is the usual kind of data obtained from diffusion cell experiments) and delivery into the skin or dermal delivery (as determined from skin accumulation data) if the optimization process is to be based on diffusion cell data.

Values of flux from the "second" application of a standard solute/vehicle after the washout period can be compared to a control value to determine if the membranes are damaged by the initial application of a drug/vehicle combination. These data are important for two reasons. First, the greater the degree of damage, the greater the degree of deviation from the assumptions that D_i and h_s are constants. If D_i and h_s are not constants because each vehicle affects membrane integrity differently, then equation 9 does not hold and the application of regular solution theory to analyze this partitioning process is not possible. Conversely, if there is little damage caused by most vehicles, then it is possible. Second, if it is possible to assess the damage caused by a particular drug/vehicle combination, it should be possible to separate the thermodynamic effects (a) of the drug/vehicle interaction, or (b) of physicochemical properties of the prodrug on the partitioning process, from the chemical or physical effects of the vehicles themselves on the integrity of the membranes.

The effects of vehicles on the transdermal delivery of four drugs were evaluated by Sloan and coworkers (7,15–17). The results for three of the drugs—theophylline (7), 6-mercaptopurine (16), and 5-fluorouracil (17)—are given in Table 1. The theoretical partition coefficients, K_i, in Table 1 were calculated assuming a δ_s value of about 10 $(cal/cm^3)^{1/2}$ (18), whereas the δ_v values were literative values (24) except for isopropyl myristate (IPM) (7). The solubility parameter values for the drug, δ_i, and the molar volumes, V_i, were all calculated using the group contribution method of Fedors (5) as illustrated by Martin and coworkers (6). Experimental P_i values were determined for the delivery of each polar drug from vehicles exhibiting a wide range of polarities from very polar (H_2O) to very nonpolar (oleic acid) through hairless mouse skin. The corresponding fluxes, J_i, and saturated concentrations, C_v, are also given in Table 1. The data from a plot of the log experimental P_i values versus δ_v for the vehicles that were examined in Table 1 approximates a parabola for each of the three drugs examined, except for the data from octanol or IPM. In those cases, the values for the second application fluxes were much higher than the control values, so those vehicles had damaged the integrity of the skin. Thus, the assumptions about D_i and h_s being constant were not valid for those vehicles.

A typical plot of log experimental P_i values versus δ_v is given in Fig. 1 for 6-mercaptopurine (6-MP). Disregarding the data from octanol and IPM (also water and glycerin because of the tendency of heterocycles to self-associate in those solvents) (16), it can be seen that the shape of the plot approximates a parabola. A plot of the log theoretical K_i values versus δ_v for the partitioning of 6-MP from those vehicles into the skin is also given in Fig. 1. The position of the minimum in the parabola and the shape of the parabola is very similar to the plot of log experimental P_i versus δ_v for the delivery of 6-MP through the skin. If the outliers in the experimental P_i are disregarded, a plot of log theoretical P_i versus δ_v

Table 1 The Effect of Single Component Vehicles on the Delivery of Drugs through Hairless Mouse Skin: Solubilities (C_v) Fluxes (J_i), Permeability Coefficients (P_i), and Theoretical Partition Coefficients (K_i)

Solvent[a]	C_v mg/cm^3	J_i[b] mg/cm^2/h	P_i[c] cm/h	log K_i[d]
Theophylline[e]				
2 IPM	0.062	0.041	0.660	1.12
4 OCT	1.70	0.547	0.320	−0.18
6 DMF	34.6	0.017	0.00049	−0.98
8 PG	8.07	0.0015	0.00019	−1.22
9 EG	7.40	0.0019	0.00026	−0.92
10 FOR	1.57	0.0037	0.0024	−0.06
6-Mercaptopurine[f]				
1 OA	0.0030	0.000043	0.014	1.57
2 IPM	0.0034	0.00060	0.176	0.90
3 DET	4.4	0.0032	0.00072	0.06
4 OCT	0.23	0.019	0.081	−0.15
5 MEG	10.0	0.00075	0.000075	−0.82
6 DMF	14.5	0.0038	0.00026	−0.82
7 DMSO	34.8	0.0021	0.000059	−1.02
8 PG	6.2	0.000093	0.000015	−1.12
9 EG	3.0	0.00010	0.000033	−0.96
10 GLY	9.7	0.000037	0.0000038	−0.49
11 FOR	9.1	0.0015	0.00016	−0.42
12 H$_2$O	0.17	0.00036	0.0021	3.76
5-Fluorouracil[g]				
1 OA	0.74	1.100	0.150	1.35
2 IPM	0.0051	0.028	5.4	0.78
4 OCT	0.60	0.440	0.73	−0.13
6 DMF	62.3	0.025	0.00041	−0.75
8 PG	16.5	0.0016	0.000097	−1.13
9 EG	19.6	0.0047	0.00024	−1.08
11 FOR	13.7	0.015	0.0011	−0.75

[a]OA = oleic acid (δ_v = 7.6), IPM = isopropyl myristate (δ_v = 8.5), DET = diethyltoluamide (δ_v = 10), OCT = 1-octanol (δ_v = 10.3), DMF = dimethylformamide (δ_v = 12.1), MEG = 2-methoxyethanol (δ_v = 12.1), DMSO = dimethyl sulfoxide (δ_v = 13.0), PG = propylene glycol (δ_v = 14.8), EG = ethylene glycol (δ_v = 16.1), GLY = glycerin (δ_v = 17.7), FOR = formamide (δ_v = 17.9), H$_2$O = water (δ_v = 23).
[b]Steady-state fluxes, n = 3.
[c]Permeability coefficients calculated from J_i/C_v.
[d]Calculated from equation 6:R = 1.98 cal/degree, T = 305°K, δ_s = 10 (cal/cm^3)$^{1/2}$; for theophylline δ_i = 14.0 (cal/cm^3)$^{1/2}$, V_i = 110 cm^3/mol; for 6-MP δ_i = 14.4 (cal/cm^3)$^{1/2}$, V_i = 81.2 cm^3/mol; for 5-FU δ_i = 15.0 (cal/cm^3)$^{1/2}$, V_i = 70.4 cm^3/mol.
[e]From Ref. 7.
[f]From Ref. 16.
[g]From Ref. 17.

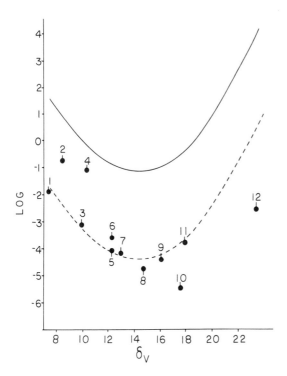

Figure 1 A plot of log experimental permeability coefficients for the delivery of 6-MP from suspensions of 6-MP in various vehicles versus the solubility parameter values of the vehicles (δ_v). Data points are labeled numerically according to designations for vehicles in Table 1. Plots of calculated log permeability coefficients (– – –) and calculated log partition coefficients (——) versus δ_v are also shown.

can be constructed from the sum of the corresponding log theoretical K_i values and the average of the differences between the log theoretical K_i values and the log experimental P_i values. A reasonably good fit between the individual log theoretical P_i values and the corresponding experimental P_i values is obtained. In addition, the average difference between log theoretical K_i and log experimental P_i corresponds to the constant in equation 9. If the thickness of the stratum corneum is assumed to be about 10 μm, then D_i is about 10^{-10} cm²/s based on the constants derived from equation 9 for most of the drugs that were evaluated. That value for D_i is about the right order of magnitude for such polar molecules.

There are four significant conclusions that can be drawn from the results of Sloan and coworkers (7,15–17) for these experiments. First, there is generally a minimum in the plot of log experimental P_i versus δ_v that corresponds to the vehicle for which $\delta_v = \delta_i$. Since drugs usually exhibit their greatest solubility in solvents for which $\delta_v = \delta_i$, there is generally an inverse relationship between the solubility of the drug in the vehicle and P_i. The relationship between solubility and J_i is not as general, but the same sort of trend exists in that relationship as well. Second, vehicles for which $\delta_v \approx \delta_s$ cause the most damage to the skin as assessed by second-application studies. Since the values for δ_v for those vehicles and δ_s are similar $[\delta \approx 9\text{–}11 \ (cal/cm^3)^{1/2}]$, the vehicles may be solubilizing a portion of the membranes that is responsible for providing the diffusional resistance to drug permeation and especially to polar drug molecules $[\delta = 13\text{–}15 \ (cal/cm^3)^{1/2}]$ because a relatively nonpolar portion of the membrane would be solubilized by such vehicles, leaving behind a more polar environment for a polar drug to diffuse through. Third, the parabolic nature of the relationship between δ_v and P_i, expected if the partitioning process obeyed regular solution theory, has been confirmed for several polar drugs. Fourth, the direct relationship between P_i and K_i, in the absence of significant damage to the membrane by the vehicle, has been established. Thus, from a knowledge of the solubilities of a drug in various vehicles, the calculated K_i, the constant from equation 9, and the flux of the drug from one vehicle, it should be possible to determine the flux of that drug from other vehicles, assuming that the vehicles do not damage the skin.

Sloan and coworkers also evaluated the effect of a binary component vehicle [oleic acid–propylene glycol (PG)] on the rates of delivery of 6-MP (16) and 5-fluorouracil (5-FU) (17) through hairless mouse skin. The results are given in Table 2. Although the individual components of the binary system caused no damage to the skins as assessed by second-application studies, all of the binary component vehicles did. There was some enhancement in the rates of delivery of 6-MP from such vehicles, but there was no enhancement in the rates for 5-FU. Thus, enhanced delivery of a drug from a binary component vehicle, even when achieved, may be due to enhanced damage to the integrity of the skin rather than enhanced partitioning into the skin.

One of the initial articles by Cohen and coworkers (18), which evaluated the effect of various solvents on the transdermal delivery of a solute, studied the delivery of alkanoic acids through porcine skin. For a series of straight chain alkanoic acid the maximum flux was observed for butyric acid $[\delta = 10.0 \ (cal/cm^3)^{1/2}]$, so the apparent δ_s was assumed to be about $10 \ (cal/cm)^{1/2}$. The delivery of propionic acid from a variety of solvents was also studied. The expected parabolic relationship between P_i and δ_v with a minimum at $\delta_v = \delta_i$ was not observed. Instead, there was a steady increase in P_i with increasing δ_v. This result may have been obtained because saturated solution could not be used.

More recently, Cohen and coworkers (19) have attempted to separate and to quantify two variables responsible for differences in flux of a solute from different vehicles: (a) The thermodynamic activity of the solute in the vehicle—the push effect; (b) the extent of alteration of the barrier function of the skin caused by the vehicle—the pull effect. Because $P_i = K_i \cdot constant$, if the experimentally

Table 2 The Effect of Binary Component Vehicles on the Delivery of Drugs through Hairless Mouse Skin: Solubility Parameters (δ_v), Solubilities (C_v), Fluxes (J_i), and Permeability Coefficients (P_i)

Solvent[a] (mole ratios)	$\delta_v{}^b$ (cal/cm³)$^{1/2}$	C_v mg/cm³	$J_i{}^c$ mg/cm²/h	P_i cm/h
6-Mercaptopurine[d]				
OA	7.6	0.0030	0.000043	0.014
OA:PG (3:1)	8.1	0.087	0.00044	0.0051
OA:PG (1:1)	9.3	0.39	0.00095	0.0024
OA:PG (1:3)	10.6	1.23	0.0016	0.0013
OA:PG (1:5)	12.0	2.25	0.0016	0.00071
OA:PG (1:14.5)	13.5	4.35	0.0019	0.00044
PG	14.8	6.2	0.000093	0.000015
5-Fluorouracil[e]				
OA	7.6	0.74	0.100	0.15
OA:PG (1:1)	9.3	0.98	0.050	0.051
OA:PG (1:3)	10.6	4.3	0.050	0.012
OA:PG (1:14.5)	13.5	11.1	0.088	0.0079
PG	14.8	16.5	0.0016	0.000097

[a]OA = oleic acid, PG = propylene glycol.
[b]Calculated on a volume fraction basis.
[c]Steady-state fluxes, n = 3.
[d]From Ref. 16.
[e]From Ref. 17.

determined ration of $P_{i,v(1)}/P_{i,v(2)}$ is equal to the theoretically determined ratio of $K_{i,v(1)}/K_{i,v(2)}$, then only thermodynamic effects are responsible for driving the flux of the solute. On the other hand, if the vehicle v(1) affects δ_s by making it more polar, then the experimental ratio $P_{i,v(1)}/P_{i,v(2)}$ will be larger than the theoretical ratio $K_{i,v(1)}/K_{i,v(2)}$. Conversely, if vehicle v(2) affects δ_s by making it more polar, then the experimental ratio will be smaller than the theoretical ratio.

The experimental results showed that P_i for the delivery of theophylline from propionic, hexanoic, octanoic, and a mixture of octanoic and hexanoic acids was inversely related to δ_v values. However, P_i for the delivery of theophylline from mixtures of alkanoic acids containing propionic acid was higher than expected based on the δ_v of the mixture. Thus, the experimental ratio of $P_{i,v(1)}/P_{i,v(2)}$ was smaller than the theoretical ratio if propionic acid was v(2) and larger if it was v(1). It was concluded that all the single-component vehicles and binary component vehicles without propionic acid exerted only a push effect on the transdermal delivery of theophylline, whereas binary component vehicles containing propionic acid exerted an additional pull effect.

Another article by Cohen and coworkers (20) evaluated the effect of alkanoic acids on the delivery of adenosine through human skin. For the delivery of adenosine from mixtures of hexanoic and propionic acid, a bell-shaped dependence of observed ln P_i on volume fraction of hexanoic acid was observed. An increase in the volume fraction of hexanoic acid in the vehicle caused an increase in the excess free energy of adenosine in the vehicle, and hence an increased push effect. On the other hand, an increase in the volume fraction of propionic acid in the vehicle caused an increase in the flux of propionic acid from the vehicle and into the skin where it caused an increase in the pull effect. A similar result was obtained from mixtures of propionic acid and isopropyl myristate.

Thus, for the transdermal delivery of drugs, the effect of vehicles on the thermodynamic driving force for the partitioning and diffusion processes has been separated from vehicle (solvent) effects on the integrity of the skin using second-application experiments or by comparing experimental P_i with theoretical K_i and P_i calculated from regular solution theory. Analysis of the results of the thermodynamic effect of vehicles on transdermal delivery suggest that such analyses have predictive value.

However, although this theoretical treatment of the partitioning process is satisfactory for evaluating the delivery of drugs from different vehicles through a membrane, there is no mechanism for evaluating the effect of the rate of chemical or enzymatic hydrolysis of prodrugs on their abilities to deliver their parent drugs through the membrane. A prodrug frequently exhibits quite different physicochemical properties compared to its parent drug, so its diffusion coefficient, D_i, may be quite different from that of its parent. Thus, the constantly changing composition of the mixture of permeants, as the prodrug hydrolyzes during the diffusion process, makes it difficult to separate the effect of changing the physicochemical properties of the prodrug from the effect of changing its chemical or enzymatic stability on the ability of the prodrug to enhance transdermal delivery. The situation is more easily analyzed if the prodrug is so stable that it permeates intact, or it is so unstable that it hydrolyzes almost immediately as it reaches the aqueous environment of the skin, and hence its different physicochemical properties affect only the partitioning process.

In the next section, we will examine the effect that rapid hydrolysis has on the use of δ values of prodrugs to describe and to predict the transdermal delivery process, and to compare those results with results form prodrugs that undergo hydrolysis more slowly during the course of their diffusion through the skin.

Prodrugs: Transdermal

In order to determine if the effect of vehicles on the transdermal delivery of a parent drug by its prodrugs can be analyzed in the same way that the effect of vehicles on the transdermal delivery of the parent drugs was analyzed in the previous section, it was first necessary to use a series of prodrugs that was stable in protic vehicles. Otherwise, the spectrum of polarities of the vehicles used in the experiments would be so limited as to almost preclude the possibility of observing any correlation. Thus, the first set of data that are analyzed are obtained from prodrugs that undergo enzymatic hydrolysis during their diffusion through the skin and not from prodrugs that hydrolyzed chemically or enzymatically immediately upon reaching the skin. The acyloxymethyl prodrugs that were evaluated exhibit ideal physicochemical properties to provide the necessary data. They are sufficiently stable in water (25) and protic vehicles such as octanol, propylene glycol, etc., that they should not hydrolyze chemically in the donor phase. On the other hand, they undergo enzymatic hydrolysis at a sufficient rate to function as prodrugs (25), yet they are also sufficiently stable even to enzymatic hydrolysis that some members of the series will diffuse through the hairless mouse skin partially intact (26).

The results from diffusion cell experiments in which the rates of delivery of 6-MP by an homologous series of S^6,9-bisacyloxymethyl-6-MP derivatives from seven different vehicles were determined (27) are given in Table 3. It is important that these results were obtained under the same conditions that the results for the delivery of 6-MP by 6-MP from these same vehicles were obtained (see Table 1). In each case, a saturated solution of the prodrug in a vehicle was applied as the donor phase, a washout period after the initial application of prodrug/vehicle was used to determine relative drug accumulation in the skin, and a second application of a standard drug/vehicle was used to determine the relative extent of damage to the skin. For each prodrug/vehicle combination examined, the damage it caused to the skin was not significantly greater than the damage caused by the drug/vehicle combination. Also, as has been noted in a previous chapter, regardless of the vehicle used in the experiment, the S^6,9-bisacetyloxymethyl and S^6,9-bispropionyloxymethyl-6-MP derivatives delivered the greatest amount of 6-MP through the skin.

When the log permeability coefficients, P_i, values for the four prodrugs, for which results from most of the seven vehicles are available (see Table 3) are plotted against the δ_v values of the vehicles in Fig. 2, several trends are observed. First, for oleic acid, isopropyl myristate, and octanol, the rank order of the P_i values is the same for the delivery of 6-MP by the four prodrugs and by 6-MP itself, with the most polar prodrug (S^6,9-bisacetyloxymethyl-6-MP) exhibiting the highest P_i value and the least polar (S^6,9-valeryloxymethyl-6-MP) the lowest P_i value. The rank order for the prodrugs remains the same when the P_i values for the delivery of 6-MP by the prodrugs from PG are considered; but the P_i values for the first three members of the series are not significantly different from each other, and the P_i value for 6-MP is much smaller than for any of the prodrugs. The rank order for the P_i values for the prodrugs and 6-MP is reversed for the three remaining more polar vehicles (glycerin, formamide, and water), although the differences among the P_i values for the delivery of 6-MP from formamide are not significant. Thus, the most polar prodrug exhibits the lowest P_i value and the least

Table 3 Solubilities (C_v) and Solubility Parameter Values (δ_i) for S^6,9-Bisacyloxymethyl-6-Mercaptopurine Derivatives: Their Rates of Delivery of 6-Mercaptopurine (J_i) and Log Permeability Coefficients (P_i) from Various Vehicles

$$S\,CH_2O(C=O)\,R$$

$$CH_2O(C=O)\,R$$

R/Vehicle[a]	δ_i^b	C_v^c	J_i^d	P_i^e
1 6-MP/IPM	14.4	0.0034	0.00060	−0.73
2 R = CH₃/IPM	13.34	0.80	0.0345	−1.36
3 R = C₂H₅/IPM	12.75	5.11	0.0352	−2.16
4 R = C₃H₇/IPM	12.29	13.8	0.0215	−2.81
5 R = C₄H₉/IPM	11.93	26.5	0.0155	−3.23
6 R = C₅H₁₁/IPM	11.63	7.56	0.00175	−3.63
7 R = C₇H₁₅/IPM	11.17	2.60	0.00019	−4.14
8 R = C(CH₃)₃/IPM	11.7	31.7	0.00548	−3.76
1 6-MP/OA	14.4	0.0030	0.000043	−1.84
2 R = CH₃/OA	13.34	1.08	0.00592	−2.26
3 R = C₂H₅/OA	12.75	11.3	0.00833	−3.13
5 R = C₄H₉/OA	11.93	69.6	0.00335	−4.32
1 6-MP/OCT	14.4	0.23	0.0186	−1.09
2 R = CH₃/OCT	13.34	1.11	0.0754	−1.17
3 R = C₂H₅/OCT	12.75	5.57	0.0853	−1.81
4 R = C₃H₇/OCT	12.29	11.50	0.0257	−2.65
1 6-MP/PG	14.4	6.2	0.000093	−4.82
2 R = CH₃/PG	13.34	2.79	0.00058	−3.68
3 R = C₂H₅/PG	12.75	8.63	0.00195	−3.65
4 R = C₃H₇/PG	12.29	9.54	0.00160	−3.76
5 R = C₄H₉/PG	11.93	8.32	0.00077	−4.03
6 R = C₅H₁₁/PG	11.63	1.71	0.00018	−3.99
1 6-MP/GLY	14.4	9.7	0.0000367	−5.42
2 R = CH₃/GLY	13.34	0.51	0.000135	−3.58
3 R = C₂H₅/GLY	12.75	0.35	0.000450	−2.88
5 R = C₄H₉/GLY	11.93	0.066	0.000290	−2.35
1 6-MP/FOR	14.4	9.1	0.00150	−3.79
2 R = CH₃/FOR	13.34	15.8	0.00259	−3.78
3 R = C₂H₅/FOR	12.75	22.3	0.00706	−3.50
5 R = C₄H₉/FOR	11.93	6.2	0.00200	−3.49
1 6-MP/H₂O	14.4	0.17	0.00036	−2.68
2 R = CH₃/H₂O	13.34	0.44	0.00158	−2.44
3 R = C₂H₅/H₂O	12.75	0.25	0.00197	−2.11
4 R = C₃H₇/H₂O	12.29	0.030	0.00081	−1.57
5 R = C₄H₉/H₂O	11.93	0.0071	0.00050	−1.15

[a]See Table 1 for definitions.
[b]Calculated from group contribution method of Fedors [5].
[c]Solubility in equivalent mg of 6-MP/ml.
[d]Flux in mg/cm²/h, n = 3.
[e]Permeability coefficient calculated from J_i/C_v.
Source: From Ref. 27.

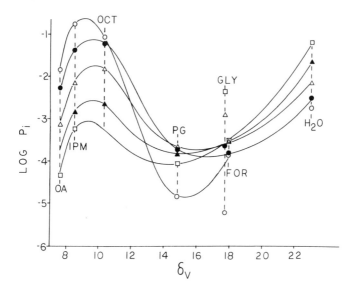

Figure 2 A plot log experimental permeability coefficients for the delivery of total 6-MP from suspensions of selected S^6,9-bisacyloxymethyl-6-MP derivatives and 6-MP in various vehicles versus the solubility parameter values of the vehicles (δ_v). The data points are for 6-MP (o), S^6,9-bisacetyloxymethyl-6-MP (•), S^6,9-bispropionyloxymethyl-6-MP (Δ), S^6,9-bisbutyryloxymethyl-6-MP (▲), and S^6,9-bisvaleryloxymethyl-6-MP (□). The vehicles are OA = oleic acid, IPM = isopropyl myristate, OCT = 1-octanol, PG = propylene glycol, GLY = glycerin, FOR = formamide, H_2O = water.

polar prodrug the highest P_i value for the delivery of 6-MP from the more polar vehicles.

Second, if we assume that the P_i values for the missing data points follow the trends for the available data, then a curve drawn through the P_i versus δ_v values for the delivery of 6-MP by one prodrug from olecic acid, IMP, octanol, PG formamide, and water is very similar to the same curve drawn for the other prodrugs (see Fig. 2). A partial curve drawn through the P_i versus δ_v values for the delivery of 6-MP by 6-MP from the same vehicles, except for water, is quite different from the curves drawn for its prodrugs. This may be expected because the functional groups contributing to the solubilities, and hence the partitioning processes, are so different in 6-MP compared to the prodrugs. The P_i values obtained for the delivery of 6-MP by the prodrugs from glycerin do not fit the curves drawn through the P_i values for the other vehicles.

Finally, log experimental P_i versus δ_v curves generated from the data in Fig. 2, but excluding the data for IPM and octanol, are not similar to theoretical K_i versus

δ_v curves generated from K_i calculated from regular solution theory (eq. 6 or 7) or from K_i obtained from the ratios of the respective saturated solubilities in Table 3; i.e., C_{OCT}/C_v (K_i or P_i curves not shown). Such curves are all much flatter than the one in Fig. 1, for instance. Thus, there is little similarity between these results for the delivery of a parent drug by its prodrugs and the results from the previous section where there was a good correlation between log theoretical K_i and log experimental P_i for the delivery of 6-MP from the same vehicles. However, the curves generated from these plots of P_i values for the prodrugs versus δ_v do exhibit a shift in their minima toward lower δ_v values as the prodrug becomes more lipidlike and exhibits a lower δ_i value. This result is expected based on the discussion in the previous section where there was a good correlation between experimental results and predictions based on regular solution theory, since it would predict minima in log P_i versus δ_v curves where $\delta_i = \delta_v$.

The relationship between P_i values for the delivery of a drug by an homologous series of prodrugs from one vehicle and the δ_i values for the prodrugs shown in Fig. 2 can be seen more clearly in Fig. 3 where the log P_i for the delivery of 6-MP by the S^6,9-bisacyloxymethyl-6-MP prodrugs from IPM, PG, and water are plotted against δ_i for the prodrugs. For IPM there is a direct relationship between δ_i values and log P_i values—the higher the δ_1 value, the more polar the prodrug and the higher the log P_i value. For water there is an inverse relationship, and for PG there is not much change in log P_i with changing δ_i. The results for oleic acid and octanol are similar to that for IPM, whereas the results for glycerin are similar to that for water, and the results for formamide are similar to that for PG (curves not shown).

The general shape of these results is a direct consequence of the relationship between P_i and K_i from equations 8 and 9 and the form of equations 6 or 7 for the calculation of K_i. For the convenience of the reader, equation 6 is repeated here.

$$\log K_i = \frac{(\delta_i - \delta_v)^2 \, v_i \, \phi_v^{\,2}}{2.3RT} - \frac{(\delta_i - \delta_s)^2 \, v_i \, \phi_s^{\,2}}{2.3RT}$$

In the case where the vehicle is IPM and $\delta_v = 8.5$ (cal/cm^3)$^{1/2}$, the substitution of smaller values for δ_i will lead to smaller values for log K_i and hence for log P_i because of the relationship between K_i and P_i from equation 9. Conversely, if water is the vehicle [$\delta_v = 23$ (cal/cm^3)$^{1/2}$], substitution of smaller values of δ_i will lead to larger values for K_i and hence for P_i. However, for an homologous series of prodrugs such as the acyloxymethyl prodrugs of 6-MP, as the value of δ_i decreases, the value of V_i increases with increasing length of the alkyl chain in the acyl portion of the promoiety. In the case of IPM, this results in a compensating effect in the evaluation of the first part of the right-hand-side of equation 6. As the square of the difference between δ_i and δ_v gets smaller, it is multiplied by an increasingly larger value for V_i, so there is a tendency for the difference between that product for one prodrug and that product for the next in a series of homologous prodrugs to be small. In those cases where log K_i have been

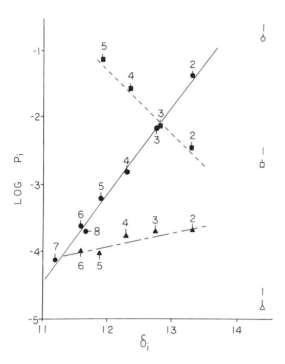

Figure 3 A plot of log experimental permeability coefficients for the delivery of total 6-MP from suspensions of S^6,9-bisacyloxymethyl-6-MP derivatives in IMP ($\bullet$) (——), water ($\blacksquare$) (– – –), and PG ($\blacktriangle$) (— –) versus the calculated solubility parameter values of the derivatives (δ_i). The data points for 6-MP are represented by (o) for IPM, by ($\square$) for water, and by ($\triangle$) for PG. Data points are labeled numerically according to structures in Table 3.

calculated from equation 6, the trend in the relationship between calculated K_i and δ_i is the same as between experimental P_i and δ_i except for the case where PG is the solvent. Then the prediction is that there should be an inverse relationship between P_i and δ_i instead of the observed slight direct relationship. Also, the absolute values calculated for K_i have no quantitative relationship to P_i. The differences between the calculated values for K_i of the individual prodrugs are much smaller than the experimental values for P_i when IPM is the vehicle, whereas they are much larger when water is the vehicle.

Although the only example of an evaluation of the abilities of an homologous series of prodrugs to deliver its parent drug form a wide variety of vehicles is the evaluation of the S^6,9-bisacyloxymethyl-6-MP series, a number of other types of prodrugs of 6-MP that exhibit a spectrum of stability in water and protic vehicles have also been evaluated, but generally only for their abilities to deliver 6-MP from IPM. The solubilities, permeability coefficients, solubility parameters, and rates of delivery of 6-MP by S^6-acyloxymethyl- (28) and S^6-(N-alkyl-N-alkoxycarbonyl)aminomethyl-6-MP derivatives (29) from IPM are given in Table 4. The S^6-acyloxymethyl-6-MP derivatives are very stable in pH 7.4 buffer (the acetyloxymethyl derivative exhibits a half-life of 114 h, whereas the butyryloxymethyl derivative exhibits a half-life of 228 h), but they undergo hydrolysis up to 100 times faster in buffer containing enzymes leached from mouse dermis. On the other hand, the S^6-(N-alkyl-N-alkoxycarbonyl) aminomethyl-6-MP derivatives are not very stable in pH 7.4 buffer (they exhibit

Table 4 Solubilities (C_v) and Solubility Parameter Values (δ_i) for S^6-Acyloxymethyl- and S^6-(N-Alkyl-N-alkoxycarbonyl)aminomethyl-6-mercaptopurine Derivatives: Their Rates of Delivery of 6-Mercaptopurine (J_i) and Log Permeability Coefficients (P_i) from IPM

Compound	$\delta_i{}^a$	$C_v{}^b$	$J_i{}^c$	Log $P_i{}^d$
1 6-MP	14.4	0.0034	0.00060	–0.73
9 R = O(C=O)CH$_3$[e]	14.4	0.16	0.0308	–0.72
10 R = O(C=O)C$_2$H$_5$[e]	13.9	0.35	0.0325	–1.03
11 R = O(C=O)C$_3$H$_7$[e]	13.5	0.50	0.0398	–1.10
12 R = O(C=O)C$_4$H$_9$[e]	13.1	0.64	0.0335	–1.28
13 R = O(C=O)C$_5$H$_{11}$[e]	12.8	0.56	0.0083	–1.83
14 R = O(C=O)C$_7$H$_{15}$[e]	12.3	0.63	0.0020	–2.50
15 R = O(C=O)C(CH$_3$)$_3$[e]	12.6	0.80	0.0094	–1.94
16 R = CH$_3$,R'=CH$_3$[f]	13.75	0.167	0.0039	–1.63
17 R = CH$_3$,R'=C$_2$H$_5$[f]	13.36	0.182	0.00058	–2.50
18 R = CH$_3$,R'=C$_4$H$_9$[f]	12.73	0.167	0.000054	–3.49
19 R = C$_2$H$_5$,R'=CH$_3$[f]	13.36	0.319	0.000058	–3.74
20 R = C$_2$H$_5$,R'=C$_2$H$_5$[f]	13.02	0.213	0.000014	–4.18
21 R = C$_4$H$_9$,R'=CH$_3$[f]	12.73	0.730	0.00020	–3.50
22 R = C$_4$H$_9$,R'=C$_4$H$_9$[f]	12.05	10.34	0.000071	–5.16

[a]Calculated from group contribution method of Fedors [5].
[b]Solubility in equivalent mg of 6-MP/ml.
[c]Flux in mg/cm^2/h, n = 3.
[d]Permeability coefficient calculated from J_i/C_v.
[e]From Ref. 28.
[f]From Ref. 29.

an average half-life of about 1.5 h), and their rates of hydrolysis are not increased in the presence of dermis enzymes. In spite of the large differences in stability, both series of prodrugs deliver only 6-MP through hairless mouse skin.

In order to determine if the difference in stability of the two types of derivatives has an effect on the relationship between log P_i and δ_i, the log P_i versus δ_i values for the two types of prodrugs from Table 4 are plotted in Fig. 4. In each case, a direct relationship between log P_i and δ_i is observed which is very similar to that observed for the plot of log P_i versus δ_i data for the S^6,9-bisacyloxymethyl-6-MP derivatives in Fig. 3. However, there is some variation in the slopes of the plots of the data obtained for each type of derivative. The slope is 1.32 for the S^6,9-bisacyl-oxymethyl derivatives, 1.18 for the S^6-acyloxymethyl derivatives, and 1.84 for the S^6-(N-alkyl-N-alkoxycarbonyl)aminomethyl derivatives. Only the slope generated from the latter data includes the log P_i versus δ_i data for 6-MP itself, as can be seen from Figs. 3 and 4. This latter result is also observed for plots of log P_i versus δ_i data for other types of prodrugs that undergo rapid chemical or enzymatic hydrolysis to their parent drugs.

Different types of N-acyl derivatives also exhibit a wide variation in chemical and enzymatic stability. For example, 1-alkylcarbonyl derivatives of 5-FU exhibit half-lives of about 3–4 min in pH 7.4 buffer (30), whereas 1-alkoxycarbonyl

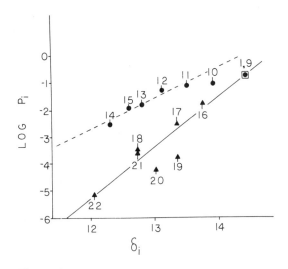

Figure 4 A plot of log experimental permeability coefficients for the delivery of 6-MP from suspensions of S^6-acyloxymethyl-6-MP (•) (– – –) and S^6-(N-alkyl-N-alkoxycar-bonyl)aminomethyl-6-MP derivatives (▲) (——) in IPM versus the calculated solubility parameter values of the derivatives (δ_i). The data point for 6-MP is represented by (▢). Data points are labeled numerically according to structures in Table 4.

derivatives exhibit half-lives of 200–500 min in pH 7.4 buffer but half-lives of only 2–3 min in 80% human plasma (31). 1-Alkylaminocarbonyl derivatives exhibit half-lives in pH 7.4 buffer (8–11 min) (32) that are intermediate in value compared to other two acyl derivatives. That anomaly is because a different mechanism of hydrolysis is operating. The latter acyl derivatives are also actually somewhat more stable in the presence of plasma than not, probably because of protein binding (32). The solubilities, solubility parameters, fluxes, and permeability coefficients for the three series of derivatives (30,33) are given in Table 5.

In order to determine if there are any differences in the relationship between log P_i and δ_i for the three series generated by the differences in their stabilities, their

Table 5 Solubilities (C_v) and Solubility Parameter Values (δ_i) for 1-Alkylcarbonyl-, 1-Alkoxycarbonyl-, and 1-Alkylaminocarbonyl-5-FU Derivatives: Their Rates of Delivery of 5-FU (J_i) and Log Permeability Coefficients (P_i) from IPM

Compound	$\delta_i{}^a$	$C_v{}^b$	$J_i{}^c$	Log $P_i{}^d$
23 5-FU[e]	15.00	0.0051	0.031	+0.79
24 R = CH$_3$[e]	14.08	2.87	1.21	−0.37
25 R = C$_2$H$_5$[e]	13.46	4.73	0.56	−0.93
26 R = C$_3$H$_7$[e]	12.97	2.26	0.168	−1.13
27 R = C$_4$H$_9$[e]	12.57	5.10	0.133	−1.58
28 R = OCH$_3$[e]	14.10	0.28	0.34	+0.08
29 R = OC$_2$H$_5$[e]	13.50	1.70	0.77	−0.35
30 R = OC$_3$H$_7$[e]	13.00	1.97	0.29	−0.83
31 R = OC$_4$H$_9$[e]	12.62	4.39	0.28	−1.20
23 5-FU[f]	15.0	0.0104	0.0043	−0.39
32 R = NHC$_4$H$_9$[f]	12.94	4.95	0.016	−2.49
33 R = NHC$_6$H$_{13}$[f]	12.29	5.84	0.014	−2.62
34 R = NHC$_8$H$_{17}$[f]	11.81	6.25	0.0057	−3.04

[a]Calculated from group contribution method of Fedors [5].
[b]Solubility in equivalent mg of 5-FU/ml.
[c]Flux in mg/cm^2/h, n = 3.
[d]Permeability coefficient calculated from J_i/C_v.
[e]From Ref. 30.
[f]From Ref. 33.

log P_i versus δ_i values from Table 5 are plotted in Fig. 5. The data from the 1-alkylaminocarbonyl derivatives is from a different laboratory (33) using a different protocol and using rats instead of mice, so that data is of a different magnitude. Only the 1-alkylcarbonyl derivatives delivered only 5-FU through skin, whereas the other two types of acyl derivatives also delivered measurable amounts of intact prodrug. Nevertheless, the slopes of the plots of log P_i versus δ_i for all three derivatives are essentially the same (0.95, 0.83, and 0.85 for **24–27**, **28–31**, and **32–34**, respectively), and a better correlation coefficient is obtained if the data for 5-FU is included in each plot. Thus, all of these types of prodrugs of 5-FU behave more like the S^6-(N-alkyl-N-alkoxycarbonyl)aminomethyl derivatives of 6-MP. This result may be a consequence of the fact that the differences in the rates of hydrolysis of the N-acyl derivatives are not sufficiently different from each other to see any difference in the log P_i versus δ_i relationships.

N-Mannich base–type prodrugs of drugs containing acidic amide and imide functional groups also hydrolyze very rapidly in the presence of water or protic vehicles. Two different categories of studies of N-Mannich bases, or aminomethyl-type prodrugs of amides and imides, are available for analysis of their abilities to deliver their parent drugs. Examples of the first category are

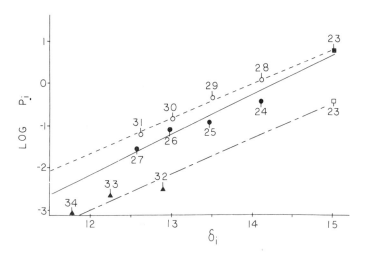

Figure 5 A plot of log experimental permeability coefficients for the delivery of total 5-FU from suspensions of 1-alkylcarbonyl-5-FU (•) (———), 1-alkoxycarbonyl-5-FU (o) (– – –), and 1-alkylaminocarbonyl-5-FU derivatives (▲) (— —) in IPM versus the calculated solubility parameter values of the derivatives (δ_i). The data points for 5-FU from the two different studies are represented by (■) [30] or by (□) [33]. Data points are labeled numerically according to structures in Table 5.

prodrugs where only an aminomethyl promoiety is incorporated into the drug. N-Mannich base prodrugs of theophylline (34), 5-FU (34), 6-MP (35), 5-fluorocytosine (36), and 5-iododeoxycytidine (37) are examples of this category. The most representative study is that of the N-Mannich bases of theophylline and 5-FU (34). A compilation of the solubilities, solubility parameters, fluxes, and permeability coefficients obtained for the delivery of theophylline and 5-FU by their N-Mannich bases is given in Table 6. A plot of the log P_i versus δ_i values is given in Fig. 6. The slope of the combined log P_i versus δ_i data, which also includes the data for theophylline and 5-FU, is 0.71 with a correlation coefficient of 0.95.

Table 6 Solubilities (C_v) and Solubility Parameter Values (δ_i) for N-Mannich Base Derivatives of Theophylline and 5-FU: Their Rates of Delivery of Theophylline and 5-FU (J_i) and Log Permeability Coefficients (P_i) from IPM

Compound	$\delta_i{}^a$	$C_v{}^b$	$J_i{}^c$	Log $P_i{}^d$
35 Theophylline	14.05	0.062	0.041	−0.18
36 R = N(CH$_3$)$_2$	12.14	8.71	0.21	−1.62
37 R = N(C$_2$H$_5$)$_2$	11.65	21.76	0.37	−1.77
38 R = H(C$_3$H$_7$)$_2$	11.27	77.59	0.36	−2.33
39 R = N(C$_4$H$_9$)$_2$	10.98	86.13	0.30	−2.46
40 R = N(CH$_2$)$_5$	12.04	11.42	0.16	−1.85
41 R = N(CH$_2$CH$_2$)$_2$O	12.35	1.05	0.11	−0.98
42 R = N(CH$_2$CH$_2$)$_2$NCH$_3$	11.99	2.84	0.09	−1.50
43 R = N(CH$_2$)$_4$	12.30	8.47	0.23	−1.57
23 5-FU	15.0	0.0051	0.022	0.63
44 R = N(CH$_2$)$_5$	11.04	6.98	0.076	−1.96
45 R = N(CH$_2$CH$_2$)$_2$O	11.46	2.53	0.11	−1.36
46 R = N(CH$_2$CH$_2$)$_2$NCH$_3$	11.00	4.27	0.013	−2.52

[a]Calculated from group contribution method of Fedors [5].
[b]Solubility in equivalent mg of theophylline or 5-FU/ml.
[c]Flux in mg/cm^2/h, n = 3.
[d]Permeability coefficient calculated from J_i/C_v.
Source: From Ref. 34.

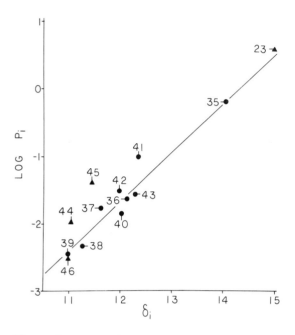

Figure 6 A plot of log experimental permeability coefficients for the delivery of theophylline and 5-FU from suspensions of N-Mannich base derivatives of theophylline (•) and 5-FU (▲) in IPM versus the calculated solubility parameter values of the derivatives (δ_i). Data points are labeled numerically according to structures in Table 6.

Examples of the second category of N-Mannich base–type prodrugs, which have been evaluated for their abilities to deliver their parent drugs, are those in which an additional promoiety is incorporated into the drug. 9-Aminomethyl derivatives of S^6-acyloxymethyl-6-MP are examples of this second category. As opposed to the N-Mannich base prodrugs where the only promoiety is the aminomethyl group, these "combination" prodrugs deliver significant amounts of intact S^6-acyloxymethyl-6-MP as well as 6-MP. The results from analysis of the diffusion cell experiments are given in Table 7, and the log P_i versus δ_v data are plotted in Fig. 7 for the delivery of total 6-MP by the series of N-Mannich bases derived from S^6-acetyloxymethyl-6-MP (38) and S^6-pivaloyloxymethyl-6-MP (39). In spite of the fact that the two S^6-acyloxymethyl derivatives that were chosen to combine with the 9-aminomethyl groups represent the two extremes in the S^6-acyloxymethyl series in terms of polarity and lipid solubilities, there is a reasonable correlation for the log P_i versus δ_i data between the two series.

Thus, it is possible to predict log P_i values for a particular member of a series of one type of prodrug if the log P_i values for two suitably distant members of the

Table 7 Solubility Parameter Values (δ_i) for N-Mannich Base Derivatives of S^6-Acetyloxymethyl-6-MP[a] and S^6-Pivaloyloxymethyl-6-MP[b]: Their Rates of Delivery of Total 6-MP (J_i) and Log Permeability Coefficients (P_i) from IPM

$$S\,CH_2O(C{=}O)\,R$$

Compound		$\delta_i{}^{c}$	$J_i{}^{d}$	Log $P_i{}^{e}$
1	6-MP	14.40	0.00060	-0.73
9	R = CH$_3$,R'=H	14.40	0.031	-0.72
47	R = CH$_3$,R'=CH$_2$N(CH$_2$CH$_2$)$_2$O	12.81	0.15	-1.22
48	R = CH$_3$,R'=CH$_2$N(CH$_2$)$_5$	12.52	0.028	-1.96
49	R = CH$_3$,R'=CH$_2$N(CH$_2$CH$_2$)$_2$NCH$_3$	12.46	0.062	-1.33
50	R = CH$_2$,R'=CH$_2$N(C$_2$H$_5$)$_2$	12.17	0.11	-2.33
51	R = CH$_3$,R'=CH$_2$N(C$_3$H$_7$)$_2$	11.78	0.072	-2.49
52	R = CH$_3$,R'=CH$_2$N(C$_4$H$_9$)$_2$	11.47	0.091	-2.15
53	R = CH$_3$,R'=CH$_2$N(C$_5$H$_{11}$)$_2$	11.22	0.065	-3.24
15	R = C(CH$_3$)$_3$,R'=H	12.60	0.0094	-1.94
54	R = C(CH$_3$)$_3$,R'=CH$_2$N(CH$_2$CH$_2$)$_2$O	11.99	0.056	-1.62
55	R = C(CH$_3$)$_3$,R'=CH$_2$N(CH$_2$)$_5$	11.78	0.048	-2.68
56	R = C(CH$_3$)$_3$,R'=CH$_2$N(CH$_2$CH$_2$)$_2$NCH$_3$	11.74	0.059	-2.21
57	R = C(CH$_3$)$_3$,R'=CH$_2$N(CH$_3$)$_2$	11.81	0.080	-2.35
58	R = C(CH$_3$)$_3$,R'=CH$_2$N(C$_2$H$_5$)$_2$	11.47	0.053	-2.97
59	R = C(CH$_3$)$_3$,R'=CH$_2$N(C$_3$H$_7$)$^2{}_2$	11.20	0.065	-2.55
60	R = C(CH$_3$)$_3$,R'=CH$_2$N(C$_4$H$_9$)$^2{}_2$	10.98	0.051	-3.37

[a]From Ref. 38.
[b]From Ref. 39.
[c]Calculated from group contribution method of Fedors [5].
[d]Flux in mg/cm^2/h, n = 3.
[e]Permeability coefficients calculated from J_i/C_v.

series are known and their solubility parameter values have been calculated. Then it is reasonably easy to determine the solubility of the member and predict a value for its rate of delivery of its parent drug.

CONCLUSIONS

The use of theoretical activity coefficients derived from regular solution theory to calculate partition coefficients, K_i, for partitioning-driven processes has been evaluated for two cases. In each case, it was assumed that there was a direct

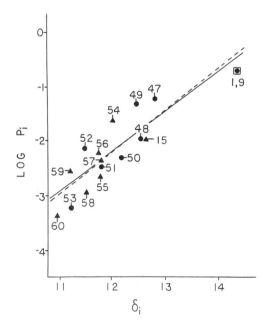

Figure 7 A plot of log experimental permeability coefficient for the delivery of total 6-MP from suspensions of N-Mannich base derivatives of S^6-acetyloxymethyl-6-MP (•) (——) and of S^6-pivaloyloxymethyl-6-MP (▲) (– – –) in IPM versus the calculated solubility parameter values for the derivatives (δ_i). The data point for 6-MP is represented by (□). Data points are labeled numerically according to structures in Table 7.

correlation between partition coefficients and permeability coefficients, P_i, for the diffusional process: $P_i = K_i$•constant. If there was a correlation between experimental P_i values obtained from the fluxes of drugs divided by their solubilities and theoretical K_i values calculated from solubility parameters, then regular solution theory could be used to describe those partitioning-driven processes.

In the first case, the effect of vehicles on the experimental P_i for the delivery of various drugs was evaluated. There was a direct correlation between the theoretical K_i and the experimental P_i for vehicles that did not damage the skin or cause aggregation of the drug in the vehicle. Also, the shapes of the plots of log experimental P_i versus the solubility parameter values of the vehicles, δ_v, approximated parabolas with minima at those points where the solubility parameter value of the drugs, δ_i, were equal to that of the vehicle. This result was predicted by the relationship between the theoretical K_i and δ_i from regular solution theory. The practical value of these results is that once the constant in, $P_i = K_i$•constant, has been determined experimentally for one vehicle, P_i can be calculated from the product of K_i for other vehicles and the constant. Fluxes can be predicted from those P_i values simply by measuring the solubility of the drug in the vehicle of interest.

In the second case, the effect of vehicles on the experimental P_i for the delivery of various drugs by their prodrugs was evaluated. Two types of prodrugs were considered. The first type was relatively stable to water and protic vehicles. Thus, vehicles exhibiting the same wide range of polarities that were used in the first case were also used in the second case. However, the parabolic relationship between log P_i and δ_v that had been observed for the delivery of 6-MP from various vehicles was not observed in the plots of log P_i versus δ_v for the delivery of 6-MP by its S^6,9-bisacyloxymethyl prodrugs from the same vehicles. In addition, there was no observed direct relationship between theoretical K_i and experimental P_i: There was no constant. On the other hand, there were clear correlations between the experimental P_i for the delivery of 6-MP by the series of prodrugs from individual vehicles and the calculated δ_i for the prodrugs. The values of P_i for the more polar prodrugs were higher than those of the less polar prodrugs for the delivery of 6-MP from lipophilic vehicles (a direct relationship), but the reverse was true when hydrophilic polar vehicles were considered (an inverse relationship).

The second type of prodrugs were ones in which the prodrugs were relatively unstable to water and protic vehicles: They hydrolyzed almost immediately upon partitioning into the skin. Thus, these prodrugs could only be evaluated in aprotic vehicles. However, the results from the evaluation of those prodrugs were the same as for the evaluation of the more stable prodrugs in the same aprotic, lipophilic vehicles. There was a direct relationship between experimental P_i and the calculated δ_i for the prodrugs.

The results from the evaluation of these two types of prodrugs suggest that regular solution theory cannot predict the flux of a drug from various vehicles when a prodrug is used, but it can predict fluxes of drug by the members of an homologous series of prodrugs from an individual vehicle.

There is not enough flux and solubility data available from the evaluation of a sufficiently large number of different types of functional groups in promoieties to be able to predict an optimal promoiety with which to deliver polar and nonpolar drugs. There is no obvious "magic" functional group or promoieties from our analysis of the available data. However, the incorporation of a tertiary amine functional group into a promoiety, either alone or in combination with another promoiety, invariably gives significant enhancement in the topical delivery of the parent drug. Also, in the two comparisons of promoieties containing carbonyl functional groups (see Tables 4 and 5), the promoiety containing an ester functional group performed better than one containing a carbamate functional group (see Table 4), whereas the promoiety containing an amide-type functional group performed better than one containing a carbamate-type or urea-type functional group (see Table 5).

REFERENCES

1. J. H. Hildebrand, *J. Am. Chem. Soc.*, 51, 66 (1929).
2. G. Scatchard, *Chem. Rev.*, 8, 321 (1931).
3. M. J. Chertkoff and A. Martin, *J. Am. Pharm. Assoc., Sci. Ed.*, 49, 44 (1960).
4. A. Martin, P. L. Wu, Z. Liron, and S. Cohen, *J. Pharm. Sci.*, 74, 638 (1985).
5. R. F. Fedors, *Polym. Eng. Sci.*, 14, 147 (1974).
6. A. Martin, P. L. Wu, and T. Velasquez, *J. Pharm. Sci.*, 74, 277 (1985).
7. K. B. Sloan, S. A. M. Koch, K. G. Siver, and F. P. Flowers, *J. Invest. Dermatol.*, 87, 244 (1986).
8. A. Martin and J. Mauger, *Am. J. Pharm. Ed.*, 52, 68 (1988).
9. S. A. Khalil and A. Martin, *J. Pharm. Sci.*, 56, 1225 (1967).
10. A. Adjei, T. Newburger, S. Stavchansky, and A. Martin, *J. Pharm. Sci.*, 73, 742 (1984).
11. S. Cohen, A. Goldschmid, G. Shtacher, S. Srebrenik, and S. Gitter, *Mol. Pharmacol.*, 11, 379 (1975).
12. E. M. Landau, J. Richter, and S. Cohen, *J. Med. Chem.*, 22, 325 (1979).
13. L. J. Mullins, *Chem. Rev.*, 54, 289 (1954).
14. P. Bustamante and E. Selles, *J. Pharm. Sci.*, 75, 639 (1986).
15. K. B. Sloan, K. G. Siver, and S. A. M. Koch, *J. Pharm. Sci.*, 75, 744 (1986).
16. R. P. Waranis, K. G. Siver, and K. B. Sloan, *Int. J. Pharm.*, 36, 211 (1987).
17. E. F. Sherertz, K. B. Sloan, and R. G. McTiernan, *J. Invest. Dermatol.*, 89, 147 (1987).
18. Z. Liron and S. Cohen, *J. Pharm. Sci.*, 73, 538 (1984).
19. R. Kadir, D. Stempler, Z. Liron, and S. Cohen, *J. Pharm. Sci.*, 76, 774 (1987).
20. R. Kadir, D. Stempler, Z. Liron, and S. Cohen, *J. Pharm. Sci.*, 77, 409 (1988).
21. R. J. Scheuplein, *J. Invest. Dermatol.*, 45, 334 (1965).
22. R. F. Rekker, *The Hydrophobic Fragment Constant.* Elsevier, New York, 1977.
23. A. Leo, C. Hansch, and D. Elkins, *Chem. Rev.*, 71, 525 (1971).
24. A. F. M. Barton, *Chem. Rev.*, 75, 731 (1975).
25. A. Buur, H. Bundgaard, and E. Falch, *Int. J. Pharm.*, 24, 43 (1985).
26. B. Mollgaard, A. Hoelgaard, and H. Bundgaard, *Int. J. Pharm.*, 12, 153 (1982).
27. R. P. Waranis and K. B. Sloan, *J. Pharm. Sci.*, 76, 587 (1987).
28. R. P. Waranis and K. B. Sloan, *J. Pharm. Sci.*, 77, 210 (1988).
29. K. G. Siver and K. B. Sloan, *J. Pharm. Sci.*, 79, 166 (1990).
30. H. D. Beall, Research toward Ph.D. thesis.
31. A. Buur and H. Bundgaard, *J. Pharm. Sci.*, 75, 522 (1986).
32. A. Buur and H. Bundgaard, *Int. J. Pharm.*, 23, 209 (1985).
33. H. Sasaki, T. Takahashi, Y. Mori, J. Nakamura, and J. Shibasaki, *Int. J. Pharm.*, 60, 1 (1990).
34. K. B. Sloan, E. F. Sherertz, and R. G. McTiernan, *Int. J. Pharm.*, 44, 87 (1988).
35. K. G. Siver and K. B. Sloan, *Int. J. Pharm.*, 48, 195 (1988).
36. S. A. M. Koch and K. B. Sloan, *Int. J. Pharm.*, 35, 243 (1987).
37. S. A. M. Koch and K. B. Sloan, *Pharm. Res.*, 4, 317 (1987).
38. A. N. Saab, K. B. Sloan, H. D. Beall, and R. Villaneuva, *J. Pharm. Sci.*, 79, 1099 (1990).
39. A. N. Saab and K. B. Sloan, *Int. J. Pharm.*, 57, 253 (1989).

6

The Effect of Partitioning and Enzymatic Hydrolysis on the Percutaneous Transport of Lipophilic Prodrugs

Russell O. Potts
Cygnus Therapeutic Systems, Redwood City, California

INTRODUCTION

The use of prodrugs to enhance drug delivery through the skin has been extensively and well reviewed (1–4). The reader is referred to those reviews for general discussions of synthetic and physical organic chemistry, pharmacokinetics, and the epidermal metabolism aspects of this topic. The results reviewed here are intended to show that the enhancement of dermal drug delivery via prodrugs is often meager and substantially less than that predicted solely on the basis of increased lipophilicity. Moreover, this predictive failure leads to insight into possible mechanistic differences between the dermal transport of the drug vs prodrug.

The rationale for the use of lipophilic prodrugs to enhance topical delivery comes from an analysis of Fick's law of diffusion (eq. 1).

$$Jss = D \times Km \times \frac{dC}{dx}$$

(1)

This law states that the steady-state flux (Jss) is proportional to the diffusion coefficient of the permeant through the barrier (D), the concentration (or more correctly, activity) gradient of permeant across the barrier (dC/dx), and the partition coefficient for the permeant between the vehicle and stratum corneum (Km). Since the stratum corneum is highly lipophilic in character, increased flux

205

should result from increased drug lipophilicity, as shown by the results of Michaels et al. (5).

For a number of compounds, especially those which are relatively polar, the stratum corneum represents the primary barrier to diffusion through the skin. Thus, chemical derivatization which renders the compound more lipophilic should increase flux. If the chemical linkage is metabolically labile, epidermal enzymes may then convert the prodrug back into the parent compound. Hence, lipophilic prodrugs have the potential to enhance the dermal delivery of polar compounds.

REVIEW OF EXPERIMENTAL RESULTS

In the past 10–15 years, lipophilic prodrugs of more than a dozen compounds have been synthesized and their delivery through human skin studied. The structures of a number of these compounds and their derivatives are shown in Table 1. In the comparisons of dermal delivery to be reviewed here, it is important to distinguish between flux and permeability coefficient measurements. When compared on the basis of the permeability coefficients (P = flux divided by the drug concentration in the vehicle), there is often a substantial increase in prodrug delivery relative to the parent compound. This effect is often due to decreased prodrug concentration in the vehicle, while flux values show little if any relative enhancement. Flux, which measures the mass of material transported through the skin, is the more therapeutically relevant parameter and thus, all enhancement values cited in this review will refer to flux.

The topical delivery of a number of prodrugs of anti-inflammatory compounds has been studied. Loftsson and Bodor studied the synthesis and delivery of methylsulfonylmethyl (MSM) and methylthiomethyl (MTM) derivatives of aspirin (6). The in vitro delivery through hairless mouse skin was measured from 2M solutions of each prodrug in polyethylene glycol (PEG 400). Their results showed that aspirin itself was 70% hydrolyzed to salicylic acid upon passage through the skin. The MSM derivative showed similar delivery relative to the parent compound, but no intact aspirin remained upon passage through the skin. Furthermore, while a twofold enhancement in delivery over aspirin was noted for the MTM derivative, only salicylate was detected in the receiver chamber. Thus, only marginal delivery enhancement was achieved and then at the expense of increased hydrolysis of aspirin.

The delivery of the N,N-diethylhydroxylamine derivative of indomethacin was studied both in vivo and in vitro (7). When 30 mM solutions of drug or prodrug in a polyethylene and liquid paraffin ointment were applied to the dermis side of hairless mouse skin mounted in a diffusion cell, only indomethacin was found in the receiver chamber. In addition, the prodrug resulted in a twofold greater delivery after 24 h than the parent compound. Several in vivo studies were performed based on the anti-inflammatory properties of indomethacin. In a rat ear burn model, dose-response results showed the prodrug to be about threefold more

Table 1 Some Lipophilic Prodrugs That Have Been Synthesized and Their Delivery Through Human Skin Studied

Prodrugs of	Structure	Ref.

Acetylsalicylic acid

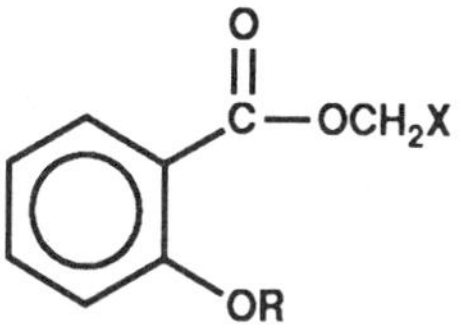

$X = -SCH_3$
$-SOCH_3$
$-SO_2CH_3$

$R = -H \text{ or } -COCH_3$

6

Indomethacin

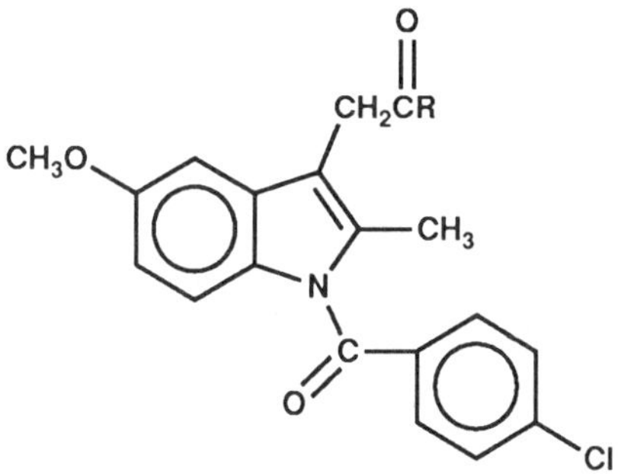

$R = -OH$
$-Cl$
$-ON(C_2H_5)_2$

7

Cromoglycic acid

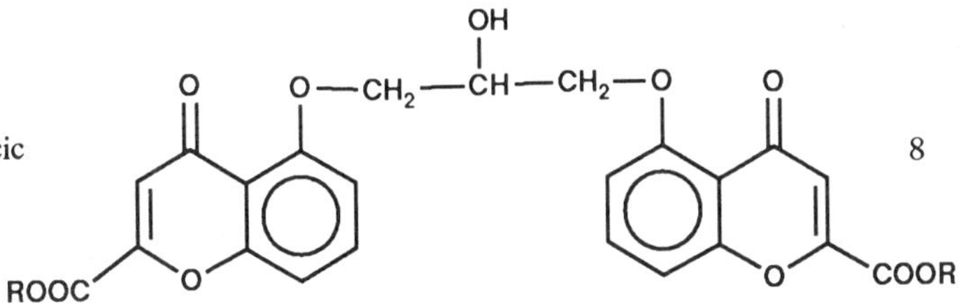

$R = $ Acyloxyalkyl esters

8

Theophylline

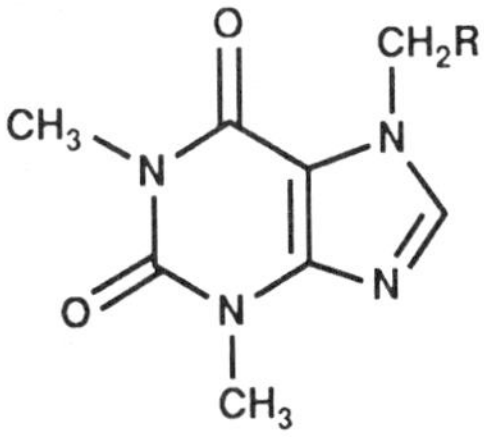

$R = -O_2C-(CH_2)_n-CH_3$

9

Table 1   (Continued)

Prodrugs of	Structure	Ref.

Estradiol

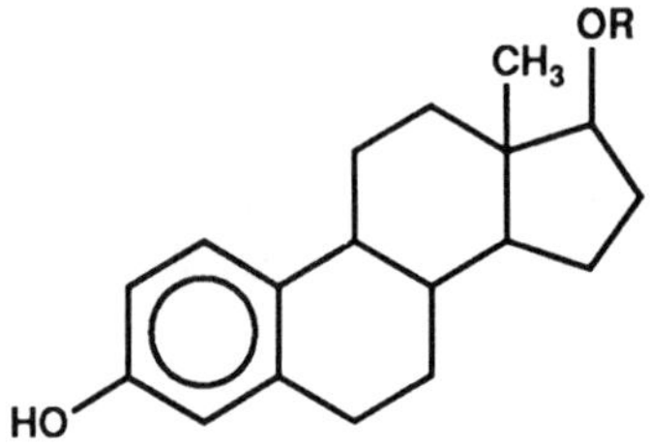

$$R = \ \overset{\overset{\textstyle O}{\|}}{-C(CH_2)_n} -CH_3$$

10

6-Mercapto-purine

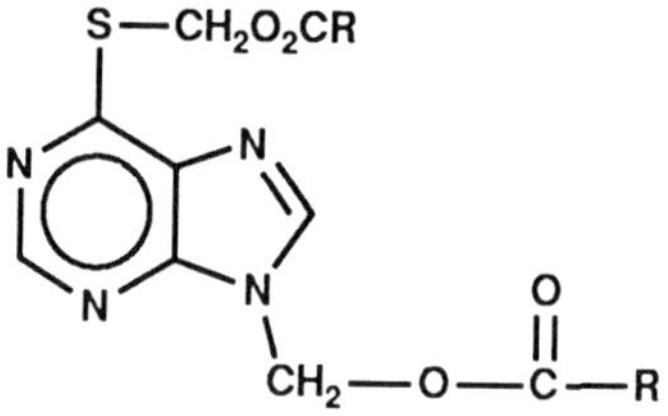

$$R = \ -(CH_2)_n -CH_3$$
$$n = 0\text{-}6$$

11

Methotrexate

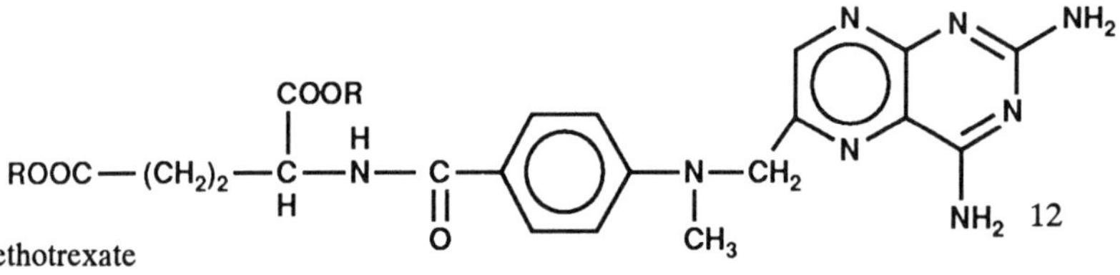

$$R = \ -CH_3$$
$$-C_2H_5$$

12

Metronidazole

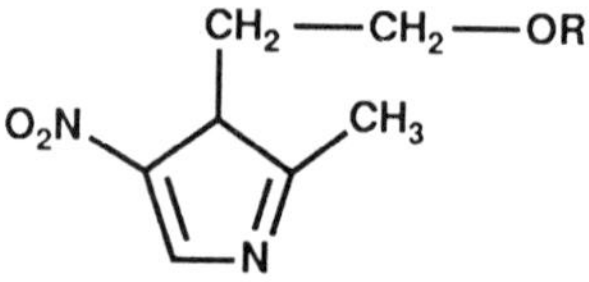

$$R = \ \overset{\overset{\textstyle O}{\|}}{C}$$

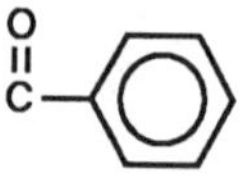

13

Table 1 (Continued)

Prodrugs of	Structure	Ref.
5-Fluoruracil		15
Vidarabine		17–22
Mitomycin C		24–25
Hydrocortisone		27

For 5-Fluorouracil:

$$R = -CH_2O-\overset{O}{\underset{\|}{C}}-CH_2CH_2CH_3$$

$$-CH_2O-\overset{O}{\underset{\|}{C}}-C-(CH_3)_3$$

For Vidarabine:

$$R = -\overset{O}{\underset{\|}{C}}-(CH_2)_3CH_3$$

For Mitomycin C:

$$R = -CH_2-\bigcirc$$

$$-\overset{O}{\underset{\|}{C}}-CH_2-\bigcirc$$

For Hydrocortisone:

$$R = -\overset{O}{\underset{\|}{C}}-(CH_2)_n-CH_3$$

$$n = 0\text{-}6$$

potent than indomethacin. In contrast, in a ultraviolet (UV) irradiation–induced erythema (sunburn) model with human volunteers, no differences were noted between prodrug and parent compound in two different vehicles. Thus, both in vivo and in vitro results showed only modestly increased delivery and efficacy with lipophilic prodrugs.

Bodor and coworkers also investigated the delivery of prodrugs of the anti-inflammatory compound cromoglycic acid (8). The in vitro delivery through hairless mouse skin was measured for a series of acyloxyalkyl diester derivatives at saturation (e.g., maximum activity) in isopropyl myristate. Results showed that a maximal sixfold flux enhancement was obtained with the hexanoyloxy-ethylidene derivative. In contrast to results predicted from Fick's law (eq. 1), further derivatization to even more lipophilic compounds resulted in lower flux. Finally, in vivo delivery was measured in hairless mice using radiolabeled compounds. These results showed that after 24 h of occlusive application, maximal delivery was again achieved with the hexanoyloxyethylidene derivative, albeit only about 50% greater than that obtained with cromolyn alone. Thus, both in vivo and in vitro results showed only modest enhancement of topical drug delivery via prodrugs. Furthermore, delivery enhancement showed a parabolic dependence on prodrug lipophilicity (as measured, for example, by the octanol/water partition coefficient).

The topical delivery of theophylline was evaluated in vivo and in vitro using 7-acyloxymethyl derivatives (9). In both in vivo and in vitro investigations, the drug or prodrugs were applied as saturated suspensions in an isopropyl myristate vehicle, thereby assuring maximum thermodynamic activity for each. In vitro results showed that maximal delivery through hairless mouse skin of about fivefold greater than the parent compound was achieved with the hydroxymethyl derivative. In contrast, the more lipophilic butyryloxymethyl and pivaloyloxy-methyl derivatives produced only about threefold enhancement. All prodrugs tested were completely hydrolyzed upon passage through the skin, except the pivaloyloxymethyl derivative, which yielded about 15% intact prodrug in the receiver chamber. Topically applied pivaloyl- and butyryloxymethyl derivatives also inhibited UV light–induced DNA synthesis in vivo in the skin of hairless mice, and, in agreement with in vitro delivery results, the latter derivative was more effective. Thus, under conditions of delivery from a common vehicle with the prodrug or drug at maximum thermodynamic activity, a series of 7-acyloxymethyl derivatives of theophylline showed a maximal fivefold flux enhancement vs the parent compound. Moreover, maximum delivery was once again achieved with a prodrug of intermediate lipophilicity.

The topical delivery of a series of 17-alkyl ester derivatives of estradiol was investigated in vitro (10). Results obtained using saturated solutions of each prodrug showed that maximal delivery through hairless mouse skin was obtained with the valerate ester, whereas esters of shorter (acetate) and longer (heptanoate and cypionate) alkyl chains were less well delivered. In all cases, complete prodrug hydrolysis was observed. Thus, delivery through the skin was best for a prodrug of intermediate lipophilicity. Interestingly, while the prodrugs resulted in delivery through the skin which was about threefold greater than that obtained with estradiol, the concentration in the skin (inferred from partitioning data) was as much as an order of magnitude greater than for the parent compound. A similar enrichment in the skin, without substantially increased delivery through the skin, was noted for all prodrugs tested. These results suggested that while partitioning into the skin was favored for prodrugs, transport out of the skin may have been rate limiting. These results also suggest that prodrug derivatization may enhance delivery into the skin. However, unless the prodrug retains pharmacological activity or is hydrolyzed in the skin, the enhanced dermal delivery may be of little therapeutic relevance.

A comparison of delivery between lipophilic derivatives and the parent compound can be complicated, for as suggested by Waranis and Sloan (11), differences in physical properties between drug and prodrug may prevent maximal delivery of both from a single vehicle. Thus, these investigators compared the delivery of 6-mercaptopurine and its S_6-9-bisacyloxyalkyl derivatives from saturated solutions in a number of vehicles spanning a broad range of solvent polarities. Their results showed that steady-state flux of 6-mercaptopurine through hairless mouse skin was maximal for the methyl or ethyl derivatives in all vehicles tested. Furthermore, delivery of both the prodrug and drug was maximal in 1-octanol, a vehicle which resulted in unspecified damage to the skin. In those vehicles producing no apparent damage to the skin, the relative flux enhancement ranged from 20-fold in propylene glycol, to about three- to fivefold in water, N,N-diethyltoluamide, formamide, and 2-methoxyethanol. Thus, under conditions of maximum thermodynamic activity (e.g., saturated solutions), in dermally compatible vehicles spanning a broad range of physical properties, the best delivery enhancement achieved was 20-fold, with other vehicles resulting in three- to fivefold enhancement.

The delivery of a number of drugs via the use of either prodrugs or penetration enhancers has also been studied. For example, McCullough and coworkers (12) investigated factors influencing the in vitro delivery of methotrexate through human skin. They compared the delivery of drug in the presence of the coapplied penetration enhancer decylmethyl sulfoxide to the delivery achieved with a dimethyl ester prodrug of methotrexate. When delivered from an aqueous vehicle at 0.05% prodrug concentration, an approximate twofold flux enhancement vs the parent compound was measured. In contrast, when methotrexate (0.05%) was delivered from an ethanol vehicle containing 2.5% of the penetration enhancer, 140-fold enhancement was achieved. Interestingly, the concentration of methotrexate in the epidermis was increased approximately 10-fold by both the penetration enhancer and prodrug, suggesting that differences in transdermal delivery resulted from differences in transport out of the epidermis. Not all penetration enhancers tested worked as well as decylmethyl sulfoxide. For example, dimethyl sulfoxide (DMSO) resulted in a more modest twofold enhancement. Comparison between prodrug and penetration enhancer results is made difficult, however, by differences in vehicles and the presence or absence of penetration enhancers. For example, did the penetration enhancer alter the drug solubility (activity) in the vehicle? Nevertheless, significantly greater delivery of methotrexate was possible with the appropriate choice of penetration enhancer than that achieved with a lipophilic prodrug.

Similarly, the in vitro delivery of metronidazole through human skin was compared for prodrugs vs penetration enhancement (13,14). Numerous alkyl ester prodrugs were studied. The results showed that a maximum flux enhancement of about twofold was achieved with the propionate and butyrate derivatives, while prodrugs with both larger and smaller octanol/water partition coefficients showed lesser enhancement. In contrast, incorporation of 1% Azone (1-dodecylazacyclo-heptan-2-one) into the propylene glycol/ethanol vehicle with the parent drug resulted in a 50-fold increase in metronidazole flux relative to delivery without this penetration enhancer. Thus, under similar experimental conditions, the penetration enhancer Azone resulted in significantly greater metronidazole delivery than that achieved via lipophilic prodrugs. Again, however, such comparisons may be misleading owing to enhancer-induced differences in drug solubility in and partitioning from the vehicle. A better method of comparison might involve pretreatment of the skin with enhancer, followed by delivery of the drug at saturation in the same vehicle as used for the prodrug.

These same investigators also evaluated the delivery of butyryl- and pivaloyloxymethyl derivatives of 5-fluorouracil (13–15). Using human skin in vitro, they demonstrated maximal delivery with a butyryl derivative, resulting in enhancement of about fivefold relative to the parent compound. Higuchi and coworkers studied the in vitro flux of 5-fluorouracil in the presence of Azone (16). Using hairless rat skin, they pretreated the skin with 3.3% Azone in saline followed by replacement of the donor phase in the diffusion cell with an aqueous solution of the drug. Their results showed a 100-fold enhancement of drug delivery using this penetration enhancer. Furthermore, since enhancement occurred following pretreatment, they concluded that the penetration enhancer altered the skin's barrier properties without affecting the drug activity in the vehicle. A comparison of prodrug vs penetration enhancers results is somewhat complicated by differences in experimental conditions. However, their comparison of enhanced flux relative to an internal control (e.g., parent compound alone) diminishes these concerns and provides a means of assessing the relative efficacy between different experimental protocols. Thus, results obtained with 5-fluorouracil again suggested that penetration enhancers were more effective than prodrugs at increasing dermal drug delivery.

Higuchi and coworkers have also studied the in vitro transport of the antiviral drug vidarabine (ara-A) and its alkyl ester prodrugs through hairless mouse skin (17–22). Their results showed a similar flux with the 5'-O-valeryl derivative.

Under closely similar experimental conditions, the delivery of ara-A was determined in the presence and absence of 3% Azone, and 100- to 1000-fold increase in drug delivery was noted with this penetration enhancer. Thus, ara-A delivery in vitro was significantly increased by the penetration enhancer Azone, whereas the use of a lipophilic prodrug resulted in little, if any, enhancement.

The topical delivery of ara-A and several ester prodrugs was also investigated in vivo (22). Following cutaneous inoculation with HSV-1 (herpes simplex virus), hairless mice showed an increase in dermal lesions to a maximum value 5 days postinfection, and complete mortality by day 7. Treatment with ara-A resulted in a 33% survival rate, but no reduction in lesions at 7 days postinfection. Treatment with ara-A plus Azone resulted in 80% survival and a one-third reduction in lesions at day 7. Application of the 5'-O-valeryl prodrug also resulted in 80% survival and a modest reduction in lesions, while the coapplication of Azone resulted in 100% survival and a 50% reduction in lesions. Finally, while application of the 2',3'-O-acetyl derivative modestly increased survival and reduced lesions, coapplication with Azone resulted in 100% survival and nearly complete reduction of dermal lesions. Thus, while prodrugs were modestly effective relative to the parent compound, maximum therapeutic efficacy was achieved with a prodrug plus the penetration enhancer. Furthermore, the therapeutic efficacy was reflected by in vitro flux results which showed little transport of either prodrug or the parent compound. The addition of Azone, however, resulted in significant in vitro delivery of all three, with the prodrugs showing the greatest net effect. These results are important from two perspectives. First, they demonstrated a correlation between in vitro flux and therapeutic efficacy. Second, they showed that the therapeutic enhancement achieved with Azone was in addition to that obtained with the prodrugs, suggesting different mechanisms for each.

An important control is missing from these experiments, however. Herpes simplex virus (HSV) is a lipid-enveloped virus which is highly susceptible to membrane-disrupting agents. In fact, Azone has been shown to have in vitro and in vivo activity against HSV-1 (23). Thus, it is not at all clear that the enhanced efficacy of ara-A and its prodrugs in the presence of Azone was at all related to increased drug delivery.

The in vitro delivery of mitomycin C was measured by Sezaki and coworkers using 1-N-benzyl, 1-N-benzylcarbonyl, and 1-N-alkyloxycarbonyl derivatives (24,25). Their results showed a three- to fivefold flux enhancement through hairless mouse skin relative to the parent compound. In contrast, under similar experimental conditions, Azone and "Azonelike" penetration enhancers resulted in a 20- to 60-fold enhancement (26). Enhancement was noted regardless of whether the skin was pretreated or the penetration enhancer was coapplied with the drug, suggesting that the effect was on the skin (e.g., barrier alteration) and not due to changes in drug activity in the vehicle.

The influence of drug derivatization and penetration enhancement on hydrocortisone flux has been studied by a number of investigators. Smith synthesized a series of 21-alkyl derivatives of differing chain length and measured their in vitro delivery through hairless mouse skin from saturated aqueous solutions (27). He demonstrated that maximum flux enhancement of about fourfold was achieved with this series of derivatives. Bodor and Sloan also investigated 17α and 21α derivatives of hydrocortisone, including several prodrugs incorporating functional group components of the penetration enhancers DMSO and dimethyl formamide in the promoiety (28). Flux was measured in vitro through hairless mouse skin following deposition of the drug or prodrug on the skin's surface. In addition, numerous in vivo measurements of topical efficacy, such as skin blanching, were studied. Nearly two dozen prodrugs were studied with a maximal two- to threefold delivery enhancement observed. Thus, only modest enhancement was achieved using a wide variety of prodrugs.

Several groups have also investigated the effects of penetration enhancers on the in vitro flux of hydrocortisone. Mirejovsky and Takruri studied a series of alkyl amides of cyclic amines along with Azone and oleic acid (29). Their results, obtained with hairless mouse skin in vitro, showed a 10- to 70-fold flux enhancement relative to hydrocortisone alone. Barry and Bennett also measured the effects of a number of penetration enhancers on the in vitro flux of hydrocortisone through human skin (30). Their results showed that 2-pyrrolidone, N-methyl-pyrrolidone, N-methylformamide, and propylene glycol, either alone or in combination with Azone or oleic acid, greatly increased hydrocortisone permeation, with relative enhancements of 50- to 1000-fold. Thus, these results show that coapplication of a variety of penetration enhancers results in significant increases in hydrocortisone delivery, in contrast to the more modest increase seen with prodrugs.

THE INFLUENCE OF VARIOUS FACTORS ON FLUX ENHANCEMENT

The results reviewed here were obtained with numerous drugs of widely divergent therapeutic and structural classes, and serve to illustrate the general finding that only modest flux enhancement is achieved via derivatization to form a lipophilic prodrug. Since prodrug delivery relies upon partitioning and hydrolysis steps, several hypotheses involving these events can be offered to explain these results.

Partitioning

Derivatization of drugs to form lipophilic prodrugs increases partitioning into the stratum corneum. Results obtained by Saket et al. showed that for hydrocortisone and cortisone an incremental decrease in free energy of 1.6 kJ/mol for stratum corneum/aqueous buffer partitioning resulted from the addition of each methylene group to the steroid n-alkyl ester (31). Similarly, increased organic/aqueous partitioning was noted with increased chain length for hydrocortisone (27,31) and mitomycin C (24,25) derivatives. Thus, there was increased partitioning into the stratum corneum with increased alkyl chain length (e.g., increased lipophilicity).

Flux results, however, obtained with n-alkyl esters of estradiol (10) and metronidazole (14) showed that maximum delivery was achieved with the propionate or butyrate derivative. Results obtained with prodrugs of 5-fluorouracil (13–15) and mitomycin C (24,25) demonstrated maximal delivery for derivatives of 5-carbon chain length, whereas shorter or longer chain delivery resulted in lower flux, even though the octanol/water partition coefficients increased with increasing chain length. This parabolic dependence of delivery on lipophilicity suggests that factors other than increased prodrug partitioning into the stratum corneum are also important in delivery. For example, increased partitioning into the stratum corneum with increased lipophilicity may be offset by decreased partitioning of the intact prodrug into the more aqueous viable epidermis. The best prodrugs, therefore, appear to have a good balance between an increase in lipid and water solubilities (11).

Further insight into the relative contribution of stratum corneum partitioning to flux enhancement can be obtained from the data of several studies of hydrocortisone and its alkyl esters. Saket et al. measured the partition coefficients (K) between human stratum corneum and saline for this series of compounds (31). Their results, summarized in Table 2, showed an increase in K with increasing chain length. Similar results were obtained for octanol/water (31) and ether/water (27) partition coefficients with this same series of compounds. Smith measured the permeability coefficients (P) for this series of compounds through both full-thickness mouse skin and samples where the stratum corneum was removed with adhesive tape (27). These results showed that the permeability coefficient for full-thickness skin (P_{ft}) increased by about 2000-fold from about 1.6×10^{-4} to 3.4×10^{-1} cm/h with increasing chain length from hydrocortisone to the valerate ester. Interestingly, owing to decreased solubility of the prodrug in the aqueous vehicle, only a sixfold increase in steady-state flux was achieved. In contrast to the results obtained with intact skin, only a 10-fold increase in permeability, from about 0.1 to 1.0 cm/h was noted with samples missing the stratum corneum ($P_{stripped}$).

The reciprocal of the permeability coefficient yields the resistance of the barrier under investigation. Furthermore, for a layered composite like the skin, the total resistance is equal to the sum of the resistances of each layer (e.g., stratum corneum, epidermis, dermis). Thus, as shown in equations 2a–2c, the resistance of the stratum corneum (R_{SC}) can be estimated from P values for skin with and without this layer.

$$\frac{1}{P_{ft}} = R_{ft} = R_{stripped} + R_{SC}$$

(2a)

$$\frac{1}{P_{stripped}} = R_{stripped}$$

(2b)

$$\frac{1}{P_{ft}} - \frac{1}{P_{stripped}} = R_{SC}$$

(2c)

Table 2 The Partition Coefficient (K) and Permeability Resistance of the Stratum
Corneum (R_{SC}) for a Series of Hydrocortisone Esters

Drug	Molecular weight	K^a	$R_{SH}(h/cm)^b$
Hydrocortisone	362	7	6.2×10^3
acetate	390	17	5.8×10^2
valerate	432	125	13
heptanoate	460	—	2.3
octanoate	474	813	—

[a]The stratum corneum/saline partition coefficient for human skin (31).
[b]The diffusive resistance of mouse stratum corneum calculated from the data of Smith (27) using equation 2c.

The values or R_{SC} calculated using equation 2c and Smith's data (27) are shown in the last column of Table 2. These results demonstrate a significant decrease in R_{SC} with increasing chain length for the series of esters studied. A comparison of the last two columns of Table 2 shows that this resistance is inversely proportional to the partition coefficient (K) of the permeant. Thus, these combined data suggest that the increased permeability coefficient resulting from increased chain length of an ester derivative is primarily due to greater partitioning of the prodrug into the stratum corneum.

In perhaps the most elegant and systematic study of the effects of derivatization on prodrug uptake by the SC, Anderson et al. have measured the group contribution values for hydrocortisone esters (32). These results showed that the addition of a CH_2 group to the ester alkyl chain resulted in a favorable free energy contribution to SC partitioning. More polar substituents such as carboxyl or amine groups, however, resulted in an unfavorable free energy contribution. These results are entirely consistent with the lipophilic nature of the SC. Interestingly, these results also showed that uptake by the intact SC increased with increased lipophilicity of the prodrug. In contrast, the flux data of Smith (27) showed that delivery through hairless mouse skin did not continuously increase with increased lipophilicity of hydrocortisone esters; a marked deviation from the predictions of Fick's law (eq. 1). One possible explanation for this discrepancy was offered by Anderson (32), who suggested that since the SC is a heterogeneous composite of polar (protein) and nonpolar (lipid) domains, the mechanism (or route) of permeation may differ for polar vs nonpolar drugs. Most drug candidates for derivatization are relatively polar compounds, whereas their prodrugs are much more lipophilic. Thus, these compounds may permeate through the SC via different routes characterized by different partition coefficients. Simple measurements of octanol/water (or even intact SC) partitioning, therefore, may not reflect the microdomain through which the drug permeates. As a result, enhanced prodrug delivery is often less than that predicted solely on the basis of "bulk" partition coefficients.

Hydrolysis

Since hydrolysis of the lipophilic prodrug to the more polar parent compound favors elimination of the compound from the SC into the underlying aqueous tissue, delivery via the prodrug route may be critically dependent upon enzymatic hydrolysis to liberate the parent compound. The modest flux enhancement seen with prodrugs may reflect the rate-limiting nature of this step. This hypothesis is supported by the results of an investigation which compared the delivery of a mitomycin C prodrug through hairless mouse and rat skin in vitro (24). These results showed that greater delivery through rat vs mouse skin correlated with greater hydrolysis of the prodrug in the rat tissue. In a subsequent study, the delivery through rat skin was compared for a series of mitomycin C prodrugs (25). The results obtained using saturated prodrug solutions showed that to a high degree, the flux and extent of prodrug hydrolysis were inversely correlated. Similarly, results obtained for the in vitro flux of 1-acyloxymethyl derivatives of 5-fluorouracil showed that maximum flux was accompanied by complete prodrug hydrolysis (14).

Delivery results obtained in the presence of an enzyme inhibitor also support the correlation between flux and prodrug hydrolysis. Smith investigated the flux of hydrocortisone alkyl esters through hairless mouse skin in the presence and absence of the esterase inhibitor p-nitrophenylacetate (27). His results showed that when a saturated aqueous solution of any of the prodrugs examined was placed in the donor chamber of an in vitro diffusion cell, only hydrocortisone was detected in the receiver chamber. If, however, the esterase inhibitor (0.01%) was added to these donor solutions, only intact prodrug was detected in the receiver. Furthermore, while the esterase inhibitor had little effect on the delivery of hydrocortisone or the acetate ester, delivery of other derivatives was progressively reduced with increasing lipophilicity. Since the inhibitor had no effect on the concentration of prodrug in the vehicle, and is unlikely to have altered the barrier properties of the stratum corneum, the decrease in flux was most likely due to aqueous tissue resistance to the uptake of unhydrolyzed compound. Stated differently, these results suggest that lipophilic derivatives are efficiently removed from the epidermis only after enzymatic hydrolysis.

Kao et al. studied the flux of benzo[a]pyrene through mouse skin in an in vitro diffusion chamber where tissue viability was prolonged by perfusion of the dermis side of the skin with organ culture medium (33). They found that only about 25% of benzo[a]pyrene passed through the skin intact, whereas the rest had been metabolized to more polar compounds. If the mice were topically or systemically treated with 2,3,7,8-tetrachlorodibenzo-p-dioxin (TCDD) for 48 h prior to sacrifice, in vitro flux increased about fourfold. Since TCDD is known to induce enzymes which metabolize benzo[a]pyrene, these results suggested that metabolism and flux were linked. Furthermore, when skin samples were subjected to a freeze-thaw cycle so that metabolic activity was lost, negligible amounts of benzo[a]pyrene passed through the skin. Thus, these results show that for a highly lipophilic compound like benzo[a]pyrene, the flux increases with the skin's ability to enzymatically form polar metabolites. These results suggest that the barrier to transport of lipophilic drugs may reside in the aqueous milieu beneath the stratum corneum where metabolic conversion to more polar, water-soluble compounds may be rate limiting to further diffusion.

Results from the author's laboratory obtained with a salicylate diester prodrug also suggest that enzymatic hydrolysis and flux are related (34,35). Using human skin in vitro, the prodrug was completely hydrolyzed upon passage through the skin to yield only salicylate in the receiver chamber. Furthermore, analysis of the delivery results showed a steady-state flux of 18 $nmol/cm^2/h$ and a lag time of about 2 min. In a separate experiment, an esterase inhibitor was added to the receiver chamber 4 h prior to initiation of the delivery experiment. Only intact prodrug was found in the receiver chamber in the presence of inhibitor. Furthermore, the flux decreased to 0.8 $nmol/cm^2/h$ and the lag time increased to over 9 h. Finally, the presence of the esterase inhibitor in the skin was demonstrated by detection of drug and prodrug in the skin. In the absence of the inhibitor, less than 10% of the material in the epidermis was the prodrug, whereas in the presence of the inhibitor, more than 90% of the intact prodrug remained. Interestingly, the total amount of salicylate in the stratum corneum was nearly the same in both experiments, suggesting that partitioning of the prodrug was not altered by the esterase inhibitor. Thus, these results suggest that the flux of lipophilic prodrugs through human skin is limited by their hydrolysis to more polar, water-soluble species.

Taken together, these combined results suggest that increased enzymatic hydrolysis of prodrugs correlates with increased delivery. Thus, while delivery of lipophilic prodrugs to the stratum corneum is enhanced, their subsequent removal into the more aqueous subadjacent tissue may be limited by the ability of resident enzymes to convert prodrugs into more polar metabolites.

CONCLUSIONS

In conclusion, results obtained for a number of polar compounds spanning a broad range of structural and therapeutic categories show that lipophilic prodrugs result in modest delivery enhancement. With rare exception, delivery enhancement is less than fivefold. These results show that while partitioning into the stratum corneum is favored by lipophilic derivatization, subsequent transport into the aqueous milieu beneath may be limited by the ability of epidermal enzymes to convert the prodrug into a more polar metabolite. Alternatively, the path of transport through the SC may differ significantly for parent compound vs prodrug. Thus, predicted flux increases based solely on "bulk" partition coefficients may be misleading.

REFERENCES

1. K. B. Sloan, *Adv. Drug Del. Rev.*, 3, 67–101 (1989).
2. S. Y. Chan and A. L. W. Po, *Int. J. Pharm.*, 55, 1–16 (1989).
3. D. A. W. Bucks, *Pharm. Res.*, 1, 148–153 (1984).
4. J. Hadgraft, in *Design of Prodrugs* (H. Bundgaard, ed.). Elsevier, Amsterdam, 1985.
5. A. S. Michaels, S. K. Chandrasekaran, and J. E. Shaw, *A.I.Ch.E.*, 21, 985 (1975).
6. T. Loftson and N. Bodor, *J. Pharm. Sci.*, 70:756–758 (1981).
7. K. B. Sloan, S. Selk, J. Haslam, L. Caldwell, and R. Shaffer, *J. Pharm. Sci.*, 73, 1734–1737 (1984).
8. N. Bodor, J. Zupan, and S. Selk, *Int. J. Pharm.*, 7, 63–75 (1980).
9. K. B. Sloan and N. Bodor, *Int. J. Pharm.*, 12: 299–313 (1982).
10. K. H. Valia, K. Tojo, and Y. W. Chien, *Drug. Dev. Ind. Pharm.*, 11, 1133–1173 (1985).
11. R. P. Waranis and K. B. Sloan, *J. Pharm. Sci.*, 76, 587–595 (1987).
12. J. L. McCullough, D. S. Snyder, G. D. Weinstein, A. Friedland, and B. Stein, *J. Invest. Dermatol.*, 66, 103–107 (1976).
13. H. Bundgaard, A. Hoelgaard, and B. Mollgaard, *Int. J. Pharm.*, 15, 295–292 (1983).
14. A. Hoelgaard and B. Mollgaard, in *Adv. Drug Deliv. Syst.* (J. M. Anderson and S. W. Kim, eds.). Elsevier, Amsterdam, 1986.
15. B. Mollgaard, A. Hoelgaard, and H. Bundgaard, *Int. J. Pharm.*, 12, 153–162 (1982).
16. Y. Morimoto, K. Sugibayashi, K. Hosaya, and W. I. Higuchi, *Int. J. Pharm.*, 32, 31–38 (1986).
17. C. D. Yu, J. L. Fox, N. F. H. Ho, and W. I. Higuchi, *J. Pharm. Sci.*, 68, 1341–1346 (1979).
18. C. D. Yu, J. L. Fox, N. F. H. Ho, and W. I. Higuchi, *J. Pharm. Sci.*, 68, 1347–1357 (1979).
19. C. D. Yu, W. I. Higuchi, N. F. H. Ho, J. L. Fox, and G. L. Flynn, *J. Pharm. Sci.*, 69, 770–772 (1980).
20. C. D. Yu, J. L. Fox, W. I. Higuchi, and N. F. H. Ho, *J. Pharm. Sci.*, 69, 772–774 (1980).
21. C. D. Yu, N. A. Gordon, J. L. Fox, W. I. Higuchi, and N. F. H. Ho, *J. Pharm. Sci.*, 69, 775–780 (1980).
22. W. M. Shannon, L. Westbrook, W. I. Higuchi, K. Sugibayashi, D. C. Baker, S. D. Kumar, J. L. Fox, G. L. Flynn, N. F. H. Ho, and R. Vaisyanathan, *J. Pharm. Sci.*, 74, 1157–1161 (1985).
23. M. F. Leonard, A. Kumar, D. L. Murray, and D. C. Beaman, *Chemotherapy*, 33, 151–156 (1987).
24. E. Mukai, K. Arase, M. Hashida, and H. Sezaki, *Int. J. Pharm.*, 25, 95–103 (1985).
25. M. Hashida, E. Mukai, T. Kimura, and H. Sezaki, *J. Pharm. Pharmacol.*, 37, 542–544 (1985).
26. H. Okamoto, M. Ohyabu, M. Hashida, and H. Sezaki, *J. Pharm. Pharmacol.*, 39, 531–534 (1987).

27. W. M. Smith, Ph.D. Thesis, University of Michigan, Ann Arbor, 1982.
28. N. Bodor and K. B. Sloan, *Int. J. Pharm.*, 15, 235–250 (1983).
29. D. Mirejovsky and H. Takuri, *J. Pharm. Sci.*, 75: 1089–1093 (1986).
30. B. W. Barry and S. L. Bennett, *J. Pharm. Pharmacol.*, 39, 535–546 (1987).
31. M. M. Saket, K. C. James, and I. W. Kellaway, *Int. J. Pharm.*, 27, 287–298 (1985).
32. B. D. Anderson, W. I. Higuchi, and P. V. Raykar, *Pharm. Res.*, 5, 566–573 (1988).
33. J. Kao, J. Hall, and J. M. Holland, *Toxicol. Appl. Pharmacol.*, 68, 206–217 (1983).
34. D. B. Guzek, A. K. Kennedy, S. C. McNeill, E. Wakshull, and R. O. Potts, *Pharm. Res.*, 6, 33–39 (1989).
35. R. O. Potts, S. M. McNeill, C. Desbonnet, and E. Wakshull, *Pharm. Res.*, 6, 119–124 (1989).

7

Improved Ocular Drug Delivery with Prodrugs

Vincent H. L. Lee
University of Southern California, Los Angeles, California

Hans Bundgaard
The Royal Danish School of Pharmacy, Copenhagen, Denmark

CONSTRAINTS IN OCULAR DRUG DELIVERY

A major problem in ocular therapeutics is the attainment of an optimal drug concentration at the site of action. The difficulty is largely due to the fact that all of the existing drugs, which were originally developed for systemic use, lack the physicochemical properties for overcoming the severe constraints imposed by the eye on drug absorption. These constraints include precorneal factors that rapidly remove drug from the conjunctival sac where it is applied and a well-designed corneal structure that restricts the passage of drug molecules. The net result is that less than 10%, and typically 1% or less, of the instilled dose is ocularly absorbed (1,2). Thus far, attempts to improve ocular drug bioavailability fall into two categories (3): those that aim at extending drug residence time in the conjunctival sac and those that aim at improving drug penetration across the cornea, the major pathway of drug entry to the internal eye.

Several factors are responsible for precorneal drug removal, including solution drainage, tear turnover, protein binding, and conjunctival and nasal absorption (4,5). Of these, solution drainage has received the most attention in terms of improvement in ocular drug bioavailability. These methods range from increasing the viscosity of the instilled solution through the incorporation of water-soluble polymers (6–9) to the incorporation of the drug in polymeric inserts that may or may not degrade with time (10–15). The advantages and disadvantages of these methods have been reviewed in detail by Lee and Robinson (3).

Table 1 Examples of Ophthalmic Drugs to Which the Prodrug Concept Has Been Applied

Parent compound	Reversible modification or linkage	Properties modified	Therapeutic usefulness	Ref.
Adrenergic agonists				
epinephrine	Dipivalyl ester	Enhanced corneal penetration 8–17 times, improved therapeutic index 10 times.	Glaucoma	50
phenylephrine	Pivalyl ester	Improved mydriatic effects (racemic prodrug 5 times, levorotatory prodrug 15 times)	Ester itself has pharmacological activity	39
	Oxazolidine	Enhanced corneal penetration 10 times, improved therapeutic index 10 times	Mydriatics (experimental)	40–42
adrenalone	Dibutyryl, dihexanoyl, and diisovaleryl esters	Mydriatic effect improved 40 times	Mydriatics, glaucoma (experimental)	51
adrenalone	Di(ethylsuccinyl) ester	Site specific delivery to ICB	Short-acting mydriatics (experimental)	52
adrenalone	Diisolvaleryl ester	Site specific delivery to ICB	Mydriatics, glaucoma (experimental)	53
terbutaline	Diisobutyryl ester (Ibuterol)	IOP reduction 100 times	None, due to tachyphylaxis	43

Adrenergic antagonists				
nadolol	Diacetyl ester	Enhanced corneal penetration 10 times	Ester itself has pharmacological activity	27
(S)-3-tert-butylamino-1-[4-[2(hydroxy)ethyl]phenoxy]-2-propanol	Acetyl ester	Enhanced corneal penetration, improved therapeutic index	Glaucoma (experimental)	54
timolol	Aliphatic and aromatic esters	Enhanced corneal penetration, improved therapeutic index	Glaucoma (experimental)	20–26
timolol and other β-blockers	(Acyloxy)alkyl carbamates	Enhanced corneal penetration	Glaucoma (experimental)	55
propranolol	Ketoximes	Prolonged IOP reduction, improved therapeutic index	Glaucoma (experimental)	56–58
Cholinergics				
pilocarpine	Long chain soft quarternary salts	Miosis and IOP reduction by 10 times	Glaucoma (experimental)	59
	Pilocarpic acid monoesters and diesters	Enhanced corneal penetration and prolonged miosis 1.5–2.5 times	Glaucoma (experimental)	28–31

Table 1 (Continued)

Parent compound	Reversible modification or linkage	Properties modified	Therapeutic usefulness	Ref.
Carbonic anhydrase inhibitors				
6-hydroxy-benzothiazole-2-sulfonamide	Pivalyl ester	Enhanced corneal penetration 46 times, IOP reduction by 8 times	None, due to long-term toxicity	45, 60
Prostaglandins				
$PGF_{2\alpha}$	Methyl, ethyl, and isopropyl esters	Enhanced corneal penetration and IOP reduction 10–30 times	Glaucoma (experimental)	33, 34, 36
	Methyl and benzyl esters	Enhanced corneal penetration 25–40 times	Glaucoma (experimental)	35, 36
PGA_2	Isopropyl ester	Enhanced corneal penetration 15 times	Glaucoma (experimental)	61

Antimetabolites				
acyclovir	2'-O-glycyl ester	Improved aqueous solubility 30 times	Antiviral agents (experimental)	46
vidarabine	5'-Monophosphate (Ara AMP)	Improved aqueous solubility 66 times	Antiviral agents (experimental)	47
idoxuridine	5'-Alkyl esters	Enhanced ocular absorption up to 4 times	Antiviral agents (experimental)	48, 49
Steroids				
prednisolone	Acetyl ester	Improved anti-inflammatory efficiency 1.5–2.0 times	Anti-inflammatory agents	62
dexamethasone	Acetyl ester	Improved anti-inflammatory efficiency 1.5–2.0 times	Anti-inflammatory agents (experimental)	63
fluorometholone	Acetyl ester	Improved anti-inflammatory efficiency 1.5–2.0 times	Anti-inflammatory agents (experimental)	64

Abbreviations: ICB = iris–ciliary body; IOP = intraocular pressure.
Source: Adapted from Ref. 356.

Corneal drug penetration is inefficient owing to a mismatch of the physicochemical properties of the drug with those of the cornea. The cornea is a trilaminate structure consisting of a hydrophilic stromal layer sandwiched between a very lipophilic epithelial layer and a much less lipophilic endothelial layer. Consequently, drugs with extremes in partition coefficient penetrate the cornea poorly. The optimal n-octanol/water partition coefficient for transcellular corneal drug penetration has been reported to be 2–3 on a logarithmic basis (16–18). This forms the basis for the selection of ophthalmic drugs for preclinical evaluation as well as for the chemical modification of those ophthalmic drugs which are hydrophilic to yield lipophilic prodrugs that are intended for conversion to the parent compounds either chemically or enzymatically in the eye.

The concept of prodrugs was formally introduced to ophthalmology in the late 1970s with the testing of dipivefrin for improvement of corneal penetration of epinephrine (19). Since then, several other ophthalmic drugs have been investigated for prodrug derivatization. They are timolol (20–26), nadolol (27), pilocarpine (28–31), prostaglandin $F_{2\alpha}$ ($PGF_{2\alpha}$) (32–36), phenylephrine (37–42), terbutaline (43), L-643,799 (a carbonic anhydrase inhibitor) (44,45), acyclovir (46), vidarabine (47), and idoxuridine (48,49). As seen in Table 1, the results in laboratory animals have been positive.

The purpose of this chapter is to review and describe the following aspects of ocular prodrugs: (a) factors to consider in prodrug design and evaluation, (b) drug properties amenable to improvement by prodrugs, and (c) factors influencing prodrug efficacy. Where appropriate, the effectiveness of prodrugs relative to the other approaches for improving ocular drug delivery will be reviewed. On the basis of this analysis, the future of prodrugs in improving ocular drug delivery will be suggested. Figure 1 shows the ocular structures pertinent to this chapter.

FACTORS TO CONSIDER IN THE DESIGN OF OCULAR PRODRUGS

In considering ophthalmic drugs for prodrug derivatization, it is necessary to consider three interrelated factors: pathways and mechanisms of ocular drug penetration, functional group(s) of the drug candidate amenable to prodrug derivatization, and properties of the enzymes responsible for activating the prodrugs. To be successful, an ocular prodrug should possess the correct lipophilicity that balances ocular against systemic drug absorption, should possess sufficient aqueous solubility and stability for formulation as eyedrops, and should be converted to the active parent drug within the eye quantitatively and at a rate consistent with the therapeutic need.

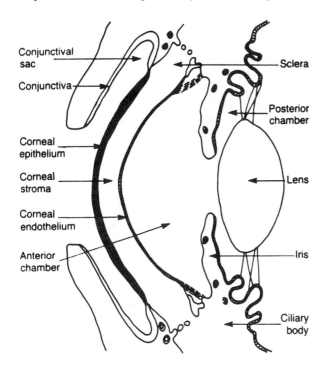

Figure 1   Structures of the anterior segment of the eye.

Pathways and Mechanisms of Ocular Drug Penetration

Corneal Route

The pathways and mechanisms by which topically applied drugs are absorbed intraocularly determine whether ocular drug absorption would benefit from prodrug derivatization. Generally, the cornea is considered as the major, but not the only, pathway of drug entry into the eye (65). For moderately lipophilic drugs such as timolol and dexamethasone, the corneal epithelium contributes 50% to the total resistance to transport, whereas the stroma and endothelium each contributes 25% (66). For hydrophilic drugs such as pilocarpine and epinephrine, the corneal epithelium can contribute even more to the total resistance. Here, much of the resistance resides in the top two cell layers (67). Thus, the corneal epithelium is a significant barrier to the penetration of all but the very lipophilic ophthalmic drugs, and it is this resistance to corneal penetration that prodrugs are designed to overcome.

There are two obvious mechanisms for drugs to move across the corneal epithelium: transcellular and paracellular diffusion. Most ophthalmic drugs appear to opt for the transcellular mechanism. Where the transcellular mechanism is untenable, the paracellular mechanism through the tight junction at the entrance of the intercellular space may assume greater quantitative importance. The stratified corneal epithelial cell layer can be characterized as a "tight" ion transporting tissue (68), having a high resistance of 12–16 k$\Omega \cdot$cm^2 (69). The tight junction which is responsible for giving rise to such a high resistance serves as a barrier not only to the paracellular diffusion of solutes, but also to the lateral diffusion of lipid-soluble solutes from the apical to the basolateral portion of the membrane (70). Integrity of the tight junction depends on Ca^{2+} (71,72) through its indirect effects on junctional elements (73) such as zonula adherens (74,75), desmosomes (76), and the Ca^{2+}-dependent adhesion molecule uvomorulin (77,78). The association of actin filaments inside the cell with the junctional complex also seems to be disrupted by low extracellular Ca^{2+} (34,75). Thus, drugs that disrupt actin filaments, such as cytochalasin B, may increase paracellular permeability (79).

The paracellular pathway is the primary route of passive ion permeation in the corneal epithelium (80). This pathway has also been proposed to be one of the two by which topically applied methanol, ethanol, and butanol are absorbed into the rabbit eye (81), the other being through putative pores in the plasma membrane of the corneal epithelial cells. The limiting size of the paracellular pathway appears to be on the order of 60 Å or less, the molecular size of glycerol (82). Evidence for the diffusion of such molecules in the aqueous space is indicated by the low values of the activation energy for transcorneal flux when compared with those for molecules using the transcellular pathway. Thus, the activation energy is 5.7 kcal mol^{-1} for water, 6.5 kcal mol^{-1} for butanol, and 4.0 kcal mol^{-1} for glycerol, when compared with values of 25.5 kcal mol^{-1} for hydrocortisone and 25.1 kcal mol^{-1} for triamcinolone acetonide (81).

Until recently, little work has been devoted to characterizing the paracellular pathway in corneal drug transport. This recent interest in the paracellular pathway was prompted by the observation that compounds of medium molecular weight such as inulin (83–85) as well as charged compounds such as sodium cromoglycate (65) and the ionized species of pilocarpine (86,87) and sulfonamides (88) could cross the cornea. It was suspected that the paracellular pathway was involved. In the case of ionizable compounds, the ionized species do not cross the cornea as efficiently as the unionized. A factor of 2–3 favoring the unionized species has been reported for pilocarpine based on in vitro corneal permeability measurements (86,87), and a factor of 4–7 has been reported for sulfonamide carbonic anhydrase inhibitors based on in vivo measurements (88).

The drug properties favoring absorption via the paracellular pathway have not been fully delineated (89). It is reasonable, however, to expect that two such principal properties may be the molecular size and charge of the drug. Grass and Robinson (82) estimated that the limiting size of a molecule undergoing paracellular diffusion is 3 nm or less. However, since the total surface area of the cornea exposed to tear that is attributable to intercellular spaces is rather small, it is unlikely that a drug would utilize the paracellular mechanism unless it is extremely water soluble. For the same reason and based on the permeability characteristics of the paracellular pathway delineated earlier, it is unlikely that prodrugs would be useful to improve the paracellular diffusion of drugs across the cornea. Nonetheless, the corneal penetration of such drugs can conceivably be improved by prodrugs that shift the absorption mechanism from para- to transcellular diffusion. This possibility has yet to be investigated in the eye, although there is preliminary supporting evidence in the absorption of 5-fluorouracil prodrugs in the rabbit colon (90).

The drug properties governing corneal drug absorption via the transcellular mechanism and which are important to consider in the design of prodrugs are well defined. They are: (a) lipophilicity, as reflected by the octanol/buffer partition coefficient, (b) pK_a, which determines the proportion of drug in its preferentially absorbed form at a given pH, and, (c) in selected cases, molecular size (81). Of these three properties, molecular size does not appear to play as important a role, since the molecular weight of most ophthalmic drugs fall within a narrow range (91).

The optimum partition coefficient for corneal drug absorption has been reported to be in the range of 10–100 (16–19), indicating that lipophilic drugs are preferred. This preference for lipophilic drugs is consistent with the lipophilic nature of the corneal epithelium (22). At the same time, drugs must also possess adequate aqueous solubility, since they must diffuse across a water-filled corneal stroma to gain access to the intraocular tissues, and since it is the initial concentration in the tear film that determines the driving force for corneal drug penetration. This inseparable importance of drug solubility and partition coefficient relative to drug absorption has been emphasized in the empirical parameter called absorption potential. This parameter, proposed by Dressman et al. (92), attempts to correlate the percent of orally administered dose absorbed into the systemic circulation with partition coefficient, aqueous solubility, fraction of drug unionized (i.e., pK_a), dose size, and volume of fluid at the absorption site. Reasonably good correlations were obtained using seven compounds, including acyclovir and prednisolone. So far, this approach has not yet been applied to predict ocular drug absorption or been considered in the design of ocular prodrugs.

Noncorneal Route

The corneal route is not the only way by which topically applied ophthalmic drugs gain access to intraocular tissues. Ahmed and Patton (93) demonstrated that certain drugs, especially the high molecular weight compounds like inulin (MW 5500), reached the iris–ciliary body by diffusion across the conjunctiva and the sclera. As much as 40% of the absorbed amount of inulin in the eye, and even larger proportions in certain ocular tissues, can be attributed to noncorneal penetration (94). Such a route appears to play an important role in the entry of topically applied MK-927, a carbonic anhydrase inhibitor, to the ciliary processes (95).

The physicochemical factors influencing drug diffusion across the sclera have been evaluated using β-blockers (96), sulfonamide carbonic anhydrase inhibitors (97), and dyes as well as drugs such as pilocarpine, penicillin G, and hydrocortisone (98). Ahmed et al. (96) reported that, as was the case in the cornea, lipophilic drugs penetrated the sclera more readily than did the hydrophilic. This suggests that in addition to diffusion across the aqueous media of the gel-like mucopolysaccharides in the sclera, partitioning into its collagen fibrils also plays a role in scleral drug diffusion. Moreover, compared with the cornea, the sclera was about 5 times more permeable to β-blockers such as penbutolol, propranolol, timolol, and nadolol (96). The same investigators also found that solute size had a more pronounced effect on scleral than on corneal permeability. In another study, Edelhauser and Maren (97) discovered that the sclera was more permeable than, or at least as permeable as, the corneal stroma to the sulfonamide carbonic anhydrase inhibitors benzolamide, bromacetazolamide, methazolamide, and ethoxzolamide. This finding is, however, opposite to that of Maurice and Polgar (98). These investigators observed that a variety of ions and solutes up to the size of serum albumin diffused across the bovine sclera about 3 times more slowly than they did in the rabbit corneal stroma.

There is limited information on drug permeability in the conjunctiva, across which the drug must pass in order to reach the sclera. Lee et al. (99) reported that conjunctival drug penetration was less sensitive to changes in drug lipophilicity than corneal drug penetration, and that scleral drug penetration was even less so. The conjunctival permeability of timolol is between the scleral and corneal permeabilities (96). The conjunctival permeability of inulin is comparable to scleral permeability but is much higher than corneal permeability (96). Interestingly, despite the higher permeability of timolol across the conjunctiva and the sclera relative to inulin (96), the extent of intraocular penetration of timolol and inulin via the noncorneal route is similar (94). This has been attributed to more extensive loss of timolol to the vasculature in the conjunctiva than inulin.

Clearly, the noncorneal route has yet to be exploited to promote intraocular drug delivery. The findings to date suggest that drugs that would benefit from this route are those that are hydrophilic and/or large, so that they can resist corneal penetration on the one hand and removal by the vasculature in the conjunctiva and the sclera on the other. It seems that drugs that opt for the noncorneal route of entry into the eye must possess a lipophilicity that directs them away from the cornea toward the conjunctiva and which, at the same time, prevents them from passing across the capillary endothelia in the lamina propia of the conjunctiva and the sclera. So far, no prodrugs have been designed to promote noncorneal drug absorption, nor has the extent of noncorneal absorption of those that are intended for improved corneal drug penetration been characterized.

Bioreversible Derivatization of Ophthalmic Drugs—Chemical Aspects

A basic requisite for the prodrug approach to be useful in solving ophthalmic drug delivery problems is the ready availability of chemical derivative types satisfying the prodrug requirements, the most prominent of these being reconversion of the prodrug to the parent drug in vivo. In recent years, several types of bioreversible derivatives have been exploited for utilization in designing prodrugs, a subject that has been reviewed extensively elsewhere (100–102). A list of prodrug forms is given in Table 2.

The majority of ophthalmic prodrugs developed up to now are esters derived from hydroxyl or carboxylic acid groups present in the parent molecules. In a number of cases, however, other strategies are required, since the drug to be modified does not contain such groups readily amenable to esterification. Even when esterification is feasible, ester prodrugs may create problems owing to chemical instability in aqueous eye drops formulations. Such cases will be discussed below along with an account of the chemistry of some newly developed nonester prodrug types that have been or may be applied to ophthalmic drugs.

Stability Problems with Ester Prodrugs

Esters of Timolol. With the aim of making prodrugs of timolol (1) to diminish the extent of systemic absorption of the drug following ocular administration, and hence its side effects, through increasing the ratio of corneal versus conjunctival/nasal penetration, a number of timolol esters have been prepared (20,21). Timolol contains a secondary amino group with a pK_a value of 9.2. Since this group is highly protonated at pH 7.4, the compound shows a low lipophilicity at physiological pH, which in turn is unfavorable for corneal absorption. Esterification of the hydroxyl group in timolol with aliphatic or aromatic acids affords a ready means to increase lipophilicity and, hence, corneal absorption. The

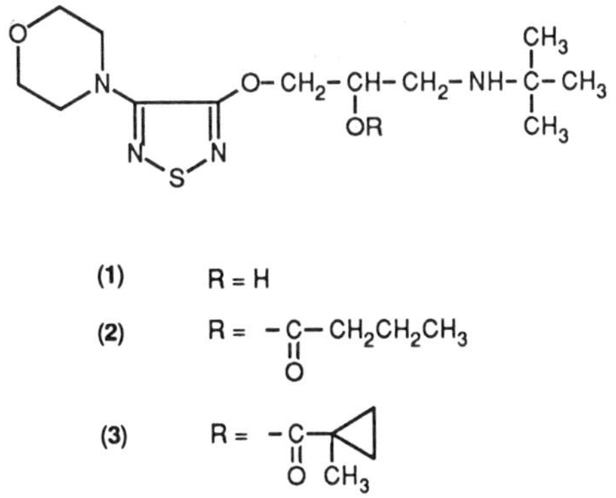

(1)   R = H

(2)   R = $-\overset{O}{\underset{\parallel}{C}}-CH_2CH_2CH_3$

(3)   R =

Table 2 Prodrug Forms of Various Functional Groups in Drug Substances

Functional group	Prodrug form	
-COOH	$-\underset{\overset{\|}{O}}{C}-OR$	Esters
	$-\underset{\overset{\|}{O}}{C}-O-\underset{\overset{\|}{R}}{C}HO-\underset{\overset{\|}{O}}{C}-R$	α-Acyloxyalkyl esters
	$-\underset{\overset{\|}{O}}{C}-NHR$	Amides
–OH	$-O\underset{\overset{\|}{O}}{C}-R$	Esters
	$-O-\underset{\overset{\|}{O}}{C}-OR$	Carbonate esters
	$-O-\underset{\overset{\|}{O}}{\overset{OH}{P}}\,_{OH}$	Phosphate esters
	–OR	Ethers
	$-O\underset{\overset{\|}{R}}{C}H-O\underset{\overset{\|}{O}}{C}-R$	α-Acyloxyalkyl ethers
–SH	$-S\underset{\overset{\|}{O}}{C}R$	Thioesters
	$-S\underset{\overset{\|}{R}}{C}H-O\underset{\overset{\|}{O}}{C}-R$	α-Acyloxyalkyl thioethers
	–S–S–R	Disulphides
$\underset{/}{\overset{\backslash}{C}}=O$	$-\underset{\overset{\|}{O}R}{C}-OR$	Ketals
	$\underset{/}{\overset{\backslash}{C}}=N-R$	Imines
	$\underset{//}{\overset{\backslash}{C}}-O\underset{\overset{\|}{O}}{C}-R$	Enol esters
	$\underset{/}{\overset{\backslash}{\underset{N}{C}}}\!\!\big\langle\!\!{\overset{O}{\,}}\,\big]$	Oxazolidines
	$\underset{/}{\overset{\backslash}{\underset{N}{C}}}\!\!\big\langle\!\!{\overset{S}{\,}}\,\big]$	Thiazolidines

Table 2 (Continued)

Functional group	Prodrug form	
$-NH_2$	$-NH-\overset{\displaystyle O}{\underset{\displaystyle \|}{C}}-R$	Amides
	$-NH-\overset{\displaystyle O}{\underset{\displaystyle \|}{C}}-OR$	Carbamates
	$-N=C\overset{\displaystyle R}{\underset{\displaystyle R}{<}}$	Imines
	$-NH-\underset{\|}{C}=\underset{\|}{C}-$	Enamines
	$-NH-CH_2-\underset{\underset{\displaystyle R}{\|}}{N}-\overset{\overset{\displaystyle O}{\|}}{C}-R$	N-Mannich bases
	$-NH-\overset{\overset{\displaystyle O}{\|}}{C}O\underset{\underset{\displaystyle R}{\|}}{C}HO-\overset{\overset{\displaystyle O}{\|}}{C}-R$	N-Acyloxyalkoxycarbonyl derivatives
$\overset{\displaystyle \backslash}{\underset{\displaystyle /}{-}}N$	$\overset{\displaystyle \backslash}{\underset{\displaystyle /}{-}}\overset{+}{N}-\underset{\underset{\displaystyle R}{\|}}{C}HO-\overset{\overset{\displaystyle O}{\|}}{C}-R$	N-Acyloxyalkyl derivatives
$R_1-\overset{\overset{\displaystyle O}{\|}}{C}-OR_2$	$R-SO_2N=C\overset{\displaystyle R_1}{\underset{\displaystyle OR_2}{<}}$	N-Sulphonyl imidates
$-SO_2NH_2$	$-SO_2N=C\overset{\displaystyle R_1}{\underset{\displaystyle OR_2}{<}}$	N-Sulphonyl imidates
	$-SO_2NH-CH_2OR$	N-Alkoxymethyl derivatives
NH-Acidic group	$-\overset{\overset{\displaystyle O}{\|}}{C}-\underset{\underset{\displaystyle R}{\|}}{N}-CH_2NR_1NR_2$	N-Mannich bases
e.g., $-\overset{\overset{\displaystyle O}{\|}}{C}-\underset{\underset{\displaystyle R}{\|}}{N}H$	$-\overset{\overset{\displaystyle O}{\|}}{C}-\underset{\underset{\displaystyle R}{\|}}{N}-CH_2OH$	N-Methylols
or heterocyclic amine	$-\overset{\overset{\displaystyle O}{\|}}{C}-\underset{\underset{\displaystyle R}{\|}}{N}-\underset{\underset{\displaystyle R_1}{\|}}{C}HO-\overset{\overset{\displaystyle O}{\|}}{C}-R_2$	N-Acyloxyalkyl derivatives

Table 3 Hydrolysis Data, Lipophilicity, and Ratio of In Vitro Corneal to Conjunctival Permeability Coefficients for Timolol and Various Timolol Esters

Ester	Half-life of hydrolysis at pH 7.4 at 37°C (h)	log P[a]	Ratio
Timolol	—	-0.04	0.34
O-Acetyl	0.47	1.12	0.62
O-Propionoyl	0.67	1.62	0.70
O-Butyryl	0.83	2.08	0.51
O-Pivaloyl	3.6	2.68	0.57
O-Hexanoyl	1.3	3.35	0.54
O-Benzoyl	2.0	2.55	0.82
O-4-Methylbenzoyl	4.9	3.11	1.27
O-4-Methoxybenzoyl	4.9	2.65	1.05
O-Cyclopropanolol	4.1	1.74	0.64
O-1'-Methylcyclopropanolol	9.9	2.22	0.77
O-Cyclohexanoyl	1.6	3.30	0.66

[a]The partition coefficient between octanol and 0.05 M phosphate buffer (pH 7.4).
Source: From Refs. 21 and 103.

task, however, turned out to be more complicated than initially thought because most esters of timolol suffered from instability in aqueous solution.

Hydrolysis data and lipophilicities of some of the esters studied are shown in Table 3. All are more lipophilic than the parent timolol. This is due to conversion of the hydroxyl group to an ester group and to reduction in pK_a values (about 8.4 for the esters vs 9.2 for timolol), affording a greater proportion of the lipophilic free base form at pH 7.4. The esters are all converted quantitatively to the parent timolol in aqueous solution at pH 1–11 as well as by enzymatic hydrolysis by eye tissue enzymes (20). The sterically unhindered straight chain aliphatic esters are especially rapidly hydrolyzed both enzymatically and chemically. The latter property is a drawback from the standpoint of formulating ready-to-use aqueous eye drops preparations with acceptable shelf-lives. The esters are most stable at pH 3–4 (Fig. 2). But even at this pH, alkyl esters such as acetate and butyrate esters show limited stability. Sterically hindered esters such as the 2-ethylbutyryl, 3,3-dimethylbutyryl, cyclopropanoyl, and 1'-methylcyclopropanoyl derivatives are, on the other hand, more stable. For these compounds it is feasible to obtain aqueous solutions with shelf-lives greater than 2 years when stored at 10–15°C (21). The greater chemical reactivity of timolol esters compared to most other simple esters has been shown to be due to an intramolecular catalytic effect by the amino group in the compounds (Scheme 1) (20).

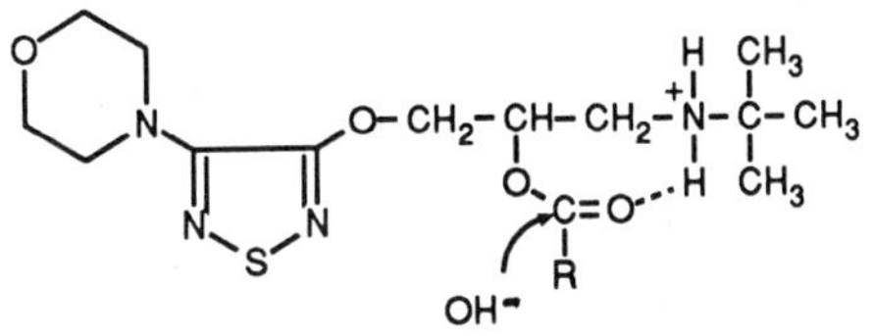

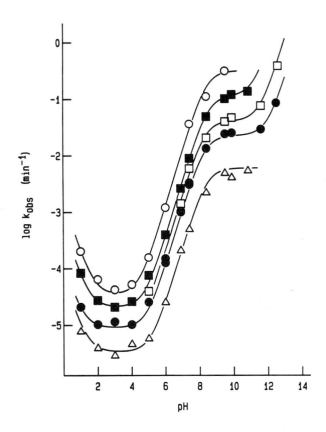

Scheme 1

Figure 2 The pH-rate profiles for the degradation of various timolol esters in aqueous solution at 37°C. Key: ○, O-acetyltimolol; ■, O-hexanoyltimolol; ●, O-pivaloyltimolol; □, O-benzoyltimolol; Δ, O-2-ethylbutyryltimolol. (From Ref. 21.)

The permeability of the timolol esters across the isolated cornea and the conjunctiva of rabbits was found to depend on both lipophilicity and enzymatic lability (22,26). Both the corneal and conjunctival permeabilities vary parabolically with the lipophilicity expressed in terms of octanol/pH 7.4 buffer partition coefficients (P), the maximal permeability being obtained for compounds with a log P value of about 2. The rates of penetration increased with increased susceptibility of the esters to undergo hydrolysis in the ocular membranes which probably can be ascribed to the fact that facile prodrug cleavage will increase the concentration gradient governing prodrug absorption.

Except for very lipophilic derivatives, the timolol esters penetrated the cornea more rapidly than timolol as a result of their increased lipophilicity. Most importantly, the increase in corneal penetration achieved with the esters was not paralleled to the same magnitude in penetration across the conjunctival membrane and hence systemic absorption, as indicated by the unequal ratios of corneal to conjunctival permeabilities shown in Table 3. Some results obtained in vivo with O-butyryl timolol (2) can illustrate this (24,25). Whereas this prodrug, as a result of increased lipophilicity, led to a four- to sixfold increase in the corneal absorption of timolol following topical administration to the rabbit, the systemic absorption of timolol was unaffected or even slightly reduced (depending on the dose) (24,25) (Table 4). Possibly, timolol already readily penetrated the conjunctival and nasal epithelia and, in turn, the underlying blood vessels. Therefore, further increase in lipophilicity did not markedly enhance the systemic absorption of timolol. It can be seen from the data in Table 4 that while the ocular absorption of the O-butyryl ester from a 15-mM solution was 5.5 times greater than that of the parent drug, the systemic absorption as reflected in plasma timolol levels was comparable. When a correspondingly lower concentration of the prodrug (3.75 mM) was used, the therapeutic index as assessed by the ratio of aqueous humor to plasma concentrations seemed to improve 15 times. Thus, it is possible to very significantly reduce the systemic absorption, and hence side effects, of timolol without reducing its concentration at its site of action in the eye by using a low dose of its butyryl ester prodrug.

Besides the improved ocular/systemic bioavailability ratio observed with O-butyryl timolol, the prodrug also shows a greatly extended duration of action in comparison with the parent timolol in an experimental animal model (104). The greater lipophilicity of the ester probably results in enhanced deposit of the prodrug in ocular tissues serving as a depot from which the active parent drug is slowly released. Just as favorable findings have been obtained with some other timolol esters such as the O-1'-methylcyclopropanoyl ester (3) (103,105). Since the latter ester shows a much higher chemical stability in aqueous solution than the O-butyryl ester, it is being considered as a lead timolol prodrug.

These investigations with timolol illustrate the difficulties in obtaining a prodrug derivative possessing adequate stability in eye drops formulations and at the same time sufficient enzymatic reactivity in order to ensure complete

Table 4 Areas Under the Concentration Time Curves (AUC) in the Plasma and Aqueous Humor, and the Ratios of These Areas (Plasma/AH) Following the Topical Instillation of 25 μl of Various Concentrations of Timolol or O-Butyryl Timolol in the Pigmented Rabbit

Concentration (μM)	Compound	AUC (μM min ± SEM)		Plasma/AH (10⁴)
		plasma	aqueous humor	
3.75	Timolol	0.51 ± 0.17	140.1 ± 23.1	36
	O-Butyryl timolol	0.42 ± 0.07	630.1 ± 47.5	7
7.5	Timolol	1.46 ± 0.15	239.5 ± 35.8	61
	O-Butyryl timolol	1.19 ± 0.18	1064.8 ± 77.5	11
11.5	Timolol	2.27 ± 0.45	311.9 ± 48.8	73
	O-Butyryl timolol	2.42 ± 0.37	1243.2 ± 104.9	19
15.0	Timolol	3.93 ± 0.52	381.9 ± 59.4	103
	O-Butyryl timolol	3.47 ± 0.58	1921.9 ± 141.7	18

Source: From Ref. 25.

conversion to the parent drug in the eye. Whereas it is well known that the chemical stability of esters is dependent on polar and steric factors within the alcohol and acyl portions, the enzymatic reactivity is less predictable. Although steric effects generally alter nonenzymatic and enzymatic hydrolysis rates in the same direction (106), the findings with the unsubstituted or substituted cyclopropanoyl esters of timolol (which are highly sterically hindered) show that this is not always the case. Because of their combination of high chemical stability and adequate enzymatic hydrolysis such esters may probably be of more general utility in prodrug design.

Amino Acid Esters. Formation of water-soluble ester prodrugs has long been recognized as an effective means of increasing the aqueous solubility of drugs containing a hydroxyl group, aiming at developing improved preparations for parenteral or ophthalmic administration. The most commonly used esters for increasing the aqueous solubility of hydroxyl-containing agents are esters containing an ionizable group; i.e., dicarboxylic acid hemiesters, phosphate esters, and α-amino acid esters (100). The ideal properties of such prodrugs are as follows.

They should possess high water solubility at the pH of optimal stability and sufficient stability in aqueous solution to allow long-term storage (>2 years) of ready-to-use solutions. Yet they should be quantitatively and rapidly converted in vivo to the active parent drug. In reality, none of these derivatives fully satisfies all these requirements. Thus, whereas α-amino acid esters or related short chain aliphatic amino acid esters are generally readily hydrolyzed enzymatically, they exhibit a very poor stability in aqueous solution, making it impossible to prepare ready-to-use solutions (100,107,108).

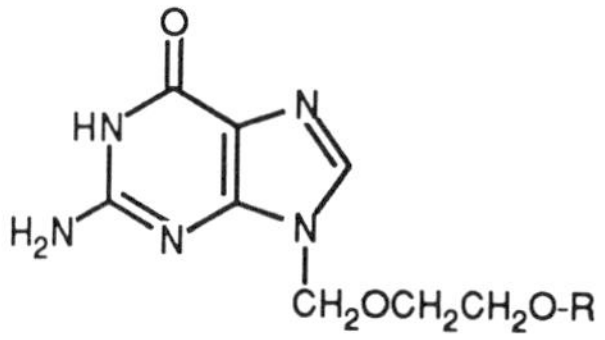

(4) R = H

(5) R = −C−CH₂NH₂

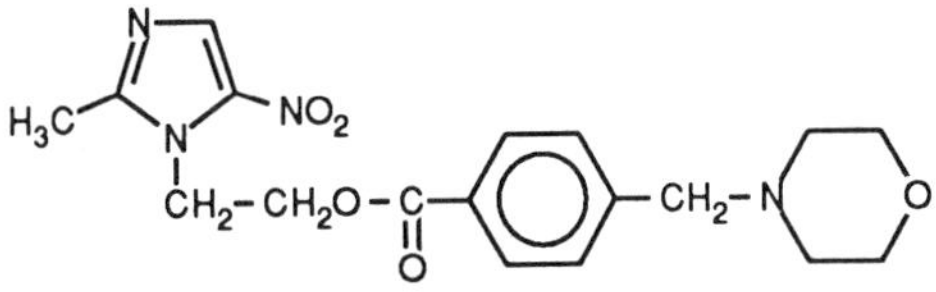

(6)

Various α-amino acid esters of the antiviral agent acyclovir (4) have been prepared to improve its corneal penetration via more water-soluble prodrugs (109). Several of such water-soluble esters were found to be almost as active as acyclovir itself in inhibiting the cytopathogenicity of herpes simplex virus types 1 and 2 in rabbit kidney cells. In particular, a 1% aqueous eye drop formulation of the glycine ester (5) was effective in the management of epithelial keratitis, stromal keratitis, and iritis (46). Because of the enhanced solubility of the glycine ester, as high as a 6% aqueous solution at pH 4–5 can be formulated. The ester is most presumably rapidly hydrolyzed by corneal enzymes, but like other α-amino acid esters, it suffers from instability in aqueous formulations.

There are two major reasons for the high instability of α-amino and short chain aliphatic amino acid esters in aqueous solution at pH values (i.e., pH 3–5) where they are most water soluble: (a) the strongly electron-withdrawing effect of the protonated amino group which activates the ester linkage toward hydroxide ion attack, and (b) intramolecular catalysis or assistance by the neighboring amino group of ester hydrolysis (108,110,111). As depicted in Scheme 2, the underlying mechanisms include intramolecular nucleophilic catalysis, intramolecular general-base catalysis, or general-base specific-base catalysis (111).

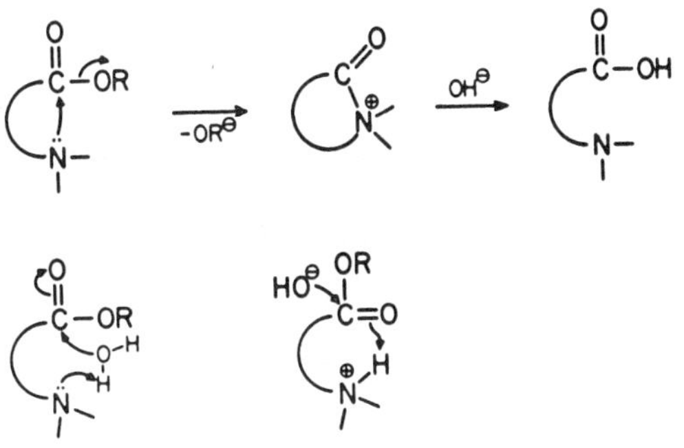

Scheme 2

It has been shown (112) that an effective and simple means to completely block the hydrolysis-facilitating effect of the amino group described above while retaining a rapid rate of enzymatic ester hydrolysis is to incorporate a phenyl group between the ester moiety and the amino group. In this way, the intramolecular catalytic reactions of the amino group as outlined in Scheme 2 are no longer possible for sterical reasons. Moreover, the ester-labilizing effect of the protonated amino group owing to its polar character is greatly diminished. Because of the requirement of a pK_a value greater than 5–6 for the amino group (to ensure good solubility), the group is not directly attached to the phenyl nucleus but separated from it by an alkylene group, in the most simple case a methylene group. Such N-substituted 3- or 4-aminomethylbenzoate esters have been found to be readily soluble in water at weakly acidic pH values and to possess very high stability in such solutions combined with high susceptibility to undergo enzymatic hydrolysis in the presence of plasma (Scheme 3) (112). Thus, the 4-(morpholinyl-methyl)benzoate ester of metronidazole possesses a shelf-life of more than 10 years in aqueous solution of pH 4 and 25°C, whereas being hydrolyzed to metronidazole in human plasma with a half-life of 0.4 min. Since the pK_a of the morpholinyl group in compound (6) is 6.1, readily water-soluble salts can be formed (113). Similar esters with the same favorable solubility, in vitro stability, and in vivo lability characteristics have been described for various corticosteroids (112), chloramphenicol (114), acyclovir (115), and other hydroxyl-containing drugs (112).

These properties regarding solubility, chemical stability, and enzymatic lability make N-substituted aminomethylbenzoate esters a promising new prodrug type for slightly soluble drugs containing an esterifiable hydroxyl group. Studies exploring the potential application of such ester prodrugs to improve the ocular delivery characteristics of slightly soluble drugs such as acyclovir and corticosteroids are certainly warranted. In this regard, it should be noted that the lipophilicity of the prodrug derivatives can readily be modified or controlled by the appropriate selection of the amino group with respect to (a) amine basicity,

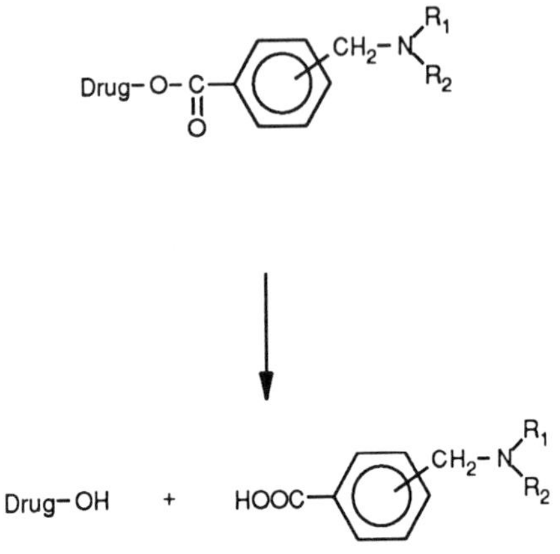

Scheme 3

and hence degree of ionization at physiological pH, and (b) hydrophobicity of the substituents on the nitrogen atom. Thus, the 4-(morpholinylmethyl)benzoate ester of acyclovir, besides being much more soluble than acyclovir in water at pH 3–5, is more lipophilic than the parent drug at pH 7.4 (112). Whereas acyclovir shows a log P value of –1.47, the value for the ester is –0.05, where P is the partition coefficient between octanol and phosphate buffer of pH 7.4.

Finally, this prodrug approach can also be applied to drugs containing an NH-acidic group, such as hydantoins, imides, secondary amides, and imidazoles, by forming N-acyloxymethyl derivatives (112,116). From such derivatives the parent drug is regenerated via a two-step reaction: enzymatic cleavage of the ester grouping followed by spontaneous and fast decomposition of the N-hydroxymethyl intermediate (100,116) (Scheme 4).

Double Prodrugs. In various cases the conversion of prodrug derivatives to the parent drug in vivo is triggered by the buffered and relatively constant value of the physiological pH of 7.4. A serious drawback of such prodrugs requiring chemical (i.e., nonenzymatic) release of the active drug is the inherent stability of the derivatives, raising some stability-formulation problems in eyedrops.

A promising means to overcome the above stability problem is cascade latentiation or the double prodrug concept (pro-prodrugs) (101,102). Thus, as outlined in Fig. 3, by derivatizing the prodrug in such a manner that an enzymatic release mechanism is required prior to the spontaneous release of the parent drug, the stability problem can be solved. An example in which this approach has successfully been applied is pilocarpic acid diesters. As will be described in a following section, these pilocarpine prodrugs are chemically highly stable and yet are easily

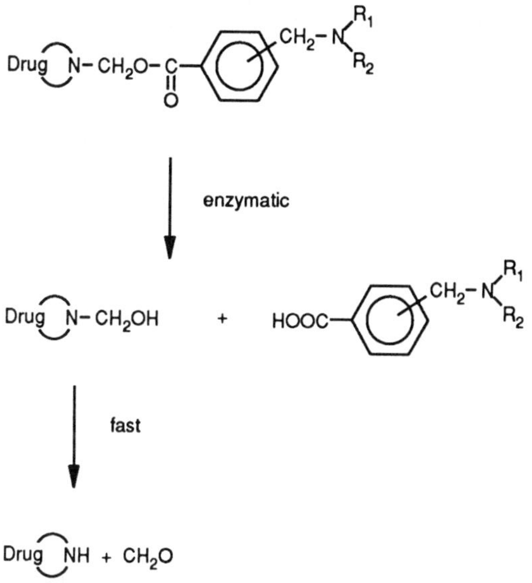

Drug N-CH₂O-C—⟨◯⟩—CH₂-N⟨R₁ R₂
                ‖
                O

enzymatic

Drug N-CH₂OH   +   HOOC—⟨◯⟩—CH₂-N⟨R₁ R₂

fast

Drug NH + CH₂O

Scheme 4

hydrolyzed in the presence of ocular esterases to pilocarpic acid monoesters, which subsequently undergo a spontaneous, enzyme-independent cyclization to yield pilocarpine.

Another example is provided by ketoximes of various β-adrenergic blocking agents such as propranolol. The bioactivation of the ketoximes proceeds via an initial hydrolysis of the oxime functionality to yield a ketone which subsequently is enzymatically reduced to afford the parent β-blocker as depicted in Scheme 5 for the ketoxime derivative (7) of propranolol (8). Being a β-amino ketone, the

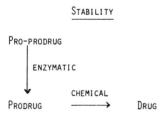

STABILITY

PRO-PRODRUG

| ENZYMATIC

              CHEMICAL
PRODRUG   ——————→   DRUG

Figure 3   Stabilization of a spontaneously decomposing prodrug by further derivatization to yield a chemically stable but enzymatically labile double prodrug.

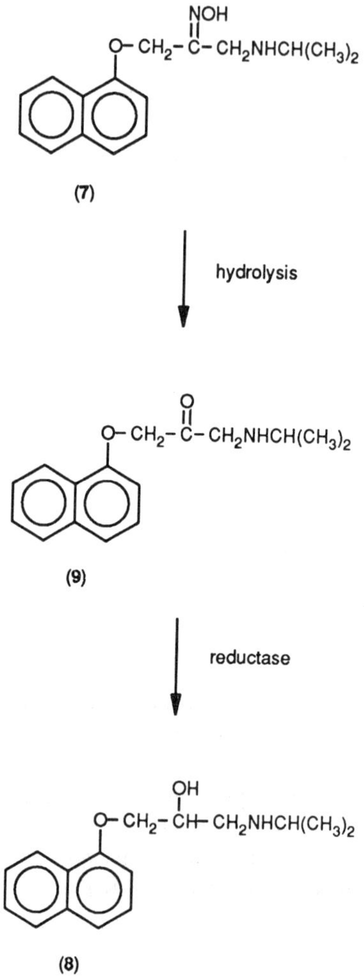

$$\underset{(7)}{\overset{\displaystyle \overset{NOH}{\underset{\|}{}}}{O-CH_2-C-CH_2NHCH(CH_3)_2}}$$

hydrolysis

$$\underset{(9)}{\overset{\displaystyle \overset{O}{\underset{\|}{}}}{O-CH_2-C-CH_2NHCH(CH_3)_2}}$$

reductase

$$\underset{(8)}{\overset{\displaystyle \overset{OH}{\underset{|}{}}}{O-CH_2-CH-CH_2NHCH(CH_3)_2}}$$

Scheme 5

intermediate (9) is chemically unstable but it can be stabilized in the form of an oxime. The reduction process has been suggested to take place in the iris–ciliary body, which implies a site-specific activation of these β-blocker prodrugs when used as antiglaucoma agents (56–58). It is not clear whether the first step in Scheme 5 is enzymatic or chemical. In rabbits, the intraocular pressure–lowering potency of the propranolol ketoxime prodrug (7) was much more pronounced and prolonged than that of propranolol itself. Moreover, administration of the prodrug to the eye of rabbits was not associated with irritation, contrary to topical administration of propranolol (56,57). The possibility that the ketoxime itself might have some intrinsic activity cannot be excluded (57).

Derivatives of Amines

N-Acyl Derivatives. N-Acylation of amines to give amide prodrugs has been used only to a limited extent owing to the relative stability of amides in vivo (100). For the same reason, the utility of carbamates as prodrug derivatives for amines is limited. This problem can, however, be circumvented by introducing an enzymatically hydrolyzable ester function in the carbamate structure. Thus, N-(acyloxy-alkoxycarbonyl) derivatives of primary or secondary amines may be readily transformed to the parent amine in vivo (55,117). Enzymatic hydrolysis of the ester moiety in such derivatives would lead to a (hydroxyalkoxy)carbonyl derivative which spontaneously decomposes to the parent amine via an unstable carbamic acid (Scheme 6).

Such (acyloxy)alkyl carbamates may be promising biolabile prodrugs for amino functional drugs, since they are neutral compounds, and since they combine high stability in aqueous solution (118) with high susceptibility to undergo enzymatic regeneration of the parent amine by ester hydrolysis (55,118,119). Thus, the derivative (**10**) of timolol shows a half-life of degradation of 1410 min in a pH 7.4 phosphate buffer at 37°C and 10 min in dog plasma (55). For primary amines, however, an intramolecular acyl transfer reaction leading to the formation of a

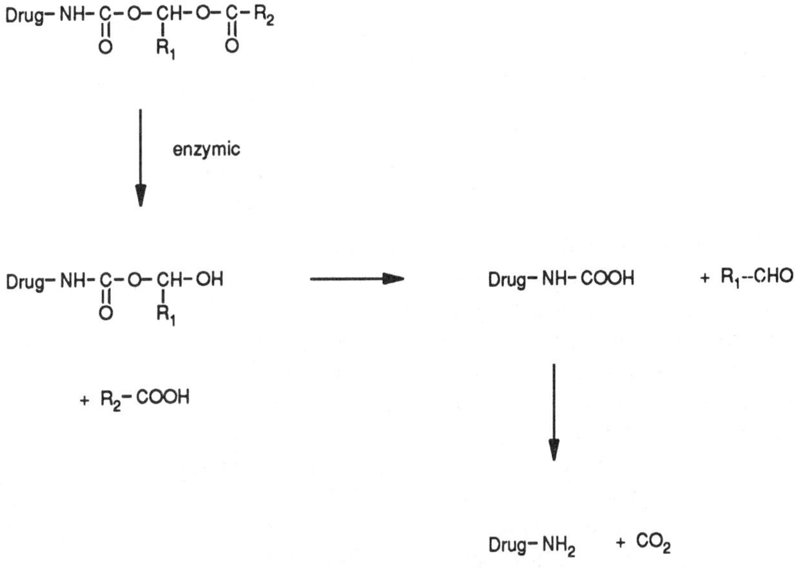

Drug– NH– C– O– CH– O– C– R$_2$
$\quad\quad\quad\ \|\quad\quad\ \|\quad\quad\ \|$
$\quad\quad\quad\ O\quad\ R_1\quad\ $O

$\downarrow$ enzymic

Drug– NH– C– O– CH– OH $\quad\longrightarrow\quad$ Drug– NH– COOH $\quad$ + R$_1$--CHO
$\quad\quad\quad\ \|\quad\quad\ \|$
$\quad\quad\quad\ O\quad\ R_1$

+ R$_2$– COOH

$\downarrow$

Drug– NH$_2$ $\quad$ + CO$_2$

Scheme 6

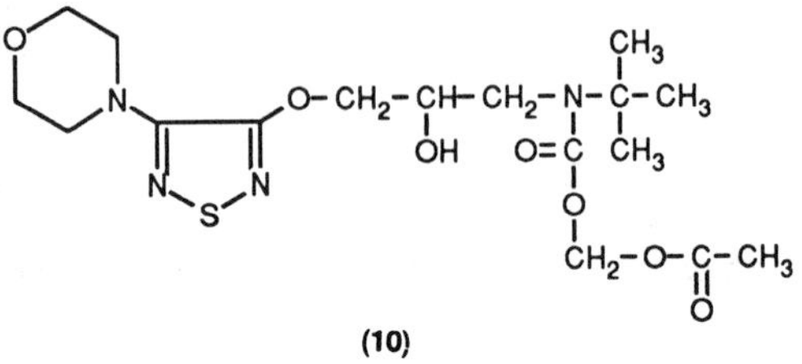

(10)

stable N-acylated parent amine, as depicted in Scheme 7, may compete with the reaction sequence in Scheme 6 at physiological pH, thus diminishing the yield of amine regenerated. Such intramolecular N-acylation is structurally impossible in the derivatives of secondary amines. Therefore, the utility of N-acyloxyalkoxycarbonyl derivatives as prodrugs of primary amines relies on a high rate of enzymatic hydrolysis to compete with the undesired intramolecular reaction. This prodrug approach has been applied to pindolol, propranolol, and betaxolol besides timolol (55) and found to be useful to improve in vitro corneal permeation. As expected, the lipophilic β-blockers do not benefit as much from prodrug derivatization as the more hydrophilic ones.

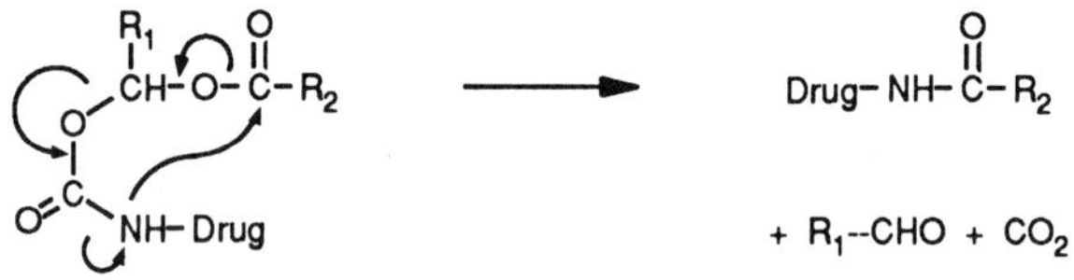

Scheme 7

Another interesting and perhaps broadly applicable prodrug type for primary and secondary amines is N-(5-substituted-2-oxo-1,3-dioxyl-4-yl)methyl derivatives (11). Such derivatives formed with the secondary amino group of the piperazinyl moiety of norfloxacin were shown to be rather chemically stable but they were readily hydrolyzed in mouse blood (120). The reaction sequence may be as outlined in Scheme 8 with initial esterase-catalyzed hydrolysis of the cyclic carbonate followed by a fast carbon-nitrogen bond cleavage to produce the parent amine and a diketone. Studies are certainly warranted to investigate the properties of this promising prodrug type in more detail. It is of interest to note that the (5-alkyl-2-oxo-1,3-dioxyl-4-yl)methyl group has also been considered as a promoiety for carboxylic acids such as ampicillin (121,122), methyldopa (123), and various angiotensin-converting enzyme inhibitors (124).

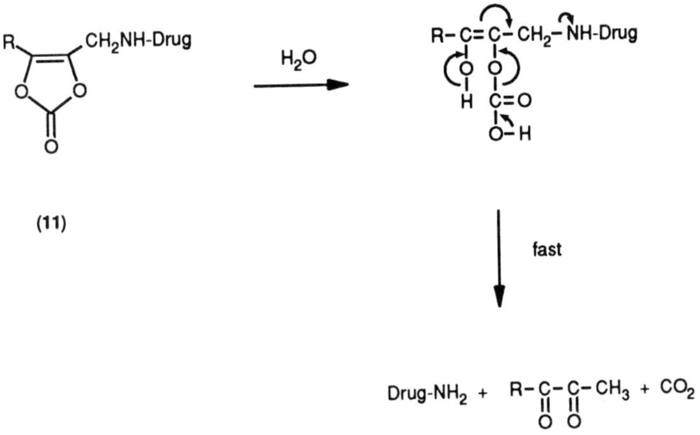

(11)

fast

$$Drug\text{-}NH_2 \ + \ R\text{-}\underset{O}{\overset{}{C}}\text{-}\underset{O}{\overset{}{C}}\text{-}CH_3 \ + \ CO_2$$

Scheme 8

Oxazolidines. Oxazolidines can be prodrug candidates for the β-aminoalcohol function which is present in several drugs, such as various sympathomimetic amines and β-blockers (125–127). Oxazolidines (**12**), which are cyclic condensation products of β-aminoalcohols and aldehydes or ketones, undergo facile and complete hydrolysis in aqueous solutions (Scheme 9). By varying the carbonyl moiety, it is possible to control the rate of formation of a given β-aminoalcohol. Thus, the following half-lives of hydrolysis for various (–)-ephedrine oxazolidines (**13**) have been found at pH 7.4 and 37°C (125,126): 5 min (benzaldehyde), 5 s (salicylaldehyde), 4 s (formaldehyde), 17 s (propionaldehyde), 30 min (pivaldehyde), 4 min (acetone), and 6 min (cyclohexanone). The hydrolysis rates at neutral and basic pH decrease with increasing steric effects of the substituents derived from the carbonyl component as well as with increasing basicity of the oxazolidines (126). The pH-rate profiles for the hydrolysis of various oxazolidines are shown in Fig. 4.

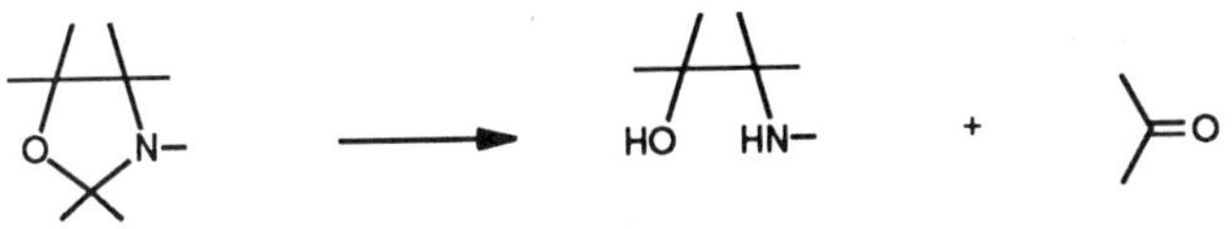

(12)

Scheme 9

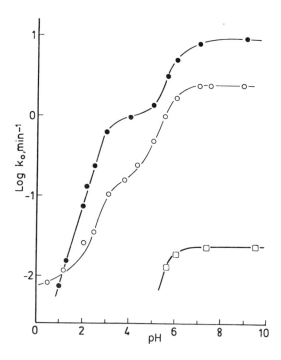

(13)

Structure-reactivity relationships have been established for the influence of the β-aminoalcohol moiety upon stability (127). Thus, the hydrolytic rates at neutral and basic pH decreased with increasing steric effects within this moiety, in particular at the α-position to the nitrogen atom, and increased with increasing electron negativity of the substituents at the β-position to the nitrogen atom (125). Obviously, such relationships may be useful for the prediction of the reactivity of

Figure 4 The pH-rate profiles for the hydrolysis of oxazolidines derived from (−)ephedrine and formaldehyde (●), propionaldehyde (○), and pivaldehyde (□) at 37°C. (From Ref. 126.)

an oxazolidine to be designed as a prodrug derivative of a drug molecule containing a β-aminoalcohol moiety or a carbonyl group.

Oxazolidines are weaker bases (pK$_a$ 6–7) than the parent β-aminoalcohols; they are therefore more lipophilic at physiological pH (126). Such increased lipophilicity may become advantageous in situations where delivery problems for β-aminoalcohol-type drugs are due to low lipophilicity, as in the case of dermal or ocular absorption. Thus, an oxazolidine prodrug (14) of phenylephrine (15) prepared from pivaldehyde (Scheme 10) has been shown to penetrate the cornea much more easily than the parent drug as a result of increased lipophilicity (40–42). In rabbits, the prodrug shows a 10-fold increased mydriatic response in comparison with topically instilled phenylephrine HCl. The greater corneal penetration allows for a 10- to 15-fold reduction in the phenylephrine dose, which leads to reduction in the systemic absorption of phenylephrine and, in turn, minimization of the undesired systemic side effects (40,41). A drawback of oxazolidines as prodrugs is their poor stability in aqueous solution. Thus, the half-life of hydrolysis of compound (14) is only 13 min at pH 7.4 and 37°C and is independent of enzymatic catalysis (40). Nevertheless, by formulating the prodrug in a non-aqueous vehicle such as sesame oil, a product with a stability sufficient for practical use can apparently be obtained (40).

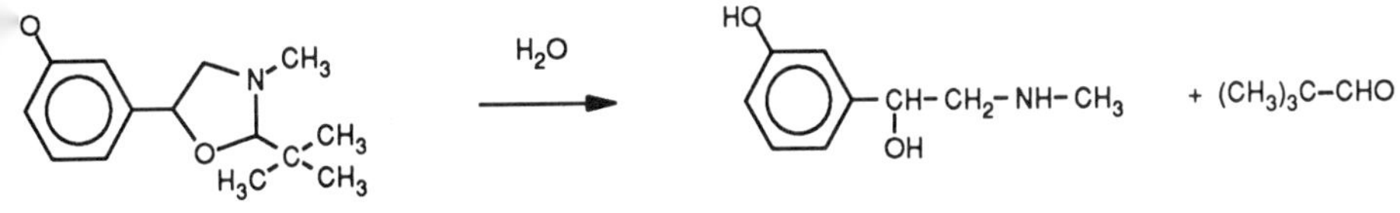

(14)   (15)

Scheme 10

A possible means to obtain an oxazolidine prodrug with good stability in aqueous solution would be further derivatization of the oxazolidine to produce compounds (double prodrugs) whose initial cleavage to oxazolidine relies on enzymatic hydrolysis. In fact, N-acylated or N-benzoylated oxazolidines derived from primary aminoalcohols are highly stable in aqueous solution, but unfortunately they are also quite resistant to enzymatic hydrolysis (128).

Derivatives of the Sulfonamide Group

As will be described in a later section, carbonic anhydrase inhibitors (CAIs) such as acetazolamide, ethoxzolamide, and methazolamide are useful for the treatment of glaucoma. Owing to limited aqueous solubility or unfavorable lipophilicity (Fig. 5), however, they are not active when administered topically to the eye and must be given orally or parenterally (129,130). In an attempt to overcome the

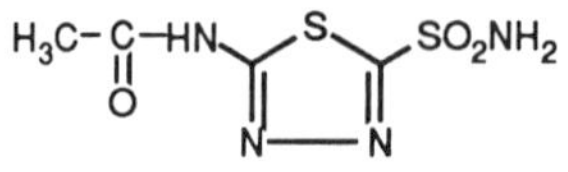

$H_3C-\overset{\overset{O}{\|}}{C}-HN$ $\underset{N\text{——}N}{\overset{S}{\diagup}}$ SO_2NH_2

S :   1.3 mg/ml

logP :   -0.51

Acetazolamide

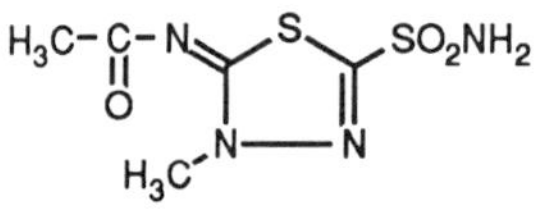

$H_3C-\overset{\overset{O}{\|}}{C}-N$ $\underset{\underset{H_3C}{N\text{——}N}}{\overset{S}{\diagup}}$ SO_2NH_2

S :   1.7 mg/ml

logP :   -0.14

Methazolamide

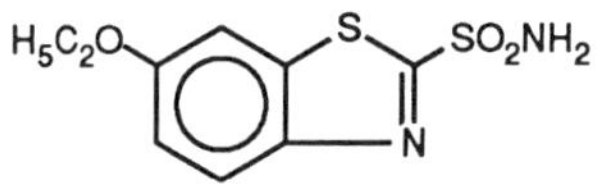

H_5C_2O $\underset{N}{\overset{S}{\diagup}}$ SO_2NH_2

S :   0.03 mg/ml

logP :   2.02

Ethoxzolamide

Figure 5   Structures of the carbonic anhydrase inhibitors acetazolamide, methazolamide, and ethoxzolamide. S refers to the solubility of the compound in aqueous buffer solution of pH 7.4 at 22°C and P is the partition coefficient between octanol and 0.02 M phosphate buffer of pH 7.4. (From Ref. 133.)

severe systemic side effects associated with this mode of therapy (131), significant activities have been undertaken to search for a new carbonic anhydrase inhibitor that would readily penetrate the cornea and which will be active in lowering intraocular pressure when topically administered to the eye (130,132).

An alternative approach to achieve ocular absorption of topically applied CAIs is development of prodrug derivatives possessing adequate water solubility and lipophilicity characteristics combined with the ability to be reconverted to the parent drug following corneal passage. Unfortunately, acetazolamide, methazolamide, and ethoxzolamide and other CAIs do not possess functional groups that are easily amenable to prodrug derivatization. The most prominent functional moiety in these drugs is the primary sulfonamide group and attempts to develop useful prodrug derivatives have, therefore, been focused on this group (133–137).

Using model sulfonamides such as p-toluenesulfonamide, several different kinds of potential prodrug derivatives for the sulfonamide group have been evaluated (133–137). The conclusions reached from these studies can be summarized as follows: N-acyl (**16**), N-alkoxycarbonyl (**17**), N-sulfonylurea (**18**), N-sulfonyl-amidine (**19**), and N-sulfonyl pseudourea (**20**) derivatives are highly stable both chemically and enzymatically, which make them unsuitable as prodrug forms. The same holds true for N-sulfonyl sulfoximines (**21**). N-Sulfonyl sulfilimines (**22**) are hydrolyzed quantitatively to yield the parent sulfonamide in aqueous solution, but at a rather slow rate at physiological pH and temperature. Hydrolysis is, however, accelerated in the presence of enzymes (134). Consequently, this derivative type deserves further consideration as a possible prodrug form.

Particular attention has been paid to N-sulfonyl imidates (**23**) (133,136). Such compounds are readily hydrolyzed in aqueous solution to yield a sulfonamide and a carboxylic acid ester (or a carbonate ester if $R_1 = OR_2$) (Scheme 11). When the sulfonyl imidate esters are derived from alcohols, the parent sulfonamide is formed quantitatively at neutral pH. Hydrolysis was found to be subject to enzymatic catalysis in plasma, and a high rate of hydrolysis is therefore expected in vivo. By varying the ester portions of the derivatives (i.e., R_1 and R_2 in formula **23**), it is readily possible to control such physicochemical properties as water solubility and lipophilicity. Thus, by introducing an ionizable amino function in the alcohol portion [e.g., $R_2 = CH_2CH_2N(CH_3)_2$], N-sulfonyl imidate esters with a high water solubility at pH 4–6 can be obtained (133). A drawback of the derivatives is, however, their limited chemical stability in aqueous solution. The sulfonyl imidate esters are most stable at weakly acidic pH values, but even at this pH, stability is so limited that eye drops formulations with practical shelf-lives cannot be made. For example, the sulfonyl imidate ester (**24**) derived from ethoxzolamide shows a half-life of hydrolysis of only 84 min at pH 3–6 and 37°C (133).

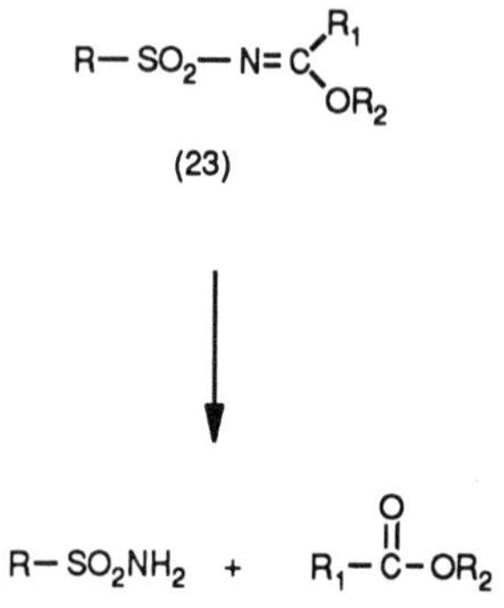

$$R-SO_2-N=C\overset{R_1}{\underset{OR_2}{\diagup}}$$

(23)

$$R-SO_2NH_2 \quad + \quad R_1-\overset{O}{\overset{||}{C}}-OR_2$$

Scheme 11

Whereas N-acyl derivatives of primary sulfonamides, as noted above, are very resistant to undergo chemical or enzymatic hydrolysis, secondary sulfonamide derivatives are more reactive and easily hydrolyzed enzymatically (135). Thus, N-acetyl-N-methyl-p-toluenesulfonamide is hydrolyzed in 80% human plasma (37°C) with a half-life of 0.5 h. In a pH 7.4 buffer solution without plasma the corresponding half-life is 192 h (135). Combined with a report that rabbit ocular tissues are capable of metabolizing N-methylacetazolamide to acetazolamide (138), this finding led to the proposal of the double prodrug approach. As depicted in Scheme 12 (134,135), sequential prodrug activation is involved whereby enzymatic hydrolysis is followed by enzymatic N-demethylation. By introducing a weakly basic amino function in the acyl part, derivatives with both good water solubility at pH 4–6 and adequate lipophilicity at pH 7.4 can be obtained readily (135). Thus far, we have not been able to confirm the ocular metabolism of

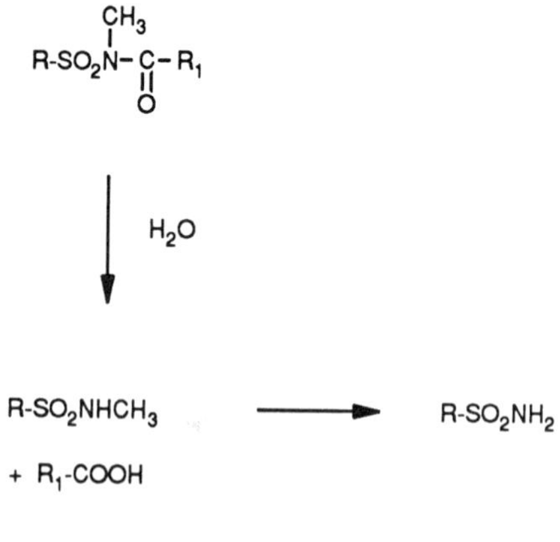

$$R-SO_2\overset{CH_3}{\underset{||}{N}}-\overset{}{\underset{O}{C}}-R_1$$

$\downarrow$ H$_2$O

R-SO$_2$NHCH$_3$ $\longrightarrow$ R-SO$_2$NH$_2$

+ R$_1$-COOH

Scheme 12

N-methylacetazolamide to acetazolamide (V. H. L. Lee and H. Bundgaard, unpublished). In fact, the inactivity of topically applied N-methylated ethoxzolamide (139) may be due to its failure to be demethylated within the eye, although poor delivery characteristics of the compound due to a very low aqueous solubility cannot be ruled out.

Properties of Enzymes Responsible for Bioconversion

An appreciation for the properties of the enzymes responsible for bioconversion, such as tissue distribution, substrate specificity, and kinetic behavior, is as important as deciding on the structural modifications of the parent drug molecule that are required in the design of prodrugs. In this section, the properties of esterases will be considered, since ester prodrugs are the most prevalent. Thus far, this information has been derived from albino and pigmented rabbits using naphthyl esters as substrates.

Tissue and Subcellular Distribution of Ocular Esterases

Esterases are present in all anterior segment tissues (140,141) except tears (142), thus ensuring that absorption of intact ester prodrugs into the eye where reconversion to the parent drugs takes place. Esterase activity is highest in the iris–ciliary body, being twice that in the cornea, where about 70% of the activity resides in the epithelium (143). The relative contribution of the esterases in the various anterior segment tissues to the conversion of the prodrug to the parent drug has not been carefully studied. Nevertheless, this is expected to be dependent on the lability of the prodrug to esterase-mediated catalysis. The corneal epithelium is probably the major conversion site for O-butyryl timolol, which is essentially completely hydrolyzed upon passage across the cornea (22), but it may assume lesser quantitative importance for O-pivaloyl timolol, which is more resistant to hydrolysis (22).

As is the case in the liver, kidney, and brain of the rat (144–147), the esterase activity in the bovine eye is predominantly microsomal (148). This amounts to about 80% in the corneal epithelium and the iris–ciliary body. By contrast, almost all of the esterase activity in the corneal stroma is cytosolic or extracellular. There are two clinical implications of these findings. First, prodrug hydrolysis would commence in the plasma membranes and/or the cytoplasm before reaching the endoplasmic reticulum. Second, the prodrug's lipophilicity can affect its rate and extent of hydrolysis while traversing a cellular layer through its influence on the rate and extent of partitioning into the endoplasmic reticulum, the principal site of subcellular hydrolysis.

Types of Ocular Esterases

Besides esterases, enzymes such as peptidases and carbonic anhydrase also possess esteraselike activity. In the albino and pigmented rabbit eyes neither peptidases nor carbonic anhydrase contributes to esterase activity, however. The exception is the iris–ciliary body, where approximately 24% of the esterase activity can be ascribed to carbonic anhydrase (140).

Two types of esterases exist in the ocular tissues of the rabbit: acetyl- (AChE) and butyrylcholinesterase (BuChE) (149). Except in the corneal epithelium, butyrylcholinesterase contributes to over 75% of the esterase activity in anterior segment tissues (149). The substrate preference of AChE and BuChE is different. Specifically, in a homologous series of model ester prodrugs (1- and 2-naphthyl esters), the rate of substrate hydrolysis decreases with increasing chain length relative to AChE, whereas varying parabolically with chain length relative to BuChE. This implies that a chain length exists at which a prodrug would be hydrolyzed equally well by both cholinesterases. This corresponds to the butyrate ester in the model prodrugs studied. It is speculated that an ester prodrug which is hydrolyzed equally well by both esterases would be desirable. This is because of the possibility that, clinically, fluctuations in the proportion of esterases in an ocular tissue may minimally affect the reconversion rate of a given prodrug. Moreover, the dominance of BuChE in most ocular tissues suggests that a prodrug which is a substrate for BuChE is preferred to one which is a substrate for AChE, since it may be less likely to affect the homeostasis of an ocular tissue by not competing as readily with acetylcholine, the physiological substrate, for hydrolysis by AChE. It is not known, however, whether prodrugs like dipivalyl epinephrine and O-butyryl timolol are substrates for AChE or BuChE.

Substrate Specificities of Ocular Esterases

Lipophilic esters appear to be hydrolyzed more readily than the hydrophilic ones. As seen in Table 5, the naphthyl esters are hydrolyzed more readily than acetyl-thiocholine (ASCh) and butyrylthiocholine (BuSCh)—the normal substrates for

Table 5 Initial Rates of Hydrolysis (nmol/min/mg protein) of Various Substrates in the Corneal Epithelial Homogenates of Albino Rabbits

Substrate	Conc. (mM)	nmol/min/mg protein[a]	Ref.
1-Naphthyl acetate	0.06	54.3 ± 0.18	150
2-Naphthyl acetate	0.06	18.9 ± 2.48	150
Dipivalyl epinephrine	0.325	2.51 ± 0.28	(V. H. L. Lee, unpublished)
Acetylthiocholine (ASCh)	0.250	5.32 ± 0.19	149
Butyrylthiocholine (BuSCh)	0.250	0.25 ± 0.01	149
Pilocarpine	25	0	(V. H. L. Lee, unpublished)
Isopilocarpine	25	0	(V. H. L. Lee, unpublished)

[a]Mean ± standard deviation.

AChE and BuChE, respectively; dipivalyl epinephrine is hydrolyzed slower than ASCh, whereas pilocarpine and isopilocarpine, being hydrophilic (151), are not hydrolyzed at all even at high substrate concentration of 25 mM. The resistance of pilocarpine to hydrolysis in vitro is not inconsistent with its ocular hydrolysis following topical solution instillation (152). This is because pilocarpine hydrolysis may be mediated by a lactonase (153), a very labile enzyme that may lose its activity during tissue homogenate preparation (154).

A means to increase the lipophilicity of an ester prodrug is to extend the number of carbon atoms in the ester side chain. Chang and Lee (150) reported that in a homologous series of 1- and 2-naphthyl esters, there existed a chain length which optimized hydrolysis and that this optimal chain length was influenced by the orientation of the ester side chain with respect to the naphthalene nucleus. Peak hydrolytic rate was reached at the caproate and the valerate esters for 1- and 2-naphthyl ester series, respectively. This finding suggests that the lipophilicity of the substrate alone does not control the rate of substrate hydrolysis and that other physicochemical properties of the parent compound may also affect the hydrolytic rate of its ester prodrug. Such a possibility has recently been confirmed in timolol prodrugs. In this instance, the aryl esters are more stable than the cycloalkyl esters and in turn than the alkyl esters (21,155).

The parabolic relationships observed in the model naphthyl ester prodrugs, which are also observed in prodrugs of timolol (155) and idoxuridine (49), indicates that there exist two chain lengths for a given rate of ester hydrolysis. There is, therefore, flexibility in selecting a prodrug candidate, especially if these esters have different lipophilicities and, therefore, corneal permeation characteristics. Moreover, as the chain length is increased beyond the optimal value, the rank order of hydrolytic rates of the esters in the different ocular tissues may be changed. For instance, in the homologous series of 1-naphthyl esters, whereas the less lipophilic esters were hydrolyzed more readily in the corneal epithelium than in the corneal stroma, the opposite was true for the more lipophilic esters (with more than 7 carbon atoms in the side chain) (150). This suggests that it may be possible to predetermine a principal site of hydrolysis for a prodrug. The clinical significance of this finding is not clear, since such an ester prodrug, by virtue of its lipophilicity, would probably be retained in the corneal epithelium where substantial ester hydrolysis may occur.

Kinetic Properties of Ocular Esterases

The BuChE in the corneal epithelium of the albino rabbit is susceptible to substrate inhibition (156), suggesting that increasing the dose of an ester prodrug may not proportionally increase the rate of delivery of the parent drug. While this enzyme is also susceptible to product inhibition, this does not occur unless the product concentration is at least 20 times higher than the substrate concentration (156). The implication is that at the therapeutic concentrations of most ester prodrugs, product inhibition is probably insignificant. Nonetheless, the diffusion rate of the product relative to its formation rate may influence the hydrolytic rate of an ester prodrug.

Ocular esterase activity is also susceptible to modulation by aromatic molecules (156), suggesting that it may be regulated by the concentration of peptides enriched in aromatic amino acid residues and by the concentration of these amino acids in the microenvironment of the enzymes. Studies by Lockridge (157) and by Chubb et al. (158) demonstrated that AChE and BuChE can hydrolyze the neuropeptides substance P (157) and enkephalins (158), both of which have been reported to be present in the eye (159–162). This finding has two clinical implications. First, these neuropeptides may spare acetylcholine from hydrolysis by AChE thereby affecting neurotransmission. Second, these neuropeptides may compete with prodrugs for hydrolysis by AChE and BuChE thereby affecting the regeneration of parent drugs from these prodrugs. This may be the explanation for the 10–30% reduction in the rate of enzymatic hydrolysis of 1-naphthyl acetate, a model prodrug, by leucine enkephalin, methionine enkephalin, and their hydrolytic fragments tyrosine and Tyr-Gly-Gly (156).

DRUG PROPERTIES AMENABLE TO MODIFICATION BY PRODRUGS

The majority of ocular prodrugs that have been investigated to date aim at improving corneal drug absorption so as to achieve one of the following five objectives: (a) to enhance the efficacy of topically applied drugs that are otherwise ineffective, as exemplified by the prodrugs of carbonic anhydrase inhibitors, steroids, antivirals, and β-blockers; (b) to reduce the incidence of systemic side effects through reduction of the instilled dose, as exemplified by the prodrugs of timolol, phenylephrine, and terbutaline; (c) to alter the duration of action, as exemplified by the prodrugs of pilocarpine and adrenalone; (d) to minimize extra-ocular side effects, as exemplified by dipivalyl epinephrine and the prodrugs of prostaglandins; and (e) to afford drug targeting, i.e., maximization of drug concentration in its target vs nontarget sites, as exemplified by divaleryl adrenolone. In the following, each of these applications will be reviewed relative to the chemistry involved, the physicochemical properties altered, and the degree to which the initial objectives are met.

Improvement in Efficacy

Most topically applied drugs used in ophthalmology are originally developed for systemic applications and are far from optimal with respect to ocular delivery characteristics. This section will examine how prodrug derivatization and other chemical modifications can be used to enhance the efficacy of such drugs as carbonic anhydrase inhibitors, steroids, antiviral agents, and β-blockers.

Carbonic Anhydrase Inhibitors

Carbonic anhydrase inhibitors such as acetazolamide, methazolamide, dichlor-
phenamide, and ethoxzolamide (163) are used orally in the treatment of glaucoma
owing to their ability to lower intraocular pressure (IOP) by reducing aqueous
humor formation. Patient compliance is poor, however, because of intolerable
systemic side effects such as numbness, tingling, malaise, anorexia, nausea,
gastrointestinal distress, and mental depression (164–166). Consequently, these
agents are used only as adjuncts in glaucoma treatment. Although systemic side
effects can be reduced by using a gastrointestinal therapeutic system based on the
osmotic pump principle (167,168), a more desirable approach seems to be the
design of CAI preparations that are topically effective.

Unfortunately, acetazolamide causes minimal or no IOP lowering when administered topically to normotensive rabbit eyes (169–171). The ineffectiveness is
probably due to its low corneal penetration and the fact that more than 99% of the
carbonic anhydrase in the ciliary processes must be inhibited to gain clinically
significant IOP reduction (172). There is now evidence that topically applied
CAIs can be rendered effective if their ocular delivery characteristics are optimized. This can be achieved by maintaining a high drug concentration at the
corneal surface. Flach et al. (173) reported that increasing the acetazolamide
concentration to 10% and administered it as a suspension was able to cause a small
but significant IOP lowering in water-loaded pigmented rabbits. Friedman et al.
(163) also showed that IOP reduction could be achieved by using soft contact
lenses presoaked in a 5% acetazolamide or a 5% methazolamide solution.

An alternative approach to vehicles is chemical modification of existing CAIs
to form labile prodrug derivatives with improved physicochemical properties.
Unfortunately, as mentioned before, acetazolamide, ethoxzolamide, and methazolamide lack functional groups that are easily amenable to prodrug derivatization. A further complication is that substitution on the sulfonamide nitrogen
usually destroys carbonic anhydrase inhibitor activity (174), unless the substituent
is enzymatically cleaved in vivo (138,139). This is illustrated by about a 1000-fold
reduction in the binding affinity of acetazolamide to the carbonic anhydrase upon
methylating its SO_2NH_2 group (138). Because of these obstacles, attempts to
produce effective prodrugs for CAIs have been met with limited success.

Aminozolamide (**29**) (see Table 6 for structure) is a CAI whose IOP-lowering
activity is critically dependent on the formation and retention of its metabolite in
the iris–ciliary body (175). The active metabolite of this CAI is 6-acetamido-2-
benzothiazole sulfonamide (**30**), which unexpectedly is ineffective when applied
topically. The site of metabolite formation has not been identified, however.
Compared with other CAIs such as trifluoromethazolamide (129) and 6-sub-
stituted 2-benzothiazole sulfonamides (139), the duration of activity of aminozolamide is 20 times longer when administered as a 3% suspension in gel form
(73) and 2 times longer when administered as a 2% suspension (176). The long
duration of this prodrug is believed to be due to the long residence time of the

Table 6 Structures of Topical Carbonic Anhydrase Inhibitors

R	Carbonic Anhydrase Inhibitor
HO	L-643,799 (**25**)
$(CH_3)_3CCOO$	L-645,151 (**26**)
CH_3CH_2O	Ethoxzolamide (**27**)
$HOCH_2CH_2O$	6-Hydroxyethoxzolamide (**28**)
NH_2	Aminozolamide (**29**)
CH_3CONH	Acetamido-2-benzothiazole sulfonamide (**30**)

metabolite in the iris–ciliary body, one of the requirements for overcoming the rapid turnover rate of carbonic anhydrase (177).

In addition to prodrugs, another focus in topical CAI research is the discovery of new analogues followed by optimization of their delivery characteristics through prodrug derivatization, if necessary (132). An example of this combination approach is the pivalyl ester (L-645,151 [**26**] in Table 6) of 6-hydroxybenzothiazole-2-sulfonamide (**25**) (L-643,799 in Table 6), an ethoxzolamide analogue, which has been found to improve the ocular hypotensive activity of the parent drug (44,45). This is presumably due to a 40-fold enhancement in corneal penetration (60,178) associated with an increase in the chloroform/pH 7.2 buffer partition coefficient from 0.01 to 56.0 (44).

The design of new CAI analogues generally aims at improving both the aqueous solubility and the partition coefficient. Improving either the aqueous solubility or lipophilicity alone, however, may not provide fruitful results. A case in point is the thiadiazolo[3,2-a]pyrimidine (**31**) and thiadiazolo[3,2-a]triazine sulfonamides (**32**), which have been found to be readily water soluble yet topically ineffective (179). The reason is that enhanced aqueous solubility occurs at the expense of reduced lipophilicity. This is to be contrasted with the topically effective n-propazolamide (**33**) (176), which was obtained by replacing the acetyl group of methazolamide with a propionyl group. In this instance, both the aqueous solubility and the partition coefficient were increased relative to the parent drug.

Maren and his associates (129,180,181) have investigated a number of analogues of acetazolamide, methazolamide, and ethoxzolamide with a wide range of aqueous solubility, lipophilicity, and carbonic anhydrase inhibition characteristics. This was a three-step process consisting of determination of first carbonic anhydrase potency, then the extent of corneal penetration, and finally IOP-lowering potency. Only those analogues with potent in vitro carbonic

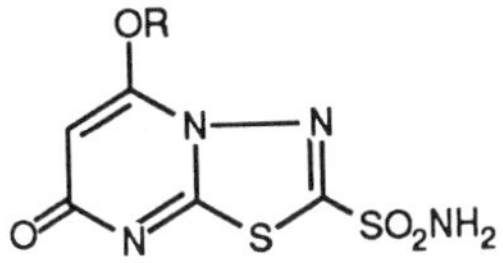

(31)

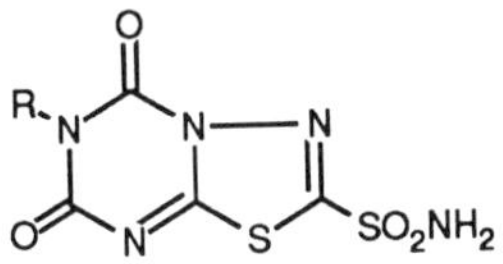

(32)

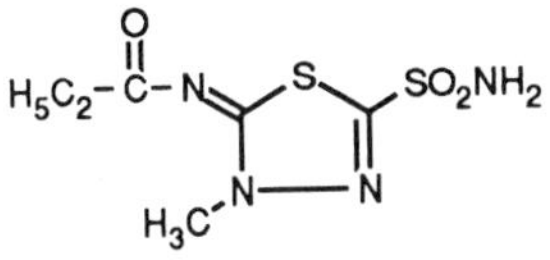

(33)

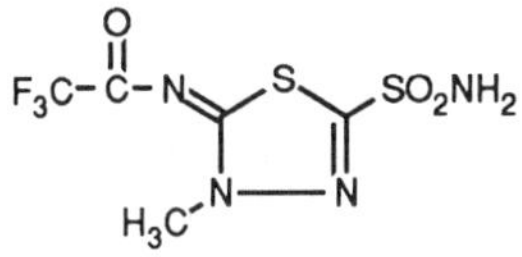

(34)

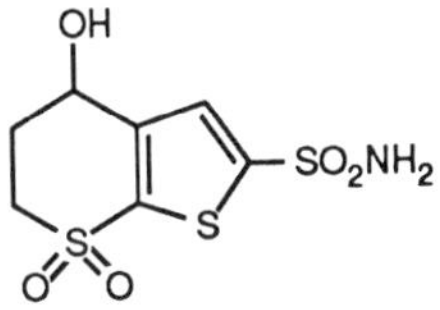

(35)

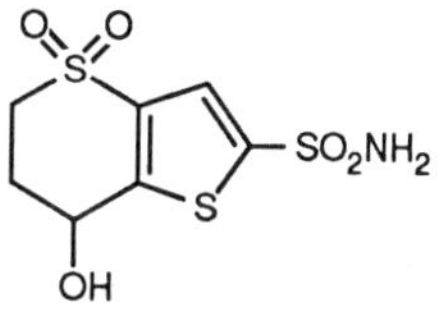

(36)

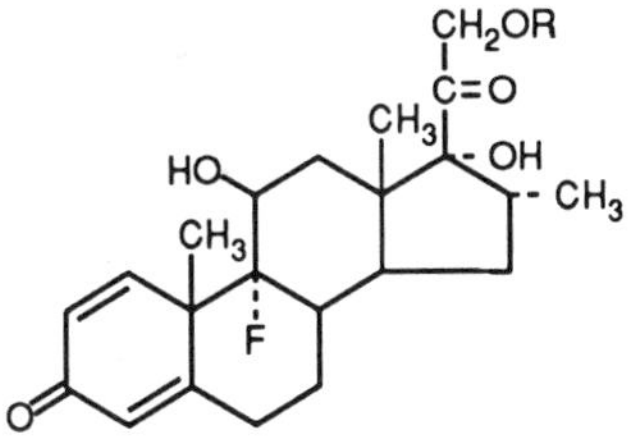

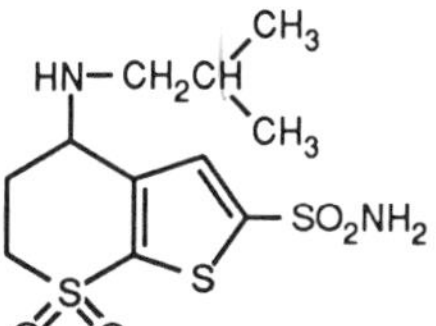

(37)

(38) R = H

(39) R = $-\underset{O}{\overset{O}{C}}-CH_3$

(40) R = $-\underset{O}{\overset{O}{P}}\overset{O^-,Na^+}{\underset{O^-,Na^+}{}}$

anhydrase inhibitory activities, as judged by I_{50} of 1–10 nM, were evaluated for their corneal penetration characteristics. In turn, only those with favorable corneal penetration characteristics were evaluated for their IOP-lowering potency. This strategy revealed trifluoromethazolamide (34) as the most potent in lowering the IOP in the albino rabbit (182,183). Its ability to lower IOP was attributed to an increase in aqueous solubility and reasonable corneal permeability of the ionized form. The ionized form of (34) was about 5 times less permeable than the unionized form, a ratio that is comparable to that of 4–7 for other sulfonamides (181) and of two for pilocarpine (184). The mechanism of corneal penetration of the ionized species is unknown but is probably mediated through the paracellular pathway.

The important physicochemical parameters governing the corneal penetration of 6-substituted ethoxzolamide analogues (Table 6) are the Hammett constant (σ) and the Hansch constant (π). The optimal region of penetration is bounded by σ of -0.2 –0.95 and π of -0.8–0.1 for functional groups substituted on the 6-position of the benzothiazole ring (185). Moreover, for those compounds possible only in suspension form, their aqueous solubility, hence dissolution rate, could be another important determinant of IOP-lowering potency. Thus, while the 6-hydroxyethoxy derivative of ethoxzolamide (28) is similar to its parent drug in corneal penetration characteristics, and in vitro carbonic anhydrase inhibition activity (185,186), it is more effective than the parent drug. This is possibly due to a faster dissolution rate of the derivative as a result of higher aqueous solubility.

None of the CAIs discussed so far possesses aqueous solubility in the 1–2% range. Consequently, they can only be formulated as suspensions or gels, which are less well accepted by patients than aqueous solutions. The poor aqueous solubility problem has now been solved in the thienothiopyran-2-sulfonamides (187). Depending on the structural features on the thienyl ring, such as the presence and position of a hydroxyl group, the oxidation state of the sulfur atom, and chirality of the hydroxyl substituent, compounds with aqueous solubility in the range of 0.03–1.5% can be obtained. Thus, compounds 35 and 36 showed a solubility of 1.3–1.5%. This is at least a factor of 10–60 improvement over ethoxzolamide (27) and (2-sulfamoyl-6-benzothiazolyl)-2,2-dimethylpropionate (26). Two of these analogues, MK-927 (dl-5,6-dihydro-4-(2-methylpropylamino)-4H-thieno(2,3b)thiopyran-2-sulfonamide-7,7-dioxide HCl) (37) and L-671,152 (S,S-5,6-dihydro-4H-4-ethylamino-6-methylthieno-[2,3-b]-thiopyran-2-sulfonamide-7,7-dioxide), have been found to lower the intraocular pressure in monkeys and rabbits with experimentally induced ocular hypertension for 6–8 h following the topical instillation of 2% solutions (188–196). MK927, the most promising topical CAI reported to date, carries an isopropylamino group of pK 5.8 and has desirable physicochemical properties: good water solubility at pH 4–5, an octanol/ buffer partition coefficient of 8 at pH 7, and a K_i value of 12 nM against human carbonic anhydrase II (193,195). The concentration of drug reaching the ciliary processes and aqueous humor is of the same order as that following parenteral administration (195). Sugrue et al. (193) reported that the ocular hypotensive effect of a 2% solution of MK-927 was greater in magnitude and longer in duration in normotensive pigmented than in albino rabbits. This was attributed to a higher drug concentration achieved in the pigmented ciliary body as MK-927 was moderately bound, through its protonated alkylamino group, to melanin pigments (197).

An important aspect in the development of ophthalmic drugs is the possible contact sensitization potential of the compounds. Thus, although several benzofuran- and indole-2-sulfonamides were found to be strong CAIs with good activity following topical administration, they showed such strong allergenic activities that further development of the compounds for clinical use was precluded (198).

Steroids

Topically applied steroids offer an effective means to control inflammations involving the external eye as well as the anterior segment. Like carbonic anhydrase inhibitors, steroids are poorly water soluble but, unlikely carbonic anhydrase inhibitors, steroids possess more favorable partition coefficients. Steroids are perhaps the first class of ophthalmic drugs to which the prodrug principle was applied. The acetate and the phosphate ester prodrugs were originally designed to enhance the corneal absorption and aqueous solubility of certain steroids, respectively. It has been proposed that a clear solution ensures better patient compliance and a more reproducible applied dose (199).

The corneal permeability of steroid prodrugs does not always correlate with their partition coefficient. Thus, in spite of similar lipophilicity (log P of ~ 2.4), dexamethasone acetate was found to permeate the cornea less readily than prednisolone acetate, prednisolone sodium phosphate, and fluorometholone (Table 7). The relatively high in vitro corneal permeability of prednisolone sodium phosphate was unexpected given that the same prodrug of another steroid, dexamethasone (**38**), did not penetrate the cornea after topical application to the uninflamed rabbit eye (204,205). In contrast to its in vitro behavior, prednisolone sodium phosphate did behave as expected following topical application to the rabbit eye, in that it afforded lower corneal and aqueous humor drug concentrations than its acetate counterpart (206,207). The discrepancy between in vitro and in vivo results may be due to the duration over which the concentration is exposed to the drug. In vitro permeability is typically measured with a solution at steady state, and the lag time in permeability is not reflected in that value. Moreover, the acetate, being dosed in the form of a suspension, may remain in the cul-de-sac longer than the aqueous solution. This is one of the two requirements to be met by a suspension for it to provide improved ocular absorption, the other being a dissolution rate that is slow enough to contribute to tear drug concentrations (201).

Another unusual characteristic of steroid prodrugs is that steroid bioavailability measurements do not always correlate with anti-inflammatory efficacy. For instance, when tested in an experimental keratitis model (208), dexamethasone acetate (**39**) showed the highest anti-inflammatory effectiveness in spite of the lowest corneal permeability (Table 8). Conversely, its phosphate counterpart (**40**), with the most favorable corneal permeability characteristics, had the lowest anti-inflammatory effectiveness. Furthermore, removing the corneal epithelium, which

Table 7 Physicochemical and Corneal Permeability Parameters of Steroids

Compound	M_r^a	Solubility (mol/L)[a]	log DC[a]	log CP (cm/s)[a] intact	log CP (cm/s)[a] deepithelized
Dexamethasone	392	2.58×10^{-4} (200)	1.83 (200)	−5.11 (17)	—
acetate	343	1.25×10^{-5} (200)	2.91 (200)	−4.42 (17)	—
phosphate	516	—		−5.21 (203)	−4.56 (203)
Prednisolone	360	6.54×10^{-4} (200)	1.62 (200) 1.10 (200)	−5.02 (203) −5.42 (17)	−5.11 (203) —
acetate	402	4.22×10^{-5} (200)	2.40 2.20	−4.50 (17)	—
phosphate	484	—	—	−5.01 (203)	−4.52 (203)
Fluorometholone	476	4.12×10^{-5} (201)	2.10 (17) 1.50 (202)	−5.01 (203)	−5.05 (203)
acetate	418	—	—	—	—

Abbreviations: M_r = molecular weight; DC, distribution coefficient; CP = corneal permeability.
[a]Numbers in parentheses are reference numbers.

Table 8 Experimental Anti-Inflammatory Effects and Corneal Bioavailability of Various 21-Substituted Dexamethasone Derivatives Following Topical Administration of 50 µl of 0.1% Suspension to Inflamed Rabbit Eye Induced by Stromal Injection of Clove Oil

Corticosteroid	Anti-inflammatory effect (%)	Corneal bioavailability (µg/min/g)
Epithelium intact		
dexamethasone acetate (**39**)	55	111
dexamethasone alcohol (**38**)	40	543
dexamethasone sodium phosphate (**40**)	19	1068
Epithelium absent		
dexamethasone acetate (**39**)	60	118
dexamethasone alcohol (**38**)	42	1316
dexamethasone sodium phosphate (**40**)	22	4642

Source: Adapted from Ref. 208.

increased the concentration of the phosphate and alcohol, did not affect their anti-inflammatory effectiveness. The lack of direct correlation between bioavailability and pharmacological activity may be explained, at least in part, by the fact that steroid prodrugs are intrinsically active, albeit less so than the parent steroid. The phosphate prodrug of dexamethasone alcohol, for instance, is only one-fifteenth as potent as dexamethasone itself in its ability to compete for binding to the glucocorticoid receptors (209).

Despite their long history of clinical use, the intraocular metabolism of the steroid prodrugs is essentially unknown. Enzymatic conversion of the prodrugs is assumed to occur in the cornea, since both esterases (143) and phosphatases (210) are present. Both Yamauchi et al. (211) and Musson et al. (212) showed that prednisolone acetate was quantitatively metabolized to its free alcohol following topical application, and Tsuji et al. (213) showed that prednisolone succinate was quantitatively hydrolyzed to prednisolone following subconjunctival injection. The fate of the other ester prodrugs is unknown.

Antivirals

Herpes simplex virus is an important etiological agent of ocular infection and a major cause of blindness in the United States. Idoxuridine (5-iodo-2'-deoxyuridine) (41), a halogenated pyrimidine derivative currently indicated in the topical treatment of herpes simplex keratitis, is poorly absorbed into the cornea, resulting in a high incidence of treatment failure unassociated with resistant viral strains (214). Promising results in corneal penetration were obtained when the 5'-ester prodrugs of idoxuridine were administered. Of the five prodrugs tested, the 5'-butyryl ester (42) was the best, improving the ocular absorption of idoxuridine about 4 times (48). Whether improved ocular absorption will increase the therapeutic efficacy of idoxuridine remains to be seen.

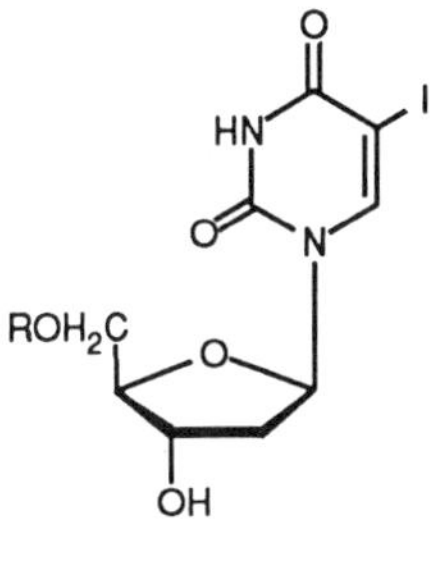

(41) R = H

(42) R = $-\overset{\text{O}}{\underset{\text{||}}{\text{C}}}\cdot CH_2CH_2CH_3$

Acyclovir (**4**), a potent and selective antiherpes drug with marked activity against herpes simplex virus types 1 (HSV-1) and 2 (HSV-2) and varicella zoster virus (214), is another antiviral that would benefit from improved ocular absorption. Probably owing to its low aqueous solubility (~0.2% at 25°C) and poor corneal penetration, this drug is not effective against stromal keratitis and iritis (215,216). It is, therefore, reasoned that corneal penetration can be improved by a more water-soluble derivative. As already mentioned in an earlier section, various amino acid esters have been synthesized and may be useful in solving the solubility problem and lead to more efficient corneal penetration (46,109).

β-Blockers

Of the large number of β-blockers that have been investigated for their effectiveness in lowering intraocular pressure (217–222), only four, namely, timolol, levobunolol, betaxolol, and metipranolol, have been approved for glaucoma treatment in the United States. A major factor limiting the clinical effectiveness of several of the other β-blockers is their inability to achieve therapeutically effective concentrations in the eye because of unfavorable lipophilicity (223–225). They are, therefore, good candidates for prodrug derivatization. So far, this approach has been investigated in detail, both preclinically and clinically, only with nadolol (**43**). Compared with the parent drug, the diacetate ester prodrug (**44**) was 20 times more lipophilic and was ocularly absorbed 10 times more readily. Yet, its ocular hypotensive effect was no better than the parent drug (27). This is surprising in light of the improvement in corneal absorption and of the fact that the diacetyl prodrug itself possesses β-adrenergic antagonistic activity. Nevertheless, an advantage this prodrug has over the parent drug is that no tolerance to it was developed in glaucoma patients over a 3-month period (226).

(**43**)   R = H

(**44**)   R = $-\overset{\text{O}}{\underset{\text{||}}{C}}-CH_3$

Alteration of Duration of Action

Pilocarpine, an antiglaucoma drug, is an example of a drug whose duration of action is brief, thereby necessitating frequent dosing of 3–6 times a day. This leads to transient peaks and valleys of pilocarpine in the eye, which in turn results in dose-related ocular side effects such as myopia and miosis (227,228). There is, therefore, a high incidence of patient noncompliance, which has been suspected to be responsible for inadequate pressure control and deterioration of vision (229,230).

In an attempt to prolong the duration of action of pilocarpine (45), Bundgaard et al. (28–31) developed various mono- and diesters of pilocarpic acid. Studies in rabbits have confirmed that several of the pilocarpic acid esters not only improve upon the ocular bioavailability of the parent drug, but also prolong its duration of action (28,31) (Fig. 6). The monoesters (46) undergo a quantitative and apparent specific base-catalyzed cyclization to pilocarpine in aqueous solution (Scheme 13). As appears from the rate data in Table 9, the various esters studied differ greatly in their rates of cyclization. Except for the sterically hindered 2-methyl-benzyl and α-methylbenzyl esters the variation of the rates of cyclization of these

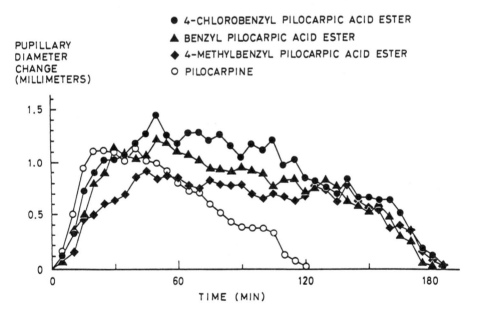

Figure 6 Plots of the average observed changes in pupillary diameters as a function of time following the instillation in rabbits of 25 µl of isotonic aqueous solutions (pH 4.75) of equimolar concentrations (0.5% pilocarpine nitrate equivalent) of the compounds indicated. Four rabbits were used in the crossover study. (From Ref. 28.)

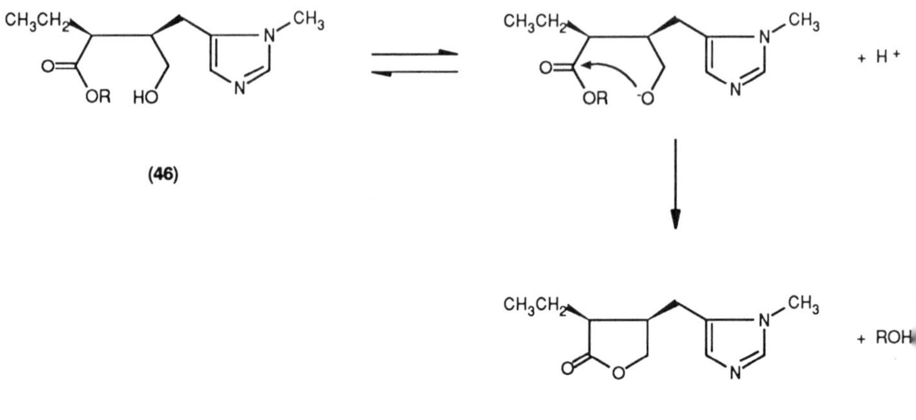

(46)

(45)

Scheme 13

Table 9 Rate Data for the Conversion of Pilocarpic Acid Monoesters (46) to Pilocarpine (45) in Aqueous Solution (37°C) and Partition Coefficients for the Compounds

Compound	$t_{1/2}^a$ (min)	log P^b
Pilocarpine		−0.15
Pilocarpic acid esters (46) R:		
Methyl[c]	95	0.07
Ethyl	510	0.58
Butyl	820	1.58
Hexyl	1105	2.56
Benzyl	50	1.82
4-Chlorobenzyl	30	2.54
4-Methylbenzyl	77	2.31
4-tert-butylbenzyl	87	3.52
Phenethyl	227	2.16
2-Methylbenzyl	139	2.27
α-Methylbenzyl	475	2.08

[a]Half-lives of lactonization at pH 7.40.
[b]Partition coefficients between octanol and 0.05 M phosphate buffer solution of pH 7.40.
[c]The data for this compound have not been reported before.
Source: From Ref. 29.

ester derivatives could be fully accounted for in terms of polar effects exhibited by the alcohol portions of the esters (29). The following correlation was found between the half-time (in min) of pilocarpine formation from these esters at pH 7.4 and 37°C and the Taft polar substituent σ*, the latter referring to R in RCH_2OH for the alcohols:

$$\log t_{1/2} = 1.44 \ \sigma^* + 2.73 \ (n = 9; \ r = 0.998)$$

It is readily evident that by appropriate variation of the alcohol portion of the esters there are ample possibilities to vary and predict the rate of ring closure, and hence to control and modify the rate of pilocarpine generation. Further studies showed that even in the presence of 75% human plasma or rabbit eye tissue homogenates, the cyclization reactions predominated entirely over hydrolysis of the pilocarpic acid esters to pilocarpic acid, which does not cyclize to pilocarpine at physiological pH. The lactonization rates observed in these media were identical to those in pure buffer solutions (29).

The pilocarpic acid esters were found to be much more lipophilic than the parent pilocarpine (see Table 9). Appropriate selection of the alcohol portion of the pilocarpic acid esters enables one to confer almost any desired degree of lipophilicity on the prodrugs.

The main drawback of these pilocarpic acid esters is their limited solution stability, making it difficult to prepare ready-to-use solutions with a not too low pH and an acceptable shelf-life (29). This problem can, however, be totally overcome by blocking the free hydroxy group in the esters by esterification. The double esters (47) thus obtained are highly stable in aqueous solutions even at pH 6–7 (shelf-lives exceeding 5 years at 25°C) and most significantly are subject to facile enzymatic hydrolysis at the O-acyl bond. It has thus been demonstrated that in the presence of human plasma or rabbit eye tissue homogenates, pilocarpine is formed from these derivatives in quantitative amounts through a sequential process involving enzymatic hydrolysis of the O-acyl bond followed by the spontaneous lactonization of the intermediate pilocarpic acid ester (Fig. 7) (Scheme 14) (30). Besides solving the stability problem of the pilocarpic acid monoesters, the pilocarpic acid diesters were found to possess even better ocular delivery characteristics (enhanced absorption and longer lasting pilocarpine activity) than the monoesters (Fig. 8) (28,31). Furthermore, the O-acylation step gives further possibilities of varying the physicochemical properties of the prodrugs. Some properties of the derivatives are given in Table 10. Although these prodrugs are highly lipophilic at pH 7.4, the basic character of the imidazole moiety in the compounds ($pK_a \sim 7$) allows the preparation of sufficiently water-soluble salts; e.g., nitrates or fumarates.

From an evaluation of the duration of action, metabolism, and ocular safety of over 20 pilocarpic acid diesters, the O-benzoyl pilocarpic acid methyl ester has been selected as having the optimal balance of properties among the derivatives tested. This compound showed no acute ocular toxicity and was nonirritating to

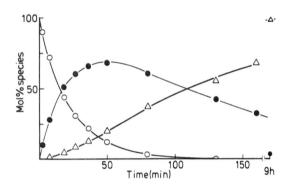

Figure 7 Time courses for O-benzoyl pilocarpic acid 4-methylbenzyl ester (O), pilocarpic acid 4-methylbenzyl ester (●), and pilocarpine (Δ) during incubation of the O-benzoyl derivative in 75% human plasma (pH 7.4) at 37°C. (From Ref. 30.)

the conjunctiva when administered repeatedly to albino rabbits (231). The compound reduced IOP significantly in both the normotensive Owl monkey and in the glaucomatous *Cynomolgus* monkey, but most importantly, it produced a much smaller miosis than a 0.5% equivalent dose of pilocarpine (231). This result suggests that a greater pilocarpine concentration is required at the pupillary muscle to cause constriction than is required at the ciliary muscle, the suggested site of action for IOP reduction.

Compared with the vehicle approach to improve bioavailability, pilocarpine prodrugs are as effective as viscous solutions (6,7), lattices (232), emulsions (233,234), and presoaked soft contact lens (235), but are less effective than gels

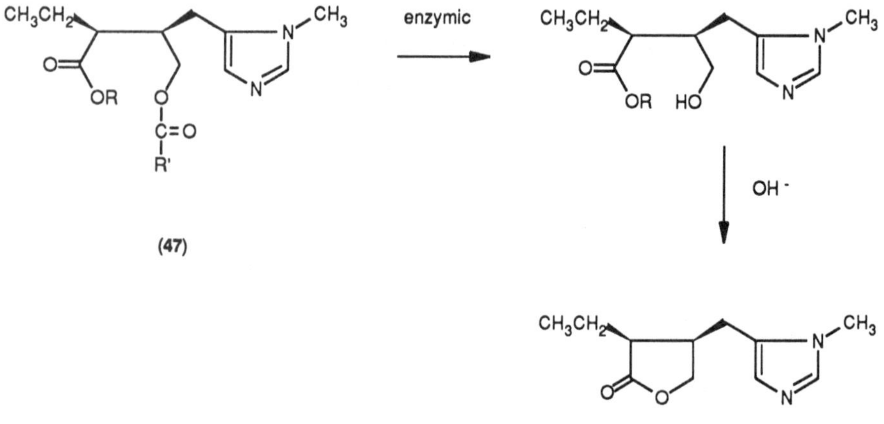

Scheme 14

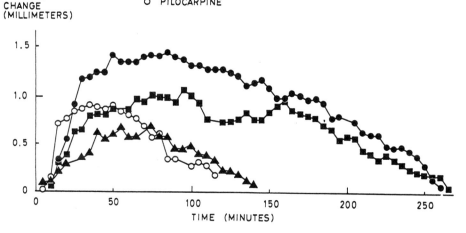

Figure 8 Plots of the average observed changes in pupillary diameters as a function of time following the instillation in rabbits of 25 μl of isotonic aqueous solutions (pH 4.75) of equimolar concentrations (0.25% pilocarpine nitrate equivalent) of the compounds indicated. Four rabbits were used in the crossover study. (From Refs. 28 and 31.)

(236), polymer matrices (237), and the Ocusert (238). In spite of these alternatives, prodrugs do offer the advantage of administration in aqueous solutions, the dosage form preferred by patients.

Reduction of Systemic Side Effects

The ultimate goal in drug management of eye diseases is to maximize exposure of the target tissues within this vital organ to the drug while sparing the remainder of the body from this agent. This would require concerted efforts to maximize its ocular absorption while minimizing its systemic absorption. While there have been numerous attempts to improve ocular drug bioavailability through prolongation of ocular contact time or improvement of corneal drug permeability (3), there have been very few attempts to deliberately modify the permissive absorption of drugs into the systemic circulation.

A number of topically applied ophthalmic drugs have been shown to be absorbed into the systemic circulation following topical application to the eye. They include timolol (239), betaxolol (240), epinephrine (241), dipivalyl epinephrine (241), phenylephrine (242), oxymetazoline (243), clonidine (244),

Table 10 Rate Data for the Hydrolysis of Various Pilocarpic Acid Diesters (**47**) to the Monoesters (**46**) at 37°C and Partition Coefficients for the Compounds

R_1	R_2	Half-lives in 75% human plasma (min)	kos[a] $(M^{-1} min^{-1})$	log P[b]
Benzyl	Benzoyl	12	3.8	4.22
4-Chlorobenzyl	Benzoyl	17	3.4	4.75
2-Phenylethyl	Benzoyl	15	3.8	4.60
4-Methylbenzyl	Benzoyl	16	4.0	4.70
4-Methylbenzyl	Acetyl	24	12.6	3.16
3-Methylbenzyl	Butyryl	5	3.5	4.09
Benzyl	Phenylacetyl	4	21.7	3.85
Benzyl	3-Chlorobenzoyl	25	14.6	4.93
Benzyl	Nicotinoyl	6	44.4	2.90
Benzyl	Butyryl	3	3.5	3.63
Benzyl	Hexanoyl	4	3.3	4.60
Methyl	Benzoyl	12	—	2.75

[a]Hydroxide ion catalytic rate constants for the overall hydrolysis.
[b]Partition coefficients between octanol and 0.05 M phosphate buffer solution of pH 7.40.
Source: From Ref. 30.

pilocarpine (245), hydrocortisone (246), flurbiprofen (247), tetrahydrocannabinol (248), and cyclosporine (249). Of these, timolol has received the most attention, mainly because of its tendency to induce severe cardiovascular and pulmonary side effects (250). This is not a trivial problem because of its popularity as an antiglaucoma medication.

Topically applied drugs enter the systemic circulation probably via the blood vessels in the conjunctival and nasal mucosae. Chang and Lee (251) demonstrated that the nasal mucosa contributed at least 70%, and as much as 100%, of the timolol systemically absorbed. This overriding importance of the nasal mucosa in systemic timolol absorption is most probably the consequence of rapid drainage of the instilled solution into the nasolacrimal duct and then the nasal cavity (252). The latter is known to offer virtually no resistance to the systemic absorption of drugs of diverse physicochemical characteristics, including alprenolol (253), metoprolol (253), and propranolol (254).

To date, punctal occlusion and eyelid closure following topical solution instillation are the only measures recommended to the patient to reduce systemic drug absorption (239,255,256). Neither approach is, however, a satisfactory long-term solution from the patient compliance standpoint. More satisfactory solutions appear to be: (a) manipulation of solution viscosity to reduce loss of the instilled dose to the nasal cavity, or (b) reducing the instilled dose in proportion to the degree of enhancement in ocular drug absorption by lipophilic prodrugs, thereby reducing the amount of drug available for systemic absorption.

The incorporation of soluble polymers into aqueous solutions to increase solution viscosity and, therefore, drug retention in the conjunctival sac, is a popular approach to enhance ocular drug absorption (3). This approach is also expected to bring about a reduction in the systemic absorption of topically applied drugs by virtue of its ability to minimize contact of the instilled dose with the nasal mucosa. Indeed, Chang et al. (24) demonstrated that isoviscous 5% poly(vinyl alcohol) and 0.2% hyaluronic acid solutions reduced the amount of timolol absorbed into the bloodstream about 2 times in the pigmented rabbit, whereas doubling the amount of timolol absorbed ocularly.

The first hint that prodrugs may be an effective means to reduce the systemic absorption of topically applied drugs was offered by dipivefrin, an epinephrine prodrug (50). As already mentioned in an earlier section, work with timolol prodrugs has provided additional evidence supporting the effectiveness of prodrugs in reducing systemic drug absorption. Chang et al. (24) demonstrated that O-butyryl timolol (**2**), a timolol ester prodrug, increased the ocular absorption of topically applied timolol 4–6 times in the pigmented rabbit, thereby allowing a corresponding reduction in the topically applied dose in either instilled volume or instilled concentration. Specifically, reducing the instilled volume of this prodrug from 25 to 5 µl allowed 9–10 times less drug to be absorbed systemically, yet providing the same drug concentrations in the aqueous humor as a 5 times higher dose of timolol (24). Similar results were obtained by reducing the instilled prodrug concentration from 15.0 to 3.75 mM (25). Since the 5-µl dose was more efficient than the 25-µl dose in terms of enhancing ocular drug absorption while simultaneously limiting systemic drug absorption, it may be possible to maximize the ratio of ocular to systemic absorption of O-butyryl timolol by using the smallest instilled volume possible or by administering it in the form of a polymeric matrix. In support of the latter, Urtti et al. (237) demonstrated that the systemic bioavailability of timolol from a silicone tubing device with a release rate of 7.2 µg h^{-1} was only 6% of that afforded by an aqueous solution.

In addition to designing prodrugs that are well absorbed ocularly, it is now possible to design prodrugs that are intrinsically poorly absorbed into the bloodstream. This approach is based on the differential lipophilic characteristics of the cornea, the conjunctiva, and presumably the nasal mucosa (257). Sasaki et al. (258) found that the conjunctiva was less lipophilic than the cornea, suggesting that it should be possible to design prodrugs of suitable lipophilicity to selectively reduce systemic drug absorption without affecting its ocular absorption. This hypothesis was confirmed for timolol with a series of alkyl, cycloalkyl, and aryl ester prodrugs following topical instillation of their solutions or suspensions to the pigmented rabbit eye (258). Except for the short chain alkyl esters, all prodrugs were less readily absorbed systemically, yet they were ocularly absorbed either equally well or better than timolol. As a result, the therapeutic index, defined as the ratio of aqueous humor to plasma timolol concentrations, was improved as much as 16 times.

Besides timolol, phenylephrine (15) is another drug that can benefit from reduction in systemic absorption. Transient hypertension and adverse cardiovascular effects frequently occur during the first 20–30 min following topical administration of a 2.5 or 10% solution of this drug for its mydriatic and capillary decongestion effects (259). Hypertension is transient, however, since phenylephrine is rapidly metabolized in the plasma within this time period (242). It is reasoned that increasing its corneal penetration through prodrug derivatization may allow dose reduction. The two prodrugs that have been investigated, the pivalate ester (48) and oxazolidine prodrugs (14), are about 10 times more potent than phenylephrine (37–41). The increase in potency afforded by the oxazolidine prodrug is consistent with the 1000-fold increase in its partition coefficient (40). As a result, a 10 times lower dose of the oxazolidine prodrug can be used, leading to a 3.5-fold reduction in the systemic absorption of phenylephrine following topical instillation (41).

The use of prodrugs to reduce the systemic absorption of ocularly applied drugs has also been applied to terbutaline, a selective β_2-agonist. Ibuterol (50), the diisobutyrate ester of terbutaline (49), was found to be 100 times more potent than its parent drug in lowering IOP in both normal and sympathectomized rabbits (43). This, coupled with a longer duration of action, suggests that both the topical dose and the dosing frequency of ibuterol can be reduced, thereby reducing systemic toxicity. While this prodrug is free of local toxicity, tachyphylaxis rapidly develops, thus limiting its therapeutic effectiveness.

Although prodrugs hold great promise in improving ocular drug delivery, they have yet to be considered routinely for improving the physicochemical characteristics of drugs originally developed for systemic use with respect to ocular absorption. Such a scenario may soon improve as a result of a recently proposed concept in ocular drug discovery. The key to this new concept is the ability of prodrugs to enhance the ocular potency of a drug candidate originally designed for systemic use but which was deliberately chosen because of its lack of systemic potency. This is, in effect, an attempt to achieve relative oculoselectivity; i.e., selective drug action in the eye without the risk of systemic complications. Therefore, the salient feature of this approach is to select a less potent drug candidate so as to minimize the incidence of systemic side effects and then to offset this loss in potency by enhancing its ocular absorption using prodrugs. Such an approach has been described by Sugrue et al. (260). These investigators

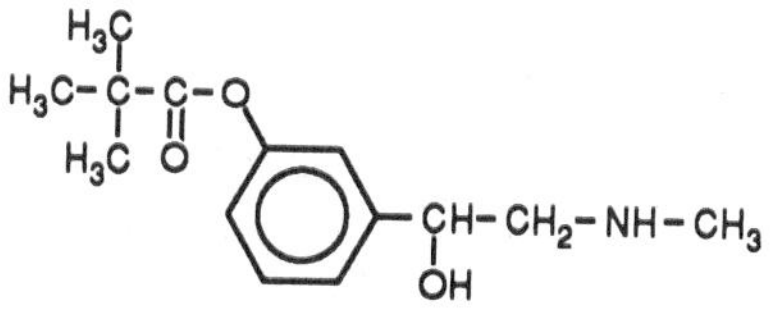

(48)

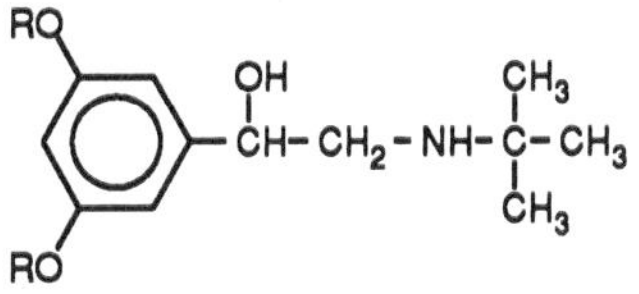

(49)   R = H

(50)   R = $-\underset{O}{\overset{}{C}}-CH(CH_3)_2$

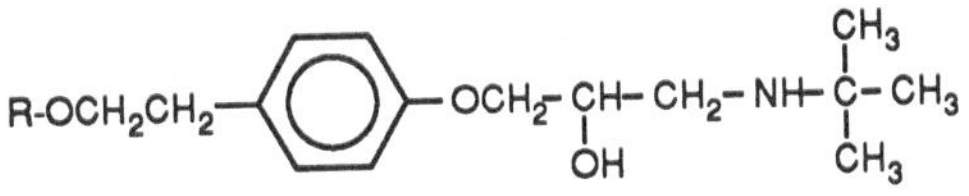

(51)   R = H

(52)   R = $-\underset{O}{\overset{}{C}}-CH_3$

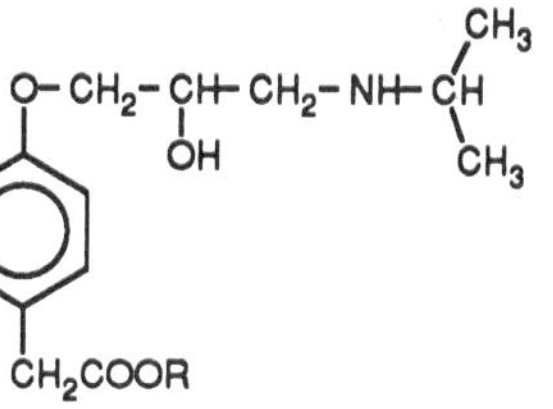

(53)   R = H

(54)   R = $-CH_2CH_2-$

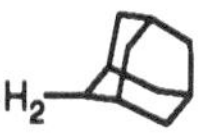

reported that L-653,328 (52), an acetate ester of the β-blocker L-652,698 (51), was as potent as timolol in lowering the intraocular pressure in the α-chymotrypsinized albino rabbit but it was at least 100 times less potent than timolol against the heart. This lack of systemic potency was consistent with the modest affinity of L-652,698, the active moiety of L-653,328, for the extraocular β-receptors.

The approach just described is akin to the soft drug approach. Soft drugs can be defined as biologically active drugs which may structurally resemble known active drugs or which could be entirely new structures, but which are all characterized by predictable in vivo destruction (metabolism) to nontoxic moieties after they achieve their therapeutic role (261). Such a concept has been applied to β-blockers (262–264) as well as to antimicrobials (265), anticholinergics (266), and steroids (267). Of the eight lipophilic esters of the acidic metabolite (53) of metoprolol tested in albino rabbits, the adamantylethyl ester (54) was the best in terms of intraocular pressure lowering potency (262) and possible low incidence of systemic side effects associated with a very fast rate of hydrolysis ($t_{1/2}$ = 7 min) to the inactive acidic metabolite (53) in human blood.

Reduction of Ocular Side Effects

Adverse effects involving the external eye, such as irritation, foreign body sensation, tearing, and reactive conjunctival hyperemia, are very prevalent in patients on epinephrine therapy. Becker and Morton (268) reported that only 20% of the patients were able to tolerate epinephrine for 4–5 years. Epinephrine (55) also suffers from other problems such as short duration of action, cardiovascular side effects, and low bioavailability (50). To circumvent these problems, a more lipophilic dipivalyl ester of epinephrine, dipivefrin (56), was synthesized (269). Because 0.1% dipivefrin solution was as effective as a 2% epinephrine solution in lowering intraocular pressure (270), it was anticipated that the incidence of extraocular side effects would be lowered. While this expectation was fulfilled when the prodrug was used on a short-term basis (271,272), its incidence of side effects was no different from that of its parent compound when used for an extended period of time (1–2 years) (273). Apparently, the incidence of epinephrine- induced extraocular side effects is related to the duration of exposure to the drug.

Local eye irritations have also been reported for prostaglandin $F_{2\alpha}$ ($PGF_{2\alpha}$) (57), which has been investigated for its ocular hypotensive effect (32). Interestingly, its methyl (58), ethyl (59), and isopropyl (60) ester prodrugs, which were designed to improve its corneal penetration, have been reported to be less irritating (34) with the additional advantage of a 10–30 times gain in IOP-lowering potency (33,34). The lower incidence of eye irritation is possibly due to the lower dose of ester prodrugs required. As is the case for $PGF_{2\alpha}$, the isopropyl ester of PGA_2 also improved the intraocular pressure lowering potency of the parent drug, the factor of improvement being about 15 (61).

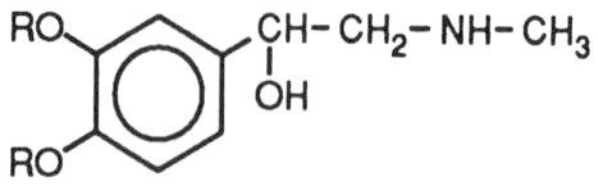

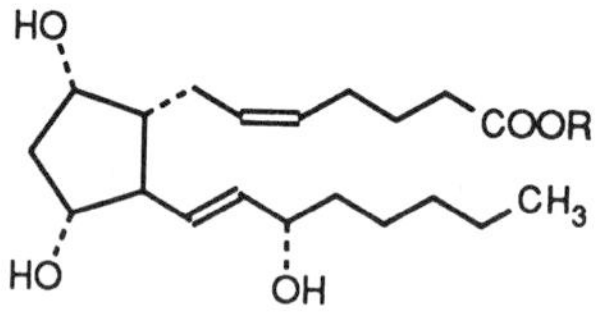

(57)   R =   H

(58)   R = $-CH_3$

(59)   R = $-CH_2CH_3$

(60)   R = $-CH(CH_3)_2$

(55)   R = H

(56)   R = $-C(=O)-C(CH_3)_3$

Drug Targeting

Maximizing the ration of target to nontarget tissue drug concentrations is a desirable goal in ocular drug therapy. Thus far, efforts to target ophthalmic drugs to specific sites have been minimal. The ophthalmic drugs that would benefit from targeting are those which cause annoying side effects upon ocular absorption. Examples are corticosteroids, which cause glaucoma and cataracts; pilocarpine, which causes miosis; epinephrine, which causes corneal staining; certain β-blockers, which cause dry eye; and antiviral compounds, which affect healthy and affected cells alike.

Drug targeting may be achieved by direct placement of the drug in the target tissue, an approach often deemed impractical, since invasive procedures are necessarily involved. A more practical approach is to modify the pharmacokinetic properties of the drug through the prodrug approach. This would require that the prodrug not be activated until it encounters a unique activating enzyme in the target site. This requirement is, however, unlikely to be met, simply because an activating enzyme like esterase is ubiquitous. An alternative approach is to exploit the differences in ratio of two or more enzymes that participate in activating the prodrug, which by necessity must be a sequentially labile prodrug. Bodor and Visor (52) exploited the marked differences in the ratio of ketone reductase (274) to esterase levels (275) among the anterior segment tissues to achieve site-specific delivery of diisovaleryl adrenalone (**62**), a bioreversible derivative of epinephrine (**55**), in the ciliary body where epinephrine is regenerated and where this drug acts. Epinephrine is regenerated only when the diester is reduced before hydrolysis occurs; no epinephrine is regenerated from adrenalone (**61**) formed from diester hydrolysis (Scheme 15). The proportion of the diester undergoing only hydrolysis vs the reduction-hydrolysis sequence, hence its duration of action, is a function of susceptibility of the ester linkage to hydrolysis (53). Thus, di(ethylsuccinyl) adrenalone (**63**), with a plasma half-life of 1 min, is anticipated to have a shorter duration of action than its diisovaleryl counterpart, which has a plasma half-life of 19 min. It is reasonable to expect that a better understanding of the enzymatic systems in the various anterior segments would enhance the usefulness of this approach to achieve drug targeting in the eye.

FACTORS INFLUENCING PRODRUG EFFICACY

The therapeutic efficacy of ester prodrugs depends ultimately on the level of esterase activity in ocular tissues, which in turn is influenced by such physiological factors as iris pigmentation and age and by such formulation factors as the presence of esterase inhibitors and preservatives.

Physiological Factors

The rate of prodrug hydrolysis is influenced by iris pigmentation. The specific effect of iris pigmentation on the rate of prodrug hydrolysis is, however,

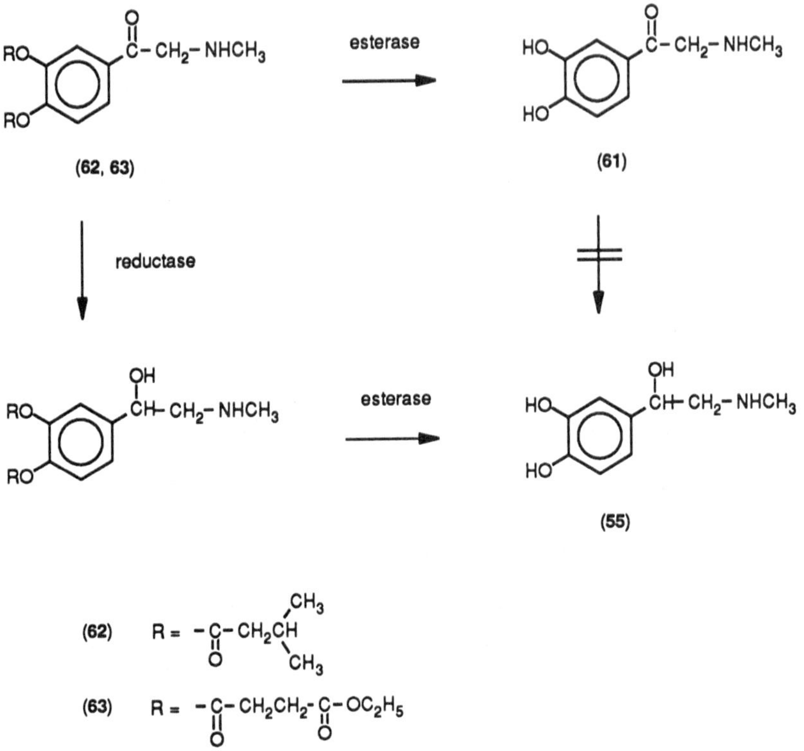

(62, 63)   (61)

reductase

(55)

(62)   R = $-\overset{\underset{\|}{O}}{C}-CH_2CH\overset{CH_3}{\underset{CH_3}{\diagup}}$

(63)   R = $-\overset{\underset{\|}{O}}{C}-CH_2CH_2-\overset{\underset{\|}{O}}{C}-OC_2H_5$

Scheme 15

influenced significantly by substrate concentration. At a concentration of 15 µM, the model ester prodrug 1-naphthyl acetate was hydrolyzed twice as fast in the cornea of the pigmented rabbit as in the albino rabbit (140). At a higher substrate concentration, however, 1-naphthyl acetate was hydrolyzed equally well in both strains of rabbits. The higher corneal esterase activity in the pigmented rabbit suggested by the 15 µM data was due to a higher activity in both the corneal epithelium and the corneal stroma, not to a higher activity in a single layer (143).

In addition to iris pigmentation, esterase activity is also dependent on age. The age at which peak esterase activity is attained is dependent on both the substrate concentration used and the iris pigmentation of the rabbit (275). Lee et al. (275) reported that the ocular esterase activity in the 6-week-old albino rabbit was 2 times higher than in the pigmented rabbit of the same age, a finding opposite to that observed in the 12-week-old age group (143). These findings suggest that both the Age and iris pigmentation of the rabbit must be considered in studies involving prodrugs and esterase activity evaluation.

The above variations in esterase activity with age and iris pigmentation affect the extent of conversion of the prodrug dipivalyl epinephrine to epinephrine in the corneal epithelium (142). It may therefore be necessary to adjust the topically applied dose of a prodrug in response to changes in corneal esterase activity. The factors that may change the esterase activity in a patient are not known. It is conceivable that chronic prodrug administration itself may stimulate esterase activity in order that the physiological role of the esterases not be unduly compromised.

Formulation Factors

Unless prodrugs are intrinsically pharmacologically active, as has been proposed for pivalyl phenylephrine (38) and diacetyl nadolol (27), their therapeutic efficacy would be anticipated to be influenced by the coadministration with an esterase inhibitor, such as echothiophate iodide and eserine sulfate. Indeed, Sasaki et al. (276) reported that in the presence of 1 mM eserine sulfate, the corneal permeation of O-butyryltimolol, 1'-methylcyclopropanoyltimolol, and O-pivaloyltimol was reduced. This was attributed to reduction in prodrug hydrolysis, which in turn caused a reduction in the concentration gradient governing prodrug absorption. An early report by Abramovsky and Mindel (277) also indicates that esterase inhibitors may influence the therapeutic efficacy of prodrugs. In this instance, the IOP-lowering response expected of 0.25% dipivalyl epinephrine in the pigmented rabbit was blunted when administered shortly after or concomitantly with 0.25% echothiophate iodide. A subsequent report by Mindel et al. (278), however, indicated that a more probable explanation was the hypertensive response rather than esterase inhibition caused by echothiophate iodide that was responsible for counteracting the hypotensive effect of dipivalyl epinephrine. Indeed, it can be calculated from the kinetic parameters for echothiophate iodide inhibition of dipivalyl epinephrine hydrolysis (279) that only 16% of the corneal esterase activity could be suppressed at the concentrations of dipivalyl epinephrine and echothiophate iodide applied. Since this was within the experimental error, suppression of the conversion of dipivalyl epinephrine to epinephrine in vivo would be difficult to detect. Clearly, the relative concentration of the prodrug and the esterase inhibitor and the relative magnitude of the Michaelis-Menten parameter (K_m) and inhibition constant (K_i) are important parameters in determining whether this potential drug-drug interaction would occur.

Because of the important role of the corneal epithelium in the penetration and conversion of the prodrug, its integrity is anticipated to affect the prodrug's efficacy. Alexander et al. (55) and Camber and Edman (36) demonstrated that deepithelizing the cornea adversely affected the corneal penetration of an (acyloxy)alkyl carbamate prodrug of timolol and the isopropyl ester of $PGF_{2\alpha}$, respectively. Chien et al. (280) obtained similar results with a number of alkyl esters of timolol except the very labile ones such as O-acetyl-, O-propionyl-, and O-butyryltimolol.

Preservatives, which are included in all multidose ophthalmic formulations to maintain sterility, are notorious for their damaging effects on the corneal epithelium (281). The popular preservatives are benzalkonium chloride and other cationic surfactants. They have been found to enhance the ocular absorption of a number of drugs varying in molecular size and lipophilicity, including pilocarpine (282), carbachol (283), prednisolone (284), homatropine (285), inulin (286), and horseradish peroxidase (287). Camber and Edman (36) have carefully compared the corneal-damaging effects of four surfactants as indicated by their influence on the corneal penetration of pilocarpine and dexamethasone in vitro. These investigators demonstrated that exposing the isolated porcine cornea to 0.01% benzalkonium chloride or 0.5% chlorobutanol for 4 h almost doubled the transcorneal flux of pilocarpine, a magnitude of increase comparable to that obtained by deepithelizing the cornea. Chlorhexidine digluconate (0.01%) and a mixture of 0.04% methyl paraben and 0.02% propyl paraben were less effective. The same rank order of effectiveness was seen in the transcorneal flux of dexamethasone, although none of the preservatives afforded the same factor of increase as the deepithelized cornea. By contrast, benzalkonium chloride reduced the corneal permeability of the isopropyl ester prodrug of $PGF_{2\alpha}$ by a factor of two, which was opposite to the 10-fold increase seen with the parent compound. The factor of reduction was, however, less than the 9-fold reduction observed with deepithelizing the cornea (36). The reason underlying the negative effect of benzalkonium chloride on the permeation of this prostaglandin prodrug has not been revealed, but it may be related to the inhibitory effect of the preservative on esterase activity or to saturation of the esterases by the higher concentration of prodrug exposed to the enzyme, as has been reported for levobunolol, which undergoes reduction during corneal penetration (274). By analogy, the observation that preservatives affect the corneal permeation of certain prodrugs raise the question of whether other ingredients in the formulation would exert a similar effect. This needs to be investigated.

ALTERNATIVES TO PRODRUGS FOR IMPROVEMENT OF CORNEAL DRUG PENETRATION

Use of Vehicles with Improved Precorneal Retention Characteristics

For many years, various attempts have been made to improve corneal drug penetration by prolonging precorneal drug retention. Of the methods investigated, the most popular is to increase solution viscosity through incorporation of soluble polymers into an aqueous solution, including poly(vinyl alcohol), poly(vinyl pyrrolidone), methylcellulose, and hydroxypropylcellulose. It is reasoned that solution drainage would be reduced as solution viscosity is increased (65,288). Chrai and Robinson (289) reported that increasing the solution viscosity from 1 to 100 cps through the incorporation of methylcellulose doubled the pilocarpine concentration in the aqueous humor of the albino rabbit as the consequence of a 10-fold reduction in the solution drainage rate constant. Similar results were obtained for timolol administered in a 5% polyvinyl alcohol solution in the pigmented rabbit (24). Such a moderate increase in ocular drug absorption, despite a significant reduction in solution drainage, is partly due to a concurrent increase in conjunctival drug absorption. While a twofold increase in corneal drug absorption may not benefit nonpotent drugs such as pilocarpine and atropine, it may be therapeutically beneficial for more potent drugs such as timolol and betaxolol.

Under proper conditions, the polymers used in viscous formulations as well as biopolymers such as collagen (10) and fibrin (11) can be fabricated into erodible inserts for placement in the cul-de-sac. These appear to be an alternative to the nonerodible Ocusert, a waferlike device programmed to release pilocarpine at a constant rate of 20 or 40 µg/h around the clock for 7 days (290). Since the pioneering work of Maichuk in 1976 (291), there has been a proliferation of erodible inserts primarily for pilocarpine and other ophthalmic drugs (10–15,290–293). In a study designed to compare gentamicin levels in the tear, sclera, and cornea from a number of dosage forms, the succinylated enzyme-solubilized collagen insert was superior to eye drops, ointments, and subconjunctival injection (10). Nevertheless, as is the case of drug-loaded soft contact lenses (294–297), water-soluble drugs are rapidly released from these hydrophilic matrices due to the leaching action of tear and the shearing action of blinking. For instance, gentamicin was released from the soluble succinylated enzyme-solubilized collagen insert much faster than the insert was dissolved (10).

In addition to sustaining drug release, another potential advantage of inserts is that owing to the placement location in the conjunctival sac they may promote drug entry to the uveal tract by diffusion across the conjunctiva-sclera laminate, the so-called noncorneal route, which has not received much attention until the past few years (83,93,95,96,298,299). Such a possibility is supported by the finding of Urtti et al. (300), who observed unequal timolol concentrations in the superior and inferior parts of the ciliary body following placement of a silicone cylindrical device in the conjunctival sac of the rabbit. In particular, timolol concentrations were higher in the part of the tissue that was closer to the site of device application. The noncorneal route deserves careful study in the future. This is because the noncorneal route may spare the various layers of the cornea from the possible ill effects of the drug and may provide drug direct access to the base of the iris anteriorly and the choroid and vitreous humor more posteriorly. The role of the noncorneal route to ocular drug absorption will be amplified upon subsequently.

Within the boundaries defined by viscous solutions and inserts are three recently developed noteworthy approaches on improving precorneal drug retention. They are bioadhesives, in situ–activated gel-forming systems, and collagen shields. The salient feature of each approach will be discussed in turn.

Bioadhesives

Bioadhesives are substances which have the ability to interact with biological materials and which are retained on the biological substrate for an extended period of time (301). The perceived advantage of bioadhesives over all the delivery systems discussed so far, except the Ocusert, is their expected markedly prolonged residence time in the conjunctival sac, since clearance would then be controlled by the much slower turnover rate of the mucus or the cell to which mucus is attached rather than by the tear turnover rate. That a variety of polymers attach directly to conjunctival tissue or to the mucin coating of this tissue has been well documented (302). In addition, evidence that such mucoadhesive polymers are retained in the eye of albino rabbits for at least 12 h to provide for sustained release of a test drug has been reported by Hui and Robinson (303). Sufficient data presently exist that certain polymers possessing the correct charge density, number of polar groups for hydrogen bonding, and balance of lipophilic to hydrophilic sections in the polymer chain are capable of good mucoadhesion in the eye. Such polymers can be used to design significantly improved ocular drug delivery systems.

A bioadhesive polymer that has gained attention as a drug delivery vehicle is hyaluronic acid. Hyaluronic acid is a natural, high molecular weight polysaccharide (304,305). A 1% solution of the sodium salt of hyaluronic acid, sodium hyaluronate (Healon), has been used as a replacement for vitreous humor in posterior segment surgery, and more dilute solutions have been tested with promising results in the treatment of a dry eye (306,307). In addition to its bioadhesive properties, sodium hyaluronate is an attractive ophthalmic drug delivery vehicle because of its high-water binding capacity, nonirritancy, increased viscosity, and pseudoplastic behavior. Based on the time course of changes in pupillary diameter, Camber et al. (308) observed a two- to threefold increase in the absorption of 1% pilocarpine hydrochloride into the albino rabbit eye when delivered in 0.2 and 0.75% sodium hyaluronate solutions. Moreover, when comparing solutions of the same viscosity, those prepared from high molecular weight sodium hyaluronate exhibited a greater miotic response than those prepared from lower molecular weight samples (308). The molecular weights studied were 0.6×10^6, 1.6×10^6, and 4.6×10^6.

In addition to their bioadhesive properties, the carboxylic anionic groups on soluble polyanionic polymers offer the opportunity of polymer salt formation with drugs containing the amine functional group. Provided that a sufficient number of anionic groups remain to exert their bioadhesive function, such a complex conceivably would be retained in the precorneal area while delivering the ionically bound drug to the target tissue within the eye at a sustained rate. Such a concept has been tested by Saettone et al. (309) using pilocarpine as the probe drug and hyaluronic acid, poly(galacturonic acid), mesoglycan (a complex mixture of mucopolysaccharides), and carboxymethylchitin as a model polyanionic polymers. All polymeric vehicles had a viscosity of about 4 Mpa/s and, except hyaluronic acid, had a pH of about 6. Using miosis as an index of bioavailability, there was a 50–100% increase in the extent of absorption and a 60% increase in the duration of action.

In Situ–Activated Gel-Forming Systems

In situ–activated gel-forming systems are those which would undergo a viscosity increase upon instillation in the eye, thereby promoting precorneal retention. Such a change in viscosity can be triggered by a change in temperature (310), pH (311), or electrolyte composition (312). Poloxamer 407 is a polymer whose solution viscosity increases when its temperature is raised to the eye temperature (310). Cellulose acetophthalate is a polymer whose solution undergoes coagulation when its native pH of 4.5 is raised by the tear fluid to pH 7.4 (311). Both systems are, however, characterized by a high polymer concentration (25% for poloxamer 407 and 30% for cellulose acetophthalate). By contrast, Gelrite, a polysaccharide, low-acetyl gellan gum (313), forms clear gels at a much lower concentration in the presence of mono- or divalent cations typically found in tear fluids (314). In fact, the concentration of sodium ions in tears, 2.6 g/L, is sufficient to cause gelation of the material upon topical instillation in the conjunctival sac.

Poloxamers are a class of thermally activated gel-forming polymers which possess several favorable properties as an ophthalmic vehicle: low toxicity, mucomimetic, and optical clarity. Poloxamer gels possess some characteristics that are ointmentlike and others that are similar to those of a viscous, aqueous solution. Miller and Donovan (310) tested a 0.25 M pilocarpine formulation in 25% poloxamer 407 instilled as a 10-μl drop against an aqueous formulation in albino rabbits. There was a 1.9-fold increase in miotic response in the gel formulation when compared with an aqueous formulation. Prolongation of contact time was probably the underlying mechanism.

In the only pH-activated system investigated to date (315), pilocarpine was adsorbed onto 0.3-μm beads of cellulose acetate hydrogen phthalate, which coagulated in the presence of a slight pH change in the cul-de-sac, thereby promoting its adsorption onto ocular surfaces. The extent of prolongation appeared to be influenced by drug loading. At 2% drug concentration, drug release was found to continue to beyond 8 h. In contrast, at 1% drug concentration, no statistically significant difference was discerned between the latex and aqueous solution or a 10% methylcellulose solution.

In the only ion-activated gel-forming system reported thus far (312), a moderate improvement in the ocular absorption of 0.34% timolol maleate was seen when administered in 0.6% Gelrite than in isoviscous hydroxyethycellulose in the albino rabbit (312). The formulation was prepared by dissolving the drug and Gelrite in 0.01 M Tris maleate buffer (pH 7) and adjusting to isotonicity with mannitol. Similar favorable results were obtained in terms of peak and duration of activity in 45 patients with intraocular pressure greater than 23 mmHg following the topical instillation of 0.008% timolol maleate in Gelrite compared to a buffer formulation (316).

Collagen Shields

The concept of using inserts to sustain drug delivery in the eye, while scientifically sound, has never found much appeal in the ophthalmology community. This trend is about to change with the recent introduction of collagen shields as a corneal bandage after radial keratotomy, keratorefractive procedures, and corneal abrasions (317,318). The shield is fabricated from porcine scleral tissue, which bears a collagen composition similar to that of the human cornea. Upon hydration by tear fluids, the shield softens and forms a clear, pliable, thin film approximately 0.1 mm in thickness, with a diameter of 14.5 mm and base curve of 9 mm that conforms to the corneal surface. Designed to slowly dissolve within 12, 24, or 72 h, the shield has stimulated much interest as a potential sustained ocular drug delivery system.

A number of water-soluble drugs have been investigated for delivery in the collagen corneal shield. These drugs include antiseptics (silver nitrate, povidone iodide, and chlorhexidine gluconate) (319), propamidine isethioniate (320), tobramycin (321), amphotericin B (322), trifluorothymidine (323), 5-fluorouracil (324), and pilocarpine (325). Typically, the drug is loaded into the collagen shield simply by soaking it in the drug solution for a period of time prior to application. In the majority of instances, there is moderate to marked improvement in the extent of ocular drug absorption. Sawusch et al. (321), for instance, observed a 30-fold improvement in the ocular absorption of tobramycin in rabbits when administered in the collagen shield, resulting in substantial reduction in the number of *Pseudomonas aeruginosa* colonies in the infected eye. Gussler et al. (323), on the other hand, observed no effect of the collagen shield in trifluorothymidine absorption into rabbit eyes, except those with preexisting corneal epithelial defects. In no instance, however, was there substantial prolongation in ocular drug absorption beyond 30 min. This is not surprising, since the drug is rapidly released from the device (324). This situation is very similar to that of soft contact lenses in their capacity as ocular drug delivery systems (326).

Clearly, the collagen shield, in its present form, is not a suitable sustained ocular drug delivery system. For it to be useful in sustained drug delivery, the existing biomaterial in the collagen shield must be modified or a new biomaterial must be used.

Use of Penetration Enhancers

In principle, because of the prominent role played by the corneal epithelium in the penetration of hydrophilic and moderately lipophilic drugs, modifying the integrity of the corneal epithelium should enhance corneal drug absorption.

This expectation is borne out in the extreme situation where the corneal epithelium is removed prior to drug administration. Under this condition, the amount of drug absorbed across the cornea is increased by a factor of 2–15 (327,328).

Although no additives has been included in ophthalmic formulations to deliberately lower the barrier function of the corneal epithelium, there exist in the very same formulations additives which can inadvertently bring about the same result. Such additives are the preservatives and the chelating agents that are required to keep formulations sterile and chemically stable. The effect of preservations on corneal drug absorption has already been discussed.

Grass and Robinson (81) were among the first to emphasize the positive effect of chelating agents on corneal drug absorption. They found that exposure of the rabbit cornea to increasing concentrations of ethylenediamine tetraacetic acid (EDTA) (0.01, 0.05, and 0.1%) in vitro caused progressive widening of the intercellular space (89) with an attendant increase in its permeability to glycerol and Na cromoglycate but not to progesterone (81), a lipophilic drug that probably crosses the corneal epithelium via the transcellular pathway. The above effect was abolished upon the addition of Ca^{2+} or Mg^{2+} to the perfusion medium (81).

The above findings support the feasibility of using penetration enhancers to promote corneal drug penetration. The use of penetration enhancers to modify the integrity of the absorptive membranes, thereby enhancing drug absorption, is an active area of research in peptide and protein drug delivery (329). Such an approach is virtually untested in ophthalmology, however, despite the striking similarity in bioavailability between ophthalmic drugs and peptide and protein drugs. To date, only two reports have hinted at the use of penetration enhancers to promote the ocular absorption of topically applied drugs (330,331). But the results were mixed—Azone was found not to affect the ocular bioavailability of topically applied levobunolol (330), whereas it promoted the ocular absorption of topically applied cyclosporine (331). In any event, before penetration enhancers can be used on a routine basis in ophthalmology, it must be established unambiguously that the changes in membrane integrity are indeed transient, are predictable, and therefore would not compromise the defense mechanisms of the eye so severely as to cause harm. Already there is evidence that the penetration enhancers themselves can penetrate the eye and may therefore lead to unknown toxicological complications. For instance, benzalkonium chloride was found to accumulate in the cornea for days (332). And EDTA was found to reach the iris–ciliary body in concentrations high enough to alter the permeability of the blood vessels in the uveal tract, indirectly accelerating drug removal from the aqueous humor (333). Moreover, repeated application of 0.5% EDTA was observed to significantly alter the corneal epithelial architecture even though a single application was well tolerated (81).

Ion Pair Formation

Ion pair formation is another approach that may be considered for facilitating corneal drug transport. In 1981, Wilson et al. reported that ion pair formation between cromolyn sodium, an organic anion, and benzalkonium chloride, an organic cation, modestly improved the absorption of both compounds in the albino rabbit eye, but that neither was transported without the other (334). Approximately 0.07% of the administered dose of cromolyn sodium and 0.7% of benzalkonium chloride were found in the aqueous humor at 30 min.

The use of ion pair formation to promote corneal drug absorption was reinvestigated in a series of recent papers by Kato et al. (335–337). These investigators found that the extent of drug ionization, hence the pH of the medium and the pK_a of the drug, and the chain length of the ion pairing agent were both important factors in determining the extent of improvement in ocular drug penetration due to ion pair formation. Thus, ion pair formation with caprylic acid enhanced the corneal penetration of bunazosin (pK_a 7.7) more than that of pilocarpine (pK_a 6.7) (335). In addition, the enhancement in corneal penetration of bunazosin by caprylic acid was more pronounced at pH 6.5 than at pH 8.0. This is indicated by the ratio of increase of 9.32 at the lower pH as compared with that of 2.28 at the higher pH. In a homologous series of saturated straight chain fatty acids, the higher homologues were more effective in enhancing the corneal absorption of bunazosin. The specific rank order was capriate (C10) > caprylate (C8) > caproate (C6) (335). Two lines of evidence implicate ion pair formation as the principal mechanism underlying the enhancement in corneal absorption by long chain fatty acids: first, the good correlation between the increase in corneal absorption of bunazosin and the increase in its partition coefficient by long chain fatty acids (335) and, second, the lack of direct effect of the long chain fatty acids on corneal epithelial integrity (337).

Thus, there is a preliminary evidence that ion pair formation may be useful in promoting corneal drug penetration under certain conditions. Nevertheless, it has yet to be resolved whether enhancement results from an increase in the availability of the drug at the corneal surface or from shielding of the charge on the drug by the ion pairing agent, thus allowing it to diffuse across the lipid environment of the corneal epithelium. As is the case of penetration enhancers, however, the ultimate usefulness of such an approach must await careful studies to verify the long-term effects of the ion pairing agents, frequently surfactant in nature, on corneal health.

Iontophoresis

Iontophoresis can be defined as a process which causes increased penetration of solute molecules into tissues by the application of a low current (milliamperes) through the tissue (338). The drug reservoir is placed at either the anode (anodal iontophoresis) or the cathode (cathodal iontophoresis) depending on the charge of the drug. This process was conceived in 1908 to drive ions across the skin, and was attempted in the ensuing years as a means to enhance corneal drug absorption (339–344). Many difficulties were encountered, however, including corneal scarring, tissue burning, and some electrical shocking of patients (345). Consequently, iontophoresis was virtually abandoned until the early 1960s when it was again used experimentally to deliver penicillin and sulfadiazine into the infected eyes of animals (346).

Two types of iontophoresis have been practiced: transcorneal and transscleral iontophoresis. Transcorneal iontophoresis has limited success in delivering drugs in high enough concentrations to the posterior segment of the eye (340–342,347). It is, however, capable of enhancing the aqueous humor concentrations of drugs such as gentamicin (347,348), tobramycin (349), vidarabine monophosphate (350), and fluorescein (348) by a factor of 25–100 when compared with topical solution instillation. The ineffectiveness of transcorneal iontophoresis in delivering drugs to the posterior segment has been attributed to the presence of an iris-lens barrier to drug diffusion from the anterior and posterior chambers to the vitreous cavity. The indirect evidence is that in aphakic rabbit eyes therapeutic levels of gentamicin were achieved in the vitreous humor for as long as 24 h following anodal iontophoresis in which a current of 0.75 mA was applied for 10 min (351). This observation prompted the investigation of transscleral iontophoresis as a means to bypass the iris-lens barrier, thereby providing therapeutic drug concentrations to the vitreous cavity and its surrounding tissues.

In transscleral iontophoresis, the device is placed over the pars plana. Burstein et al. (352) noted that the electrode position relative to the retina affected the proportion of drug reaching the vitreous vs the aqueous humor. When the electrode was placed within 3 mm of the limbus, virtually no gentamicin was recovered in the vitreous humor of the rabbit eye. More posterior placement of the electrode, avoiding external ocular muscles, was necessary to target delivery of the drug to the vitreous humor.

Other factors influencing the efficiency of transscleral iontophoresis are the current density and duration of application. Both have been investigated by Barza et al. (353) in the rabbit using ticarcillin, cefazolin, and gentamicin as model compounds. The diameter of the electrode used was 1 mm. There was a threshold current, which was 0.1 mA for ticarcillin and cefazolin and 1 mA for.gentamicin (353). The concentration of drug in the vitreous humor at 3 h correlated with the current intensity (0.1–2.0 mA) and with the duration of iontophoresis (1–10 min) but not with drug concentration, which was relatively high. This was 25–100 mg/ml for ticarcillin and gentamicin and 62.5–250.0 mg/ml for cefazolin. This lack of dependence on drug concentration is to be expected, since all the current will then be carried by the drug molecules, making the current itself the limiting factor (348).

There are at least two concerns associated with the use of iontophoresis. First, depending on the drug, there is a significant degree of variability in the drug concentration between eyes and with a given eye after repeated treatments (354). This is relatively small for cefazolin (353), but it is as much as 10- to 20-fold for ticarcillin (353) and gentamicin (353,354). There is also the possibility of loss in effectiveness during chronic therapy. Thus, the mean concentration of gentamicin in the vitreous humor was found to decline progressively with repeated treatments, being 50% as great after the fifth as after the first treatment (354). It is unclear if this was an artifact due to the loss of antibiotic during repeated sampling.

The second concern is that of safety, which has been addressed by Hughes and Maurice (348), but which has not been systematically studied. Current densities up to 20 mA/cm^2 applied to the rabbit cornea for 5 min have been found to be well tolerated (348), but possible changes in the anterior and posterior segment tissues have not been determined. Small burns over the area where the current is applied are common (354). This may be due to alterations in solution pH during ionto-phoresis. Whether these changes are fully reversible is as yet unknown. There is recent evidence that excised human skin fails to fully recover upon cessation of iontophoresis at 0.16 mA/cm^2 for 1 h (355).

CONCLUSIONS

Drug development for ocular diseases has traditionally relied on drugs originally developed for systemic use. Unfortunately, few of them are optimal for ocular absorption. This is because they possess few of the physicochemical properties that are required to overcome the constraints imposed by the eye on drug absorption, which are far more severe than those imposed by the skin or by the gastrointestinal tract. Such constraints include a short residence time, a narrow pH range that can be tolerated, a highly impermeable cornea, a small surface area for corneal absorption, and a much larger surface area for systemic drug loss. Past attempts to improve ocular drug bioavailability have focused primarily on improving precorneal drug retention. Overcoming the poor permeability of the cornea has been considered only recently. Results to date indicate that this objective may be met by perturbing the permeability of the cornea with penetration enhancers, or by improving the lipophilicity of the drug through ion pair formation or prodrug derivatization. Of these approaches, the prodrug approach is the best developed and probably holds the most promise from the standpoint of versatility and safety.

The current interest in penetration enhancers as a means to promote drug absorption elsewhere raises the interesting but, in the authors' opinion, remote possibility of using prodrugs in combination with penetration enhancers to further augment ocular drug absorption. In any event, the full potential of prodrugs in ocular drug delivery is far from realized pending investigations on its other applications. These include modifying the duration of drug action, reducing the extent of systemic drug absorption, reducing the incidence of ocular side effects, and maximizing the ratio of drug concentrations in the target to nontarget tissues. To this end, future work must be directed toward a thorough understanding of the metabolic enzymes and related biochemical aspects of the eye that are crucial to the activation of prodrugs and toward the design of carrier moieties that are biocompatible with the ocular tissues. Other equally important issues are the influence of age, disease states, and vehicle composition on the efficacy of prodrugs and the selection of an animal model required in their assessment.

ACKNOWLEDGMENT

This work was supported in part by a grant (EY-03816) from the National Institutes of Health, Bethesda, Maryland, a grant from the Lundbeck Foundation, Copenhagen, Denmark, and the Gavin S. Herbert Professorship.

REFERENCES

1. J. W. Shell, *Surv. Ophthalmol.*, 29, 117 (1984).
2. N. L. Burstein and J. A. Anderson, *J. Ocular Pharmacol.*, 1, 309 (1985).
3. V. H. L. Lee and J. R. Robinson, *J. Ocular Pharmacol.*, 2, 67 (1986).
4. V. H. L. Lee and J. R. Robinson, *J. Pharm. Sci.*, 68, 673 (1979).
5. A. G. Thombre and K. J. Himmelstein, *J. Pharm. Sci.*, 73, 219 (1984).
6. S. S. Chrai and J. R. Robinson, *J. Pharm. Sci.*, 63, 1218 (1974).
7. T. F. Patton and J. R. Robinson, *J. Pharm. Sci.*, 64, 1312 (1975).
8. M. F. Saettone, B. Giannaccini, A. Teneggi, P. Savigni, and N. Tellini, *J. Pharm. Pharmacol.*, 34, 464 (1982).
9. M. F. Saettone, B. Giannaccini, S. Ravecca, F. La Marca, and G. Tota, *Int. J. Pharm.*, 20, 187 (1984).
10. S. E. Bloomfield, T. Miyata, M. W. Dunn, N. Bueser, K. H. Stenzel, and A. L. Rubin, *Arch. Ophthalmol.*, 96, 885 (1978).
11. S. Miyazaki, K. Ishii, and M. Takada, *Chem. Pharm. Bull.*, 30, 3405 (1982).
12. I. M. Katz and W. M. Blackman, *Am. J. Ophthalmol.*, 83, 728 (1977).
13. L. Salminen, A. Urtti, H. Kujari, and M. Juslin, *Graefs Arch. Clin. Exp. Ophthalmol.*, 221, 96 (1983).
14. G. M. Grass, J. Cobby, and M. C. Makoid, *J. Pharm. Sci.*, 73, 618 (1984).
15. M. F. Saettone, B. Giannaccini, P. Chetoni, G. Galli, and E. Chiellini, *J. Pharm. Pharmacol.*, 36, 229 (1984).
16. K. Kishida and T. Otori, *Jpn. J. Ophthalmol.*, 24, 251 (1980).
17. R. D. Schoenwald and R. L. Ward, *J. Pharm. Sci.*, 67, 786 (1978).
18. R. D. Schoenwald and H. S. Huang, *J. Pharm. Sci.*, 72, 1266 (1983).
19. A. I. Mandell, F. Stentz, and A. E. Kitabchi, *Ophthalmology*, 85, 268 (1978).
20. H. Bundgaard, A. Buur, S. C. Chang, and V. H. L. Lee, *Int. J. Pharm.*, 33, 15 (1986).
21. H. Bundgaard, A. Buur, S.-C. Chang, and V. H. L. Lee, *Int. J. Pharm.*, 46, 77 (1988).
22. S. C. Chang, H. Bundgaard, A. Buur, and V. H. L. Lee, *Invest. Ophthalmol. Vis. Sci.*, 28, 487 (1987).
23. H. Sasaki, D. S. Chien, K. Lew, H. Bundgaard, and V. H. L. Lee, *Invest. Ophthalmol. Vis. Sci.*, 29(Suppl.), 83 (1988).

24. S.-C. Chang, D.-S. Chien, H. Bundgaard, and V. H. L. Lee, *Exp. Eye Res.*, 46, 59 (1988).
25. S.-C. Chang, H. Bundgaard, A. Buur, and V. H. L. Lee, *Invest. Ophthalmol. Vis. Sci.*, 29, 626 (1988).
26. D.-S. Chien, H. Bundgaard, A. Buur, and V. H. L. Lee, *J. Ocular Pharmacol.*, 4, 137 (1988).
27. E. Duzman, C. C. Chen, J. Anderson, M. Blumenthal, and H. Twizer, *Arch. Ophthalmol.*, 100, 1916 (1982).
28. H. Bundgaard, E. Falch, C. Larsen, G. L. Mosher, and T. J. Mikkelson, *J. Med. Chem.*, 28, 980 (1985).
29. H. Bundgaard, E. Falch, C. Larsen, and T. J. Mikkelson, *J. Pharm. Sci.*, 75, 36 (1986).
30. H. Bundgaard, E. Falch, C. Larsen, G. Mosher, and T. J. Mikkelson, *J. Pharm. Sci.*, 75, 775 (1986).
31. G. L. Mosher, H. Bundgaard, E. Falch, C. Larsen, and T. J. Mikkelson, *Int. J. Pharm.*, 39, 113 (1987).
32. L. Z. Bito, A. Draga, J. Blanchs, and C. B. Camras, *Invest. Ophthalmol. Vis. Sci.*, 24, 312 (1983).
33. L. Z. Bito, *Exp. Eye Res.*, 38, 181 (1984).
34. L. Z. Bito and R. A. Baroody, *Exp. Eye Res.*, 44, 217 (1987).
35. O. Camber, P. Edman, and L. I. Olsson, *Int. J. Pharm.*, 29, 259 (1986).
36. O. Camber and P. Edman, *Int. J. Pharmaceut.*, 37, 27 (1987).
37. M. V. W. Bergamini, D. L. Murray, and P. D. Krause, *Invest. Ophthalmol. Vis. Sci.*, 20(Suppl.), 187 (1979).
38. J. S. Mindel, S. T. Shaikewitz, and S. M. Podos, *Arch. Ophthalmol.*, 98, 2220 (1980).
39. S. S. Yuan and N. Bodor, *J. Pharm. Sci.*, 65, 929 (1976).
40. D. S. Chien and E. D. Schoenwald, *Biopharm. Drug Disp.*, 7, 453 (1986).
41. R. D. Schoenwald, J. C. Folk, V. Kumar, and J. G. Piper, *J. Ocular Pharmacol.*, 3, 333 (1987).
42. D.-S. Chien and R. D. Schoenwald, *Pharm. Res.*, 7, 476 (1990).
43. T. L. Phipps, D. E. Potter, and J. M. Rowland, *J. Ocular Pharmacol.*, 2, 225 (1986).
44. A. Bar-Ilan, N. I. Pessah, and T. H. Maren, *J. Ocular Pharmacol.*, 2, 109 (1986).
45. M. F. Sugrue, P. Gautheron, C. Schmitt, M. P. Viader, P. Conquet, R. L. Smith, N. N. Share, and C. A. Stone, *J. Pharmacol. Exp. Ther.*, 232, 534 (1985).
46. P. C. Maudgal, K. D. Clercq, J. Descamps, and L. Missotten, *Arch. Ophthalmol.*, 102, 140 (1984).
47. D. Pavan-Langston, R. D. North, P. A. Geary, and A. Kinkel, *Arch. Ophthalmol.*, 94, 1585 (1976).
48. M. M. Narurkar and A. K. Mitra, *Pharm. Res.*, 6, 887 (1989).
49. M. M. Narurkar and A. K. Mitra, *Pharm. Res.*, 5, 734 (1988).
50. D. A. McClure, in *Prodrugs as Novel Drug Delivery System* (T. Higuchi and V. Stella, eds.). American Chemical Society, Washington, D.C., 1975, p. 224.
51. N. Bodor, J. Kaminski, and R. Roller, *Int. J. Pharm.*, 1, 189 (1978).
52. N. Bodor and G. Visor, *Exp. Eye Res.*, 38, 621 (1984).
53. N. Bodor and G. Visor, *Pharm. Res.*, 1, 168 (1984).
54. M. F. Sugrue, P. Gautheron, J. Grove, P. Mallorga, and M. P. Viader, *Invest. Ophthalmol. Vis. Sci.*, 28, 267 (1987).

55. J. Alexander, R. Cargill, S. R. Michelson, and H. Schwam, *J. Med. Chem.*, 31, 318 (1988).
56. N. Bodor, A. Elkoussi, M. Kano, and T. Nakamura, *J. Med. Chem.*, 31, 100 (1988).
57. A. A. El-Koussi and N. Bodor, *Int. J. Pharm.*, 53, 189 (1989).
58. N. Bodor and L. Prokai, *Pharm. Res.*, 7, 723 (1990).
59. N. Bodor, in *Design of Biopharmaceutical Properties Through Prodrugs and Analogs* (E. B. Roche, ed.). American Pharmaceutical Association, Washington, D.C., 1977, p. 98.
60. H. Schwam, S. R. Michelson, J. M. Sondey, and R. L. Smith, *Invest. Ophthalmol. Vis. Sci.*, 25, 180 (1984).
61. L. Z. Bito, O. C. Miranda, M. R. Tendler, and B. Resul, *Exp. Eye Res.*, 50, 419 (1990).
62. H. M. Leibowitz and A. Kupferman, *Invest. Ophthalmol. Vis. Sci.*, 13, 757 (1974).
63. H. M. Liebowitz, A. Kupferman, R. H. Stewart, and R. L. Kimbrough, *Am. J. Ophthalmol.*, 86, 418 (1978).
64. A. Kupferman, A. P. Berrospi, and H. A. Leibowitz, *Arch. Ophthalmol.*, 100, 640 (1982).
65. V. H. L. Lee, J. Swarbrick, R. E. Stratford, and K. W. Morimoto, *J. Pharm. Pharmacol.*, 35, 445 (1983).
66. H. S. Huang, R. D. Schoenwald, and J. L. Lach, *J. Pharm. Sci.*, 72, 1272 (1983).
67. R. L. Shih and V. H. Lee, *J. Ocular Pharmacol.*, 6, 329 (1990).
68. E. Fromter and J. Diamond, *Nature*, 235, 9 (1972).
69. W. S. Marshall and S. D. Klyce, *J. Membr. Biol.*, 73, 275 (1983).
70. G. Van Meer and K. Simons, *E.M.B.O. J.*, 5, 1455 (1986).
71. A. Martinez-Palomo, I. Meza, G. Beaty, and M. Cereijido, *J. Cell Biol.*, 87, 736 (1980).
72. D. R. Pitelka, B. N. Taggart, and S. T. Hamamoto, *J. Cell Biol.*, 96, 613 (1983).
73. B. R. Stevenson and D. A. Goodenough, *J. Cell Biol.*, 98, 1209 (1984).
74. T. Volberg, B. Geiger, J. Kartenbeck, and W. W. Franke, *J. Cell Biol.*, 102, 1832 (1986).
75. T. Volk and B. Geiger, *J. Cell Biol.*, 103, 1451 (1986).
76. F. M. Watt, D. L. Mattey, and D. R. Garrod, *J. Cell Biol.*, 99, 2211 (1984).
77. K. Boller, D. Vestweber, and R. Kemler, *J. Cell Biol.*, 100, 327 (1985).
78. B. Gumbiner and K. Simons, *J. Cell Biol.*, 102, 457 (1986).
79. J. L. Madara, D. Barenberg, and S. Carlson, *J. Cell Biol.*, 102, 2125 (1986).
80. S. D. Klyce and C. E. Crosson, *Curr. Eye Res.*, 4, 323 (1985).
81. G. M. Grass and J. R. Robinson, *J. Pharm. Sci.*, 77, 3 (1988).
82. G. M. Grass and J. R. Robinson, *J. Pharm. Sci.*, 77, 15 (1988).
83. V. H. L. Lee, L. W. Carson, and K. A. Takemoto, *Int. J. Pharm.*, 29, 43 (1986).
84. N. Keller, D. Moore, D. Carper, and A. Longwell, *Exp. Eye Res.*, 30, 203 (1980).
85. R. E. Stratford, M. A. Redell, D. C. Yang, and V. H. L. Lee, *Curr. Eye Res.*, 2, 377 (1983).
86. M. Francoeur, I. Ahmed, S. Sitek, and T. F. Patton, *Int. J. Pharm.*, 16, 203 (1983).
87. A. K. Mitra and T. J. Mikkelson, *J. Pharm. Sci.*, 77, 771 (1988).
88. L. M. Jankowska, A. Bar-Ilan, and T. H. Maren, *Invest. Ophthalmol. Vis. Sci.*, 27, 29 (1986).
89. P. Ashton and V. H. L. Lee, *Pharm. Res.*, 6(Suppl.), S90 (1989).
90. A. Buur, A. Yamamoto, and V. H. L. Lee, *J. Contr. Rel.*, 14, 43 (1990).

91. E. J. Lien, A. A. Alhaider, and V. H. L. Lee, *J. Parent. Sci. Technol.*, 36, 86 (1982).
92. J. B. Dressman, G. L. Amidon, and D. Fleisher, *J. Pharm. Sci.*, 74, 588 (1985).
93. I. Ahmed and T. F. Patton, *Invest. Ophthalmol. Vis. Sci.*, 26, 584 (1985).
94. I. Ahmed and T. F. Patton, *Int. J. Pharm.*, 38, 9 (1987).
95. S. R. Michelson, H. Schwam, J. J. Baldwin, P. Mallorga, G. S. Ponticello, R. L. Smith, and M. F. Sugrue, *Invest. Ophthalmol. Vis. Sci.*, 30(Suppl.), 24 (1989).
96. I. Ahmed, R. D. Gokhale, M. V. Shah, and T. F. Patton, *J. Pharm. Sci.*, 76, 583 (1987).
97. H. F. Edelhauser and T. H. Maren, *Arch. Ophthalmol.*, 106, 1110 (1988).
98. D. M. Maurice and J. Polgar, *Exp. Eye Res.*, 25, 577 (1977).
99. V. H. L. Lee, P. Ashton, H. Bundgaard, and D. K. Heuer, *Invest. Ophthalmol. Vis. Sci.*, 31(Suppl.), 403 (1990).
100. H. Bundgaard, in *Design of Prodrugs* (H. Bundgaard, ed.). Elsevier, Amsterdam, 1985, p. 1.
101. H. Bundgaard, in *Bioreversible Carriers in Drug Design. Theory and Application* (E. B. Roche, ed.). Pergamon Press, New York, 1987, p. 13.
102. H. Bundgaard, *Adv. Drug Delivery Rev.*, 3, 39 (1989).
103. V. H. L. Lee, *J. Controlled Rel.*, 11, 79 (1990).
104. D. E. Potter, D. J. Shumate, H. Bundgaard, and V. H. L. Lee, *Curr. Eye Res.*, 7, 755 (1988).
105. H. Sasaki, D.-S. Chien, H. Bundgaard, and V. H. L. Lee, *Pharm. Res.*, 5(Suppl.), S164 (1988).
106. M. Charton, in *Design of Biopharmaceutical Properties Through Prodrugs and Analogs* (E. B. Roche, ed.), American Pharmaceutical Association, Washington, D.C., 1977, p. 228.
107. H. Bundgaard, C. Larsen, and P. Thorbek, *Int. J. Pharm.*, 18, 67 (1984).
108. H. Bundgaard, C. Larsen, and E. Arnold, *Int. J. Pharm.*, 18, 79 (1984).
109. L. Colla, E. DeClercq, R. Busson, and H. Vanderhaeghe, *J. Med. Chem.*, 26, 602 (1983).
110. A. J. Kirby and G. J. Lloyd, *J. Chem. Soc. Perkin Trans.*, 2, 1748 (1976).
111. T. C. Bruice and S. J. Benkovic, *Bioorganic Mechanisms.* Vol. 1. W. A. Benjamin, New York, 1966, p. 134.
112. H. Bundgaard, E. Falch, and E. Jensen, *J. Med. Chem.*, 32, 2503 (1989).
113. E. Jensen, H. Bundgaard, and E. Falch, *Int. J. Pharm.*, 58, 143 (1990).
114. E. Jensen and H. Bundgaard, *Int. J. Pharm.*, 70, 137 (1991).
115. E. Bundgaard, E. Jensen, and E. Falch, *Pharm. Res.*, 8, 1087 (1991).
116. H. Bundgaard, E. Jensen, E. Falch, and S. B. Pedersen, *Int. J. Pharm.*, 64, 75 (1990).
117. J. Alexander, Eur. Pat. Appl. No. 130,119 (1985).
118. U. S. Gogate, A. J. Repta, and J. Alexander, *Int. J. Pharm.*, 40, 235 (1987).
119. U. S. Gogate and A. J. Repta, *Int. J. Pharm.*, 40, 249 (1987).
120. F. Sakamoto, S. Ikeda, H. Kondo, and G. Tsukamoto, *Chem. Pharm. Bull.*, 33, 4870 (1985).
121. F. Sakamoto, S. Ikeda, and G. Tsukamoto, *Chem. Pharm. Bull.*, 32, 2241 (1984).
122. N. Awata, K. Noumi, Y. Vemura, A. Takadi, and T. Aoyama, *Jpn. J. Antibiot.*, 38, 1785 (1985).

123. W. S. Saari, W. Halczenko, D. W. Cochran, M. R. Dobrinska, W. C. Vincek, D. C. Titus, S. L. Gaul, and C. S. Sweet, *J. Med. Chem.*, 27, 713 (1984).
124. G. C. Rovnyak, Ger. Offen. 3,410,847 (1984).
125. H. Bundgaard and M. Johansen, *Int. J. Pharm.*, 10, 165 (1982).
126. M. Johansen and H. Bundgaard, *J. Pharm. Sci.*, 72, 1294 (1983).
127. A. Buur and H. Bundgaard, *Int. J. Pharm.*, 18, 325 (1984).
128. A. Buur and H. Bundgaard, *Arch. Pharm. Chem. Sci. Ed.*, 15, 76 (1987).
129. T. H. Maren, L. Jankowska, G. Sanyal, and H. F. Edelhauser, *Exp. Eye Res.*, 36, 457 (1983).
130. T. H. Maren, *Drug Dev. Res.*, 10, 255 (1987).
131. B. R. Friedland and T. H. Maren, *Handbook Exp. Pharmacol.*, 69, 279 (1984).
132. M. F. Sugrue, *Pharmacol. Ther.*, 43, 91 (1989).
133. J. D. Larsen and H. Bundgaard, *Int. J. Pharm.*, 51, 27 (1989).
134. J. D. Larsen and H. Bundgaard, *Int. J. Pharm.*, 37, 87 (1987).
135. J. D. Larsen, H. Bundgaard, and V. H. L. Lee, *Int. J. Pharm.*, 47, 103 (1988).
136. H. Bundgaard and J. D. Larsen, *J. Med. Chem.*, 31, 2066 (1988).
137. J. D. Larsen and H. Bundgaard, *Acta Pharm. Nord.*, 1, 31 (1989).
138. M. W. Duffel, I. S. Ing, T. M. Segarra, J. A. Dixson, C. F. Barfknecht, and R. D. Schoenwald, *J. Med. Chem.*, 29, 1488 (1986).
139. R. D. Schoenwald, M. G. Eller, J. A. Dixson, and C. F. Barfknecht, *J. Med. Chem.*, 27, 810 (1984).
140. V. H. L. Lee, *J. Pharm. Sci.*, 72, 239 (1983).
141. R. Weinkam, J. Miller, and M. Rann, *Invest. Ophthalmol. Vis. Sci.*, 31(Suppl.), 582 (1990).
142. M. A. Redell, D. C. Yang, and V. H. L. Lee, *Int. J. Pharm.*, 17, 299 (1983).
143. V. H. L. Lee, K. W. Morimoto, and R. E. Stratford, Jr., *Biopharm. Drug Disp.*, 3, 291 (1982).
144. J. Bernshon, K. D. Barron, P. F. Dollin, A. R. Hess, and M. T. Hedrick, *J. Histochem. Cytochem.*, 14, 455 (1966).
145. W. S. Schwark and D. J. Ecobichon, *Can. J. Physiol. Pharmacol.*, 46, 207 (1968).
146. A. Amar-Costesec, H. Beaufay, M. Wibo, D. Thines-Sempoux, E. Feytmans, M. Robbi, and J. Berthet, *J. Cell Biol.*, 61, 201 (1974).
147. W. Junge, E. Heymann, K. Krish, and H. Hollandt, *Arch. Biochem. Biophys.*, 165, 749 (1974).
148. V. H. L. Lee, D. S. Iimoto, and K. A. Takemoto, *Curr. Eye Res.*, 2, 869 (1983).
149. V. H. L. Lee, S. C. Chang, C. M. Oshiro, and R. E. Smith, *Curr. Eye Res.*, 4, 1117 (1985).
150. S. C. Chang and V. H. L. Lee, *Curr. Eye Res.*, 2, 651 (1983).
151. J. S. Sieg and J. R. Robinson, *J. Pharm. Sci.*, 65, 1816 (1976).
152. V. H. L. Lee, H. W. Hui, and J. R. Robinson, *Invest. Ophthalmol. Vis. Sci.*, 19, 210 (1980).
153. P. O. Ellis, K. Littlejohn, and R. A. Deitrich, *Invest. Ophthalmol.*, 11, 747 (1972).
154. W. N. Fishbein and S. P. Bessman, *J. Biol. Chem.*, 241, 4835M (1966).
155. V. H. L. Lee, M. A. Reinoso, D.-S. Chien, and H. Bundgaard, *Proc. Int. Symp. Control. Rel. Bioact. Mat.*, 15, 264 (1988).

156. V. H. L. Lee and R. E. Smith, *J. Ocular Pharmacol.*, 1, 269 (1985).
157. O. Lockridge, *J. Neurochem.*, 39, 106 (1982).
158. I. W. Chubb, E. Ranieri, G. H. White, and A. J. Hodgson, *Neuroscience*, 10, 1369 (1983).
159. S. Baba and Y. Miyachi, *Acta Soc. Ophthalmol. Jpn.*, 85, 1267 (1981).
160. Y. Shimizu, *Cell. Mol. Biol.*, 28, 103 (1982).
161. H. Björkland, L. Olson, and A. Sieger, *Med. Biol.*, 61, 280 (1983).
162. A. B. Tullo, P. Keen, W. A. Blyth, T. J. Hill, and D. L. Easty, *Invest. Ophthalmol. Vis. Sci.*, 24, 596 (1983).
163. Z. Friedman, R. C. Allen, and S. M. Raph, *Arch. Ophthalmol.*, 103, 963 (1985).
164. W. M. Grant, in *Symposium on Ocular Drug Therapy* (I. H. Leopold, ed.). Mosby, St. Louis, 1973, p. 19.
165. D. L. Epstein and W. M. Grant, *Arch. Ophthalmol.*, 95, 1378 (1977).
166. D. L. Epstein and W. M. Grant, in *Symposium on Ocular Therapy* (I. H. Leopold and R. P. Burns, eds.). Wiley, New York, 1979, p. 51.
167. F. Theeuwes and W. Bayne, *J. Pharm. Sci.*, 66, 1388 (1977).
168. F. Theeuwes, W. Bayne, and J. McGuire, *Arch. Ophthalmol.*, 96, 2219 (1978).
169. R. H. Foss, *Am. J. Ophthalmol.*, 36, 336 (1955).
170. H. Green and I. H. Leopold, *Am. J. Ophthalmol.*, 40, 137 (1955).
171. J. Gloster and E. S. Perkins, *Br. J. Ophthalmol.*, 39, 647 (1955).
172. T. H. Maren, *Physiol. Rev.*, 47, 595 (1967).
173. A. J. Flach, J. S. Peterson, and K. A. Seligmann, *Am. J. Ophthalmol.*, 98, 66 (1984).
174. T. H. Maen, *J. Pharmacol. Exp. Ther.*, 117, 385 (1956).
175. M. L. Putnam, R. D. Schoenwald, M. W. Duffel, C. F. Barfknecht, T. M. Segarra, and D. A. Campbell, *Invest. Ophthalmol. Vis. Sci.*, 28, 1373 (1987).
176. T. H. Maren, A. Bar-Ilan, K. C. Caster, and A. R. Katritzky, *J. Pharmacol. Exp. Ther.*, 241, 56 (1987).
177. T. H. Maren, A. L. Parcell, and M. N. Malik, *J. Pharmacol. Exp. Ther.*, 130, 389 (1960).
178. J. Grove, P. Gautheron, B. Plazonnet, and M. F. Sugrue, *J. Ocular Pharmacol.*, 4, 279 (1988).
179. A. R. Katritzky, K. C. Caster, T. H. Maren, C. W. Conroy, and A. Bar-Ilan, *J. Med. Chem.*, 30, 2058 (1987).
180. T. H. Maren and L. Jankowska, *Curr. Eye Res.*, 4, 399 (1985).
181. L. M. Jankowska, A. Bar-Ilan, and T. H. Maren, *Invest. Ophthalmol. Vis. Sci.*, 27, 29 (1986).
182. A. Bar-Ilan, N. I. Pessah, and T. H. Maren, *Invest. Ophthalmol. Vis. Sci.*, 25, 1198–1205.
183. A. Stein, R. Pinke, T. Krupin, E. Glabb, S. M. Podos, J. Serle, and T. H. Maren, *Am. J. Ophthalmol.*, 95, 222 (1983).
184. M. Francoeur, I. Ahmed, S. Sitek, and T. F. Patton, *Int. J. Pharm.*, 16, 203 (1983).
185. M. G. Eller, R. D. Schoenwald, J. A. Dixson, T. Segarra, and C. F. Barfknecht, *J. Pharm. Sci.*, 74, 155 (1985).

186. M. G. Eller, R. D. Schoenwald, J. A. Dixson, T. Segarra, and C. F. Barfknecht, *J. Pharm. Sci.*, 74, 525 (1985).
187. G. S. Ponticello, M. B. Freedman, C. N. Habeker, P. A. Lyle, H. Schwam, S. L. Varga, M. A. Christy, W. C. Randall, and J. J. Baldwin, *J. Med. Chem.*, 30, 591 (1987).
188. R. F. Wang, J. B. Serle, S. M. Podos, and M. F. Sugrue, *Invest. Ophthalmol. Vis. Sci.*, 29(Suppl.), 16 (1988).
189. M. F. Sugrue, P. Gautheron, J. Grove, P. Mallorga, H. Schwam, M. P. Viader, J. J. Baldwin, and G. S. Ponticello, *Invest. Ophthalmol. Vis. Sci.*, 29(Suppl.), 81 (1988).
190. R. F. Wang, J. B. Serle, S. M. Podos, C. H. Severin, and M. F. Sugrue, *Invest. Ophthalmol. Vis. Sci.*, 39, 99 (1989).
191. M. F. Sugrue, P. Mallorga, H. Schwam, J. J. Baldwin, and G. S. Ponticello, *Invest. Ophthalmol. Vis. Sci.*, 30, 99 (1989).
192. H. Bourgeois, A. Bron, E. Lippa, J.-L. George, D. Sirbat, P. Lesure, J.-F. Maurin, C. Clineschmidt, F. Brunner-Ferber, and J. Royer, *Invest. Ophthalmol. Vis. Sci.*, 31, 233 (1990).
193. M. F. Sugrue, P. Gautheron, J. Grove, P. Mallorga, M. P. Viader, H. Schwam, J. J. Baldwin, M. E. Christy, and G. S. Ponticello, *J. Ocular Pharmacol.*, 6, 9 (1990).
194. J. J. Baldwin, G. S. Ponticello, P. S. Anderson, M. E. Christy, M. A. Mureko, W. C. Randall, H. Schwam, M. F. Sugrue, J. P. Springer, P. Gautheron, J. Grove, P. Mallorga, M.-P. Viader, B. M. McVeener, and M. A. Navia, *J. Med. Chem.*, 32, 2510 (1989).
195. T. H. Maren, A. Bar-Ilan, C. W. Conroy, and W. F. Brechue, *Exp. Eye Res.*, 50, 27 (1990).
196. E. J. Higginbotham, M. A. Kass, E. A. Kippa, R. L. Batenhost, D. L. Panebianco, and J. T. Wilensky, *Arch. Ophthalmol.*, 108, 65 (1990).
197. P. Mallorga, E. R. Reiss, G. S. Ponticello, J. J. Baldwin, and M. F. Sugrue, *Invest. Ophthalmol. Vis. Sci.*, 30, 445 (1989).
198. S. L. Graham, J. M. Hoffman, P. Gautheron, S. R. Michelson, T. H. Scholz, H. Schwam, K. L. Shepard, A. M. Smith, R. L. Smith, J. M. Sondey, and M. F. Sugrue, *J. Med. Chem.*, 33, 749 (1990).
199. L. Apt, A. Henrick, and L. M. Silverman, *Am. J. Ophthalmol.*, 87, 210 (1979).
200. A. T. Florence, in *Techniques of Solubilization of Drugs* (S. H. Yalkowsky, ed.), Marcel Dekker, New York, 1981, p. 40.
201. H.-W. Hui and J. R. Robinson, *J. Pharm. Sci.*, 75, 280 (1986).
202. G. M. Grass and J. R. Robinson, *J. Pharm. Sci.*, 73, 1021 (1984).
203. D. S. Hull, J. E. Hine, H. F. Edelhauser, and R. A. Hyndiuk, *Invest. Ophthalmol.*, 13, 457 (1974).
204. W. V. Cox, A. Kupferman, and H. M. Leibowitz, *Arch. Ophthalmol.*, 88, 308 (1972).
205. W. V. Cox, A. Kupferman, and H. M. Leibowitz, *Arch. Ophthalmol.*, 88, 549 (1972).
206. A. Kupferman, M. V. Pratt, K. Suckewer, and H. M. Leibowitz, *Arch. Ophthalmol.*, 91, 373 (1974).
207. A. Kupferman and H. M. Leibowitz, *Arch. Ophthalmol.*, 91, 377 (1974).

208. H. M. Leibowitz and A. Kupferman, *Int. Ophthalmol. Clin.*, 20, 117 (1980).
209. J. R. Polansky and R. N. Weinreb, in *Pharmacology of the Eye* (M. L. Sears, ed.). Springer-Verlag, Berlin, 1984, p. 459.
210. J. Sugar, R. M. Burde, A. Sugar, S. R. Waltman, K. J. Kripalani, I. Weliky, and B. Becker, *Invest. Ophthalmol.*, 11, 890 (1972).
211. H. Yamauchi, H. Kito, and K. Uda, *Jpn. J. Ophthalmol.*, 19, 339 (1975).
212. D. G. Musson, A. M. Bidgood, and O. Olejnik, *J. Ocular Pharmacol.*, 7, 175 (1991).
213. A. Tsuji, I. Tamai, and K. Sasaki, *Ophthalmic Res.*, 19, 322 (1987).
214. H. J. Schaeffer, L. Beauchamp, P. De Miranda, G. B. Elion, D. J. Bauer, and P. Collins, *Nature*, 272, 583 (1972).
215. H. E. Kaufman, E. D. Varnell, Y. M. Centifanto, and S. D. Rheinstrom, *Antimicrob. Agents Chemother.*, 14, 842 (1978).
216. E. D. Varnell and H. E. Kaufman, in *Herpetic Eye Diseases* (R. Sundmacher, ed.). Bergmann-Verlag, Munich, 1981, p. 303.
217. C. Schmitt, V. J. Lotti, and J. C. Le Douarec, *Albrecht von Graefes Arch. Klin. Ophthalmol.*, 217, 167 (1981).
218. L. Bonomi, S. Perfetti, R. Bellucci, F. Massa, and E. Noya, *Albrecht von Graefes Arch. Klin. Ophthalmol.*, 217, 175 (1981).
219. J. A. Nathanson, *Curr. Eye Res.*, 4, 191 (1985).
220. M. Araie and M. Takase, *Graefes Arch. Clin. Exp. Ophthalmol.*, 222, 259 (1985).
221. A. R. Berrospi and H. M. Leibowitz, *Arch. Ophthalmol.*, 100, 943 (1982).
222. T. Wandel, A. D. Charap, R. A. Lewis, L. Partamian, S. Cobb, J. C. Lue, G. D. Novack, R. Gaster, J. Smith, and E. Duzman, *Am. J. Ophthalmol.*, 101, 298 (1986).
223. F. E. Ros, H. C. Innemee, and P. A. van Zwieten, *Albrecht von Graefes Arch. Klin. Exp. Ophthalmol.*, 208, 235 (1978).
224. F. E. Ros, H. C. Innemee, and P. A. van Zwieten, *Doc. Ophthalmol.*, 48, 291 (1979).
225. L. Bonomi, S. Perfetti, E. Noya, R. Bellucci, and F. Massa, *Albrecht von Graefes Arch. Klin. Exp. Ophthalmol.*, 210, 1 (1979).
226. E. Duzman, N. Rosen, and M. Lazar, *Br. J. Ophthalmol.*, 67, 668 (1983).
227. V. A. Place, M. Fisher, S. Herbst, L. Gordon, and R. C. Merrill, *Am. J. Ophthalmol.*, 80, 706 (1975).
228. H. S. Brown, G. Meltzer, R. C. Merrill, M. Fisher, C. Feerre, and V. A. Place, *Arch. Ophthalmol.*, 94, 1716 (1976).
229. P. A. Granström, *Br. J. Ophthalmol.*, 66, 464 (1982).
230. S. E. Norell and P. A. Granström, *Br. J. Ophthalmol.*, 64, 137 (1980).
231. R. J. Weinkam, H. Bundgaard, E. WaldeMussie, G. Ruiz, B. Feldmann, J. Dino, and I. Ismail, *Pharm. Res.*, 7, S-64 (1990).
232. R. Gurny, T. Boye, and H. Ibrahim, *J. Controlled Rel.*, 2, 353 (1985).
233. U. Ticho, M. Blumenthal, S. Zonis, A. Gal, I. Blank, and Z. W. Mazor, *Br. J. Ophthalmol.*, 63, 45 (1979).
234. Z. Mazor, U. Ticho, U. Rehany, and L. Rose, *Br. J. Ophthalmol.*, 63, 48 (1979).
235. J. R. Robinson and S. P. Eriksen, in *Soft Contact Lenses* (M. Ruben, ed.). Wiley, New York, 1978, p. 265.

236. W. F. March, R. M. Stewart, A. I. Mandell, and L. A. Bruce, *Arch. Ophthalmol.*, 100, 1270 (1982).
237. A. Urtti, J. D. Pipkin, G. Rork, T. Sendo, U. Finne, and A. J. Repta, *Int. J. Pharm.*, 61, 241 (1990).
238. M. F. Armaly and K. R. Rao, *Invest. Ophthalmol. Vis. Sci.*, 12, 491 (1973).
239. T. Kaila, R. Huupponen, and L. Salminen, *J. Ocular Pharmacol.*, 2, 365 (1986).
240. J. R. Polansky and J. A. Alvarado, *Curr. Eye Res.*, 4, 267 (1985).
241. J. A. Anderson, *Arch. Ophthalmol.*, 98, 350 (1980).
242. V. Kumar, R. D. Schoenwald, W. A. Barcellos, D. S. Chien, J. C. Folk, and T. A. Weingeist, *Arch. Ophthalmol.*, 104, 1189 (1986).
243. E. Duzman, J. A. Anderson, J. B. Vita, J. C. Lue, C. C. Chen, and I. Leopold, *Arch. Ophthalmol.*, 101, 1122 (1983).
244. C. H. Chiang and R. D. Schoenwald, *J. Pharmacokinet. Biopharm.*, 14, 175 (1986).
245. A. Urtti, L. Salminen, and O. Miinalainen, *Int. J. Pharm.*, 23, 147 (1985).
246. R. G. Janes and J. F. Stiles, *Am. J. Ophthalmol.*, 56, 84 (1963).
247. D. D. S. Tang-Liu, S. S. Liu, and R. J. Weinkam, *J. Pharmacokinet. Biopharm.*, 12, 611 (1984).
248. C. W. N. Chiang, G. Barnett, and D. Brine, *J. Pharm. Sci.*, 72, 136, (1983).
249. M. W. Mosteller, B. M. Gebhardt, A. M. Hamilton, and H. E. Kaufman, *Arch. Ophthalmol.*, 103, 101 (1985).
250. W. L. Nelson, F. T. Fraunfelder, J. M. Sills, J. B. Arrowsmith, and J. N. Kuritsky, 1978-1985, *Am. J. Ophthalmol.*, 102, 606 (1986).
251. S. C. Chang and V. H. L. Lee, *J. Ocular Pharmacol.*, 3, 159 (1987).
252. S. S. Chrai, T. F. Patton, A. Mehta, and J. R. Robinson, *J. Pharm. Sci.*, 62, 1112 (1973).
253. G. S. M. J. E. Duchateau, J. Zuidema, W. M. Albers, and F. W. H. M. Merkus, *Int. J. Pharm.*, 34, 131 (1986).
254. A. Hussain, S. Hirai, and R. Bawarshi, *J. Pharm. Sci.*, 69, 1411 (1980).
255. T. J. Zimmerman, K. S. Kooner, A. S. Kandarakis, and L. P. Ziegler, *Arch. Ophthalmol.*, 102, 551 (1984).
256. M. S. Passo, E. A. Palmer, and E. M. van Buskirk, *Ophthalmology*, 91, 1361 (1984).
257. H. Sasaki, D. S. Chien, and V. H. L. Lee, *Pharm. Res.*, 5, S98 (1988).
258. H. Sasaki, H. Bundgaard, and V. H. L. Lee, *Invest. Ophthalmol. Vis. Sci.*, 30(Suppl.), 25 (1989).
259. V. Kumar, R. D. Schoenwald, D. S. Chien, A. J. Packer, and W. W. Choi, *Am. J. Ophthalmol.*, 99, 180 (1985).
260. M. F. Sugrue, P. Gautheron, J. Grove, P. Mallorga, M.-P. Viader, J. P. Baldwin, G. S. Ponticello, and S. L. Varga, *Invest. Ophthalmol. Vis. Sci.*, 29, 776 (1988).
261. N. Bodor, *Med. Res. Rev.*, 4, 449 (1984).
262. N. Bodor and A. ElKoussi, *Curr. Eye Res.*, 7, 369 (1988).
263. N. Bodor, A. A. El-Koussi, M. Kano, and M. M. Khalifa, *J. Med. Chem.*, 31, 1651 (1988).
264. N. Bodor, Y. Oshiro, T. Loftsson, M. Katovich, and W. Caldwell, *Pharm. Res.*, 1, 120 (1984).

265. N. Bodor, R. Woods, C. Raper, P. Kearney, and J. J. Kaminski, *J. Med. Chem.*, 23, 474 (1980).
266. N. Bodor, J. J. Kaminski, and S. Selk, *J. Med. Chem.*, 23, 469 (1980).
267. N. Bodor and M. Varga, *Exp. Eye Res.*, 50, 183 (1990).
268. B. Becker and W. R. Morton, *Arch. Ophthalmol.*, 66, 219 (1961).
269. A. Hussain and J. E. Truelove, *J. Pharm. Sci.*, 65, 1510 (1976).
270. M. B. Kaback, S. M. Podos, T. S. Harbin, Jr., A. Mandell, and B. Becker, *Am. J. Ophthalmol.*, 81, 768 (1976).
271. M. E. Yablonski, D. H. Shin, A. E. Kolker, M. Kass, and B. Becker, *Arch. Ophthalmol.*, 95, 2157 (1977).
272. A. N. Kohn, A. P. Moss, N. A. Hargett, R. Ritch, H. Smith, Jr., and S. M. Podos, *Am. J. Ophthalmol.*, 87, 196 (1979).
273. J. Theodore and H. M. Leibowitz, *Am. J. Ophthalmol.*, 88, 1013 (1979).
274. V. H. L. Lee, D. S. Chien, and H. Sasaki, *J. Pharmacol. Exp. Ther.*, 246, 87 (1988).
275. V. H. L. Lee, E. Stratford, Jr., and K. W. Morimoto, *Int. J. Pharm.*, 13, 183 (1983).
276. H. Sasaki, M. A. Reinoso, H. Bundgaard, and V. H. L. Lee, *Pharm. Res.*, 5, S-177 (1988).
277. I. Abramovsky and J. S. Mindel, *Arch. Ophthalmol.*, 97, 1937 (1979).
278. J. S. Mindel, A. M. Koeingsberg, A. B. Kharlamb, J. Goldfarb, and J. Orellana, *Arch. Ophthalmol.*, 100, 147 (1982).
279. J. A. Anderson, J. B. Richman, and J. S. Mindel, *Arch. Ophthalmol.*, 102, 913 (1984).
280. D. S. Chien, H. Bundgaard, and V. H. L. Lee, *Invest Ophthalmol. Vis. Sci.*, 28(Suppl.), 71 (1987).
281. K. Green, J. M. Chapman, Jr., L. Cheeks, M. R. Clayton, M. Wilson, and A. Zehir, *J. Toxicol. Cutan. Ocular Toxicol.*, 6, 89 (1987).
282. T. J. Mikkelson, S. S. Chrai, and J. R. Robinson, *J. Pharm. Sci.*, 62, 1942 (1973).
283. V. F. Smolen, J. M. Clevenger, E. J. Williams, and H. W. Bergdolt, *J. Pharm. Sci.*, 62, 958 (1973).
284. K. Green and S. J. Downs, *Invest. Ophthalmol.*, 13, 316 (1974).
285. R. M. Kassem, A. E. M. El-Nimr, H. A. Salama, and R. M. Khalil, *Effect of Quarternary Ammonium Compounds on the Mydriatic Activity of Homatropine in Man.* Proc. 3rd Int. Conf. Pharm. Technol., A.P.G.I., Paris, 1983, pp. 275–280.
286. N. Keller, D. Moore, D. Carper, and A. Longwell, *Exp. Eye Res.*, 30, 203 (1980).
287. A. M. Tonjum, *Acta Ophthalmol.*, 52, 650 (1974).
288. A. Ludwig and M. V. Ooteghem, *Int. J. Pharm.*, 54, 95 (1989).
289. S. S. Chrai and J. R. Robinson, *J. Pharm. Sci.*, 63, 1218 (1974).
290. J. W. Shell and R. W. Baker, *Ann. Ophthalmol.*, 6, 1037 (1974).
291. Y. F. Maichuk, in *Ocular Therapy* (I. H. Leopold and R. P. Burns, eds.). Wiley, New York, 1976, pp. 1–16.
292. M. A. Attia, M. A. Kassem, and S. M. Safwat, *Int. J. Pharm.*, 47, 21 (1988).
293. R. Vasantha, P. K. Sehgal, and K. P. Rao, *Int. J. Pharm.*, 47, 95 (1988).
294. S. R. Waltman and H. E. Kaufman, *Invest. Ophthalmol.*, 9, 250 (1970).
295. Y. T. Maddox and H. N. Burstein, *Ann. Ophthalmol.*, 4, 789 (1972).

296. B. Becker, C. Assef, J. Hartstein, and S. Podos, *Am. J. Ophthalmol.*, 63, 336 (1972).
297. M. Ruben and R. Watkins, *Br. J. Ophthalmol.*, 59, 455 (1975).
298. M. G. Doane, A. D. Jense, and C. H. Dohlman, *Am. J. Ophthalmol.*, 85, 383 (1978).
299. D. S. Chien, D. D. S. Tang-Lui, and C. Gluchowski, *Invest. Ophthalmol. Vis. Sci.*, 31(Suppl.), 403 (1990).
300. A. Urtti, T. Sendo, J. D. Pipkin, G. Rork, and A. J. Repta, *J. Ocular Pharmacol.*, 4, 335 (1988).
301. J. R. Robinson and S. H. S. Leung, *CRC Crit. Rev. Ther. Drug Carrier Sys.*, 5, 21 (1988).
302. K. Park and J. R. Robinson, *Int. J. Pharm.*, 19, 107 (1984).
303. H. W. Hui and J. R. Robinson, *Int. J. Pharm.*, 26, 203 (1985).
304. E. A. Balazs and P. Band, *Cosmet. Toiletries*, 99, 65 (1984).
305. W. D. Comper and T. C. Laurent, *Physiol. Rev.*, 58, 255 (1978).
306. F. M. Polack and M. T. Niece, *Cornea*, 1, 133 (1982).
307. J. C. Stuart and J. G. Linn, *Ann. Ophthalmol.*, 17, 190 (1985).
308. O. Camber, P. Edman, and R. Gurny, *Curr. Eye Res.*, 6, 779 (1987).
309. M. F. Saettone, D. Monti, M. T. Torracca, P. Chetoni, and B. Giannaccini, *Drug Dev. Ind. Pharm.*, 15, 2475 (1989).
310. S. C. Miller and M. D. Donovan, *Int. J. Pharm.*, 12, 147 (1982).
311. R. Gurny, H. Ibrahim, A. Aebi, P. Buri, C. G. Wilson, N. Washington, P. Edman, and O. Camber, *J. Controlled Rel.*, 6, 367 (1987).
312. A. Rozier, C. Mazuel, J. Grove, and B. Plazonnet, *Int. J. Pharm.*, 57, 163 (1989).
313. C. Mazuel and M. C. Friteyre, Composition pharmaceutique de type a transition de phase liquide-gel. French Patent Application FR.2588189 A1. Date 87-04-10. Filing Fr. 8514689 date 85-10-03.
314. R. Moorhouse, G. T. Colegrove, P. A. Sandford, J. K. Baird, and K. S. Kan, in *Solution Properties of Polysaccharides* (D. A. Brandt, ed.). Washington, D.C., 1981, p. 111.
315. R. Gurny, *Pharm. Acta Helv.*, 56, 130 (1981).
316. R. Vogel, S. F. Kulaga, J. K. Laurence, R. L. Gross, B. G. Haik, D. Karp, M. Koby, and T. J. Zimmerman, *Invest. Ophthalmol. Vis. Sci.*, 31(Suppl.), 404 (1990).
317. G. J. Shaker, S. Ueda, J. A. LoCascio, and J. V. Aquavella, *Invest. Ophthalmol. Vis. Sci.*, 30, 1565 (1989).
318. B. A. Weissman, N. A. Brennan, D. A. Lee, and I. Fatt, *Invest. Ophthalmol. Vis. Sci.*, 31(Suppl.), 334 (1990).
319. M. B. Eswein, T. P. O'Brien, M. S. Osato, and D. B. Jones, *Invest. Ophthalmol. Vis. Sci.*, 31(Suppl.), 452 (1990).
320. D. Desai, J. Thomas, J. H. Rockey, and D. Sahm, *Invest. Ophthalmol. Vis. Sci.*, 31(Suppl.), 421 (1990).
321. M. R. Sawusch, T. P. O'Brien, J. D. Dick, and J. D. Gottsch, *Am. J. Ophthalmol.*, 106, 279 (1988).
322. S. D. Schwartz, S. A. Harrison, R. E. Engstrom, Jr., R. E. Bawden, D. A. Lee, and B. J. Mondino, *Invest. Ophthalmol. Vis. Sci.*, 31(Suppl.), 558 (1990).

323. J. R. Gussler, P. Ashton, W. S. Van Meter, and T. J. Smith, *Invest. Ophthalmol. Vis. Sci.*, 31(Suppl.), 485 (1990).

324. I. Finkelstein, G. E. Trope, I. A. Menon, L. Spero, D. S. Rootman, and G. Heathcote, *Invest. Ophthalmol. Vis. Sci.*, 31(Suppl.), 591 (1990).

325. J. T. Jacob-LaBarre and H. E. Kaufman, *Invest. Ophthalmol. Vis. Sci.*, 31(Suppl.), 485 (1990).

326. P. P. Ellis, M. Matsumura, and M. A. Rendi, *Curr. Eye Res.*, 4, 1041 (1985).

327. D. S. Hull, J. E. Hine, H. F. Edelhauser, and B. A. Hyndiuk, *Invest. Ophthalmol.*, 13, 457 (1984).

328. O. Camber and P. Edman, *Int. J. Pharm.*, 39, 229 (1987).

329. V. H. L. Lee, A. Yamamoto, and U. B. Kompella, *CRC Crit. Rev. Drug Carriers Sys.*, 8, 91 (1991).

330. D. D.-S. Tang-Liu and P. J. Burke, *Pharm. Res.*, 5, 238 (1988).

331. C. Newton, B. M. Gebhardt, and H. E. Kaufman, *Invest. Ophthalmol. Vis. Sci.*, 29, 208 (1988).

332. E. J. Champeau and H. F. Edelhauser, in *The Preocular Tear Film in Health, Disease, and Contact Lens Wear* (F. J. Holly, ed.). Dry Eye Institute, Lubbock, Texas, 1986, p. 292.

333. G. M. Grass, R. W. Wood, and J. R. Robinson, *Invest. Ophthalmol. Vis. Sci.*, 26, 110 (1985).

334. C. G. Wilson, E. Tomlinson, S. S. Davis, and O. Olejnik, *J. Pharm. Pharmacol.*, 31, 749 (1981).

335. A. Kato and S. Iwata, *J. Pharmacobiodyn.*, 11, 115 (1988).

336. A. Kato and S. Iwata, *J. Pharmacobiodyn.*, 11, 181 (1988).

337. A. Kato and S. Iwata, *J. Pharmacobiodyn.*, 11, 330 (1988).

338. P. Tyle, *Pharm. Res.*, 3, 318 (1986).

339. G. Erlanger, *Ophthalmologica*, 128, 232 (1954).

340. L. Von Sallmann, *Arch. Ophthalmol.*, 31, 1 (1944).

341. L. Von Sallmann, *Arch. Ophthalmol.*, 34, 195 (1945).

342. I. H. Leopold, *Arch. Ophthalmol.*, 33, 211 (1945).

343. L. Von Sallman, *Trans. Am. Ophthalmol. Soc.*, 45, 570 (1947).

344. L. Von Sallman, *Am. J. Ophthalmol.*, 25, 1292 (1942).

345. R. Harris, in *Therapeutic Electricity and Ultraviolet Radiation* (E. Licht, ed.). New Haven, 1967, p. 156.

346. D. L. Larsen and A. S. Rapperport, *Plast. Reconstr. Surg.*, 36, 547 (1965).

347. R. E. Grassman, D. F. Chu, and D. A. Lee, *Invest. Ophthalmol. Vis. Sci.*, 31, 909 (1990).

348. L. Hughes and D. M. Maurice, *Arch. Ophthalmol.*, 102, 1825 (1984).

349. G. S. Rootman, J. A. Hobden, J. A. Jantzen, J. R. Gonzalez, R. J. O'Callaghan, and J. M. Hill, *Arch. Ophthalmol.*, 106, 262 (1988).

350. J. M. Hill, L. P. Gangarosa, D. S. Hull, C. L. Tuggle, K. Bowman, and K. Green, *Invest. Ophthalmol. Vis. Sci.*, 17, 473 (1978).

351. P. H. Fishman, W. M. Jay, P. Rissing, J. M. Hill, and R. K. Shockley, *Invest. Ophthalmol. Vis. Sci.*, 25, 343 (1984).

352. N. L. Burstein, I. H. Leopold, and D. B. Bernacchi, *J. Ocular Pharmacol.*, 1, 363 (1985).
353. M. Barza, C. Peckman, and J. Baum, *Ophthalmology*, 93, 133 (1986).
354. M. Barza, C. Peckman, and J. Baum, *Invest. Ophthalmol. Vis. Sci.*, 28, 1033 (1987).
355. R. R. Burnette and B. Ongpipattanakul, *J. Pharm. Sci.*, 77, 132 (1988).
356. V. H. L. Lee and V. H. K. Li, *Adv. Drug Deliv. Rev.*, 3, 1 (1989).

Index